Diversity and Inclusion in Qu

Marcus L. Martin • Sheryl Heron
Lisa Moreno-Walton • Michelle Strickland
Editors

Diversity and Inclusion in Quality Patient Care

Your Story/Our Story – A Case-Based Compendium

Second Edition

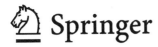 Springer

Editors
Marcus L. Martin
Office for Diversity and Equity and
Department of Emergency Medicine
University of Virginia
Charlottesville, VA
USA

Lisa Moreno-Walton
Department of Medicine
Louisiana State University
New Orleans, LA
USA

Sheryl Heron
Department of Emergency Medicine
Emory University School of Medicine
Atlanta, GA
USA

Michelle Strickland
Office for Diversity and Equity
University of Virginia
Charlottesville, VA
USA

ISBN 978-3-319-92761-9   ISBN 978-3-319-92762-6   (eBook)
https://doi.org/10.1007/978-3-319-92762-6

Library of Congress Control Number: 2018952073

Printed on acid-free paper

This Springer imprint is published by the registered company Springer Nature Switzerland AG
The registered company address is: Gewerbestrasse 11, 6330 Cham, Switzerland

"A powerful narrative of voices, Your Story/ Our Story should help all people – doctors, nurses, patients, and our communities – understand and reflect on the role bias plays in our lives. Whether we are patients or providers, a must read for us to understand and bring forth solutions to create a healthy environment."

—Kenny Leon
Tony Award-winning director and producer
True Colors Theatre Company

"This sentinel book, edited by experts in the field, not only examines the damaging impact of unconscious bias on patient care, but on the professional development and effectiveness of healthcare professionals and trainees. The chapters in this book are ideal training cases and discussions relevant for medical education seminars and simulations. They supply not only realistic scenarios, but credible solutions for managing knowledge gaps and establishing equity in health care. A must read for practitioners, educators and consumers alike."

—Richard Carmona, M.D., M.P.H., F.A.C.S.
17th Surgeon General of the United States
Distinguished Professor at the
University of Arizona

"As medical care becomes a global concern, the role of unconscious bias, cultural competency, and attitudes of inclusion becomes imperative for discussion in healthcare practice and education. This book takes several steps in raising awareness and proposing solutions that can lead to a decrease in the disparities we now see around the world. Access to care is more than just being able to get to the place where care is given. It means getting to the person who has the ability to understand the problem and the motivation to leverage the resources to fix it. For healthcare providers who want to be that person, this book is a tool towards getting there."

—Lee Wallis
Immediate Past President of the
International Federation of Emergency
Medicine and Past President of the African
Federation of Emergency Medicine

Preface

Diversity and Inclusion in Quality Patient Care: Your Story/Our Story—A Case-Based Compendium expands upon our first textbook, *Diversity and Inclusion in Quality Patient Care*. It illuminates the narratives of individual's experiences with biases in various healthcare environments and settings. This textbook is to be used as an educational resource by all levels of healthcare providers, patients, and those who serve and advocate for them. Our editors have extensive backgrounds in clinical and academic health care as well as leadership and expertise in equity, diversity, and inclusion. The three editors who published the original book (Drs. Martin, Heron, and Moreno-Walton; *Diversity and Inclusion in Quality Patient Care*), during the journey from student to full professorship, have experienced many of the scenarios you will be reading. In addition, they have mentored countless healthcare professionals through their individual journeys. This book considers the stories of students, nurses, residents, advanced practice providers, staff, and physicians in the various stages of their professional lives, as well as the patients they serve.

We recognize that a tremendous knowledge gap exists in research on the impact of implicit bias in health care. However, the significance on individuals of the various microaggressions they experience daily in seeking or providing care must be addressed and cannot be ignored.

Included in the 69 chapters are pre-case and case-based content written to provide an in-depth understanding of biases as well as real-life scenarios of race, culture, sexual orientation, religion, gender, disability, and other unique human attributes. Above all, our teaching cases recognize the influence of unconscious bias, also known as implicit bias, microaggressions, and the sensitive approach of healthcare providers to the diverse groups they will encounter. The names of the providers and patients have been changed to protect confidentiality; however, the circumstances are authentic.

The proliferation of literature on unconscious bias and microaggressions has raised public awareness. Biases are bidirectional and include patients, families, communities, providers, and trainees. This case-based compendium addresses how healthcare providers can respond with professionalism and dignity to unconscious bias and microaggressions and these lessons extend to patients, families, and train-ees within their environments where biased assumptions and attitudes exist.

Big journeys begin with small steps. Each chapter in this book provides a step toward your/our understanding that we all have biases. We hope that the *Diversity and Inclusion in Quality Patient Care: Your Story/Our Story—A Case-Based Compendium* will inspire you to take these steps toward change.

Charlottesville, VA, USA   Marcus L. Martin
Atlanta, GA, USA   Sheryl Heron
New Orleans, LA, USA   Lisa Moreno-Walton
Charlottesville, VA, USA   Michelle Strickland

Acknowledgments

The editors acknowledge the support of the University of Virginia Office for Diversity and Equity (UVA ODE), which provided invaluable assistance in the development of this book.

We specifically acknowledge the efforts of Lindy Steiner, Stephanie Bossong, Emmanuel Agyemang-Dua, DJ Cunningham, and Gail Prince-Davis for their research efforts and assistance with editing.

In addition to serving as one of our editors, Michelle Strickland provided outstanding project management and communications with authors and the publisher.

Three of the editors are founding members of the Academy for Diversity and Inclusion in Emergency Medicine (ADIEM) which is within the Society for Academic Emergency Medicine (SAEM), committed to eliminating healthcare disparities by recognizing the role that implicit biases and microaggressions play.

Your Story/Our Story would not be possible without the strong contributions of the many authors dedicated to providing culturally competent care while addressing disparities and bias in health care.

Contents

Contributors

David A. Acosta, M.D. Association of American Medical Colleges, Washington, DC, USA

Kevin Adams, M.Div., Ph.D., B.C.C. Chaplaincy Services and Pastoral Education, University of Virginia Health System, Charlottesville, VA, USA

Rebecca Adrian, M.Div., B.C.C., A.C.P.E. Chaplaincy Services and Pastoral Education, University of Virginia Health System, Charlottesville, VA, USA

Emmanuel Agyemang-Dua, M.P.H. University of Virginia, Charlottesville, VA, USA

Kumar Alagappan, M.D. The University of Texas MD Anderson Cancer Center, Houston, TX, USA

Reem Alhawas, M.B.B.S. George Washington University School of Medicine and Health Sciences, Washington, DC, USA

Imam Abdulrahman Bin Faisal University School of Medicine, Dammam, Saudi Arabia

Tareq Al-Salamah, M.B.B.S., M.P.H. University of Maryland School of Medicine, Baltimore, MD, USA

Emergency Department, University of Maryland Capital Region Health, Cheverly, MD, USA

Emergency Department, King Saud University, Riyadh, Saudi Arabia

Jessica Aviles, M.D. Integrated Residency in Emergency Medicine, University of Connecticut, Farmington, CT, USA

Loraine Bacchus, Ph.D., M.A., B.Sc. London School of Hygiene and Tropical Medicine, Faculty of Public Health and Policy, Department of Global Health and Development, London, UK

Jacqueline S. Barnett, D.H.Sc., M.S.H.S., PA-C. Department of Community and Family Medicine, Duke University School of Medicine, Durham, NC, USA

Tanya Belle, M.D. Emergency Medicine Residency Program, University of Connecticut, Storrs, CT, USA

Mildred Best, M.S.S., M.Div., B.C.C., A.C.P.E. Chaplaincy Services and Pastoral Education, University of Virginia Health System, Charlottesville, VA, USA

Charlie Borowicz, B.S. University of Pittsburgh, Pittsburgh, PA, USA

Stephanie Bossong, B.S. University of Virginia, Charlottesville, VA, USA

J. Bridgman Goines, M.D. Department of Emergency Medicine, Emory University School of Medicine, Atlanta, GA, USA

Michael K. Brown, D.O. Department of Emergency Medicine, Virginia Commonwealth University, Richmond, VA, USA

Camille Burnett, Ph.D., M.P.A., R.N., B.Sc.N. University of Virginia School of Nursing, Charlottesville, VA, USA

Caron Campbell, M.D. Einstein College of Medicine, Bronx, NY, USA

Laura Castillo-Page, Ph.D. Diversity Policy and Programs, Organizational Capacity Building. Association of American Medical Colleges (AAMC), Washington, DC, USA

Christian A. Chisholm, M.D., F.A.C.O.G. University of Virginia, Charlottesville, VA, USA

Erika Phindile Chowa, M.D. Department of Emergency Medicine, Emory University, Atlanta, GA, USA

Amy Cohee, M.D. University of Virginia, Charlottesville, VA, USA

Vanessa Cousins, M.D. Department of Emergency Medicine, Emory University, Atlanta, GA, USA

Esteban Cubillos-Torres, M.D University of Virginia School of Medicine, Charlottesville, VA, USA

DeVanté J. Cunningham, M.P.H. Clinical Psychology, Montclair State University, Montclair, NJ, USA

Xi Damrell, M.D Kaweah Delta Emergency Medicine Residency Program, Visalia, CA, USA

Adrian D. Daul, M.D., M.P.H. Department of Emergency Medicine, Emory University School of Medicine, Atlanta, GA, USA

Julie Deters, M.S.N., F.N.P., R.N. University of Northern Colorado, Greeley, CO, USA

Jeffrey Druck, M.D. University of Colorado School of Medicine, Aurora, CO, USA

Erick A. Eiting, M.D., M.P.H., M.M.M., F.A.C.E.P. Icahn School of Medicine at Mount Sinai, New York, NY, USA

David B. Kriser Department of Emergency Medicine, Mount Sinai Beth Israel, New York, NY, USA

Ugo A. Ezenkwele, M.D., M.P.H. Department of Emergency Medicine, Mount Sinai Queens, Mount Sinai School of Medicine, New York, NY, USA

Malika Fair, M.D., M.P.H. Health Equity Partnerships and Programs, Diversity Policy and Programs, Association of American Medical Colleges, Washington, DC, USA

Kevin Ferguson, M.D. Touro University at St. Joseph Medical Center, Stockton, CA, USA

Maria Ramos-Fernandez, M.D., M.Sc., F.A.C.E.P. Emergency Medicine Residency Program, University of Puerto Rico, San Juan, PR

Mekbib Gemeda, M.A. Eastern Virginia Medical School, Norfolk, VA, USA

Michael Gisondi, M.D. Department of Emergency Medicine, Stanford University School of Medicine, Stanford, CA, USA

Paolo Grenga, M.D. University of Rochester Medical Center, Rochester, NY, USA

Trevor Halle, M.D. University of Rochester Medical Center, Rochester, NY, USA

Jan Hargrave, B.S., M.S. The University of Texas MD Anderson Cancer Center, Houston, TX, USA

Marianne Haughey, M.D., F.A.A.E.M. CUNY School of Medicine, Department of Emergency Medicine, SBH Health System, New York, NY, USA

Albert Einstein College of Medicine, Bronx, NY, USA

Sheryl Heron, M.D., M.P.H. Emory University School of Medicine, Atlanta, GA, USA

Marquita Hicks, M.D. The University of Alabama at Birmingham, Birmingham, AL, USA

Mikhail C. S. S. Higgins, M.D., M.P.H. Boston University School of Medicine, Boston, MA, USA

Cherri D. Hobgood, M.D. Department of Emergency Medicine, Indiana University School of Medicine, Indianapolis, IN, USA

Lynne Holden, M.D. Einstein College of Medicine, Bronx, NY, USA

Sarah Jamison, M.D. CUNY School of Medicine, Department of Emergency Medicine, SBH Health System, New York, NY, USA

Jamie L. W. Kennedy, M.D., F.A.C.C. Cardiovascular Medicine, University of Virginia Health System, Charlottesville, VA, USA

R. Lane Coffee Jr, Ph.D., M.S. Department of Emergency Medicine, Indiana University School of Medicine, Indianapolis, IN, USA

Timothy Layng, D.O. Department of Emergency Medicine, Virginia Commonwealth University, Richmond, VA, USA

Aisha Liferidge, M.D., M.P.H. George Washington University School of Medicine and Health Sciences, Washington, DC, USA

Simiao Li, M.D., M.S. Department of Emergency Medicine, The Ohio State University Wexner Medical Center, Columbus, OH, USA

Bernard L. Lopez, M.D., M.S. Sidney Kimmel Medical College of Thomas Jefferson University, Thomas Jefferson University, Philadelphia, PA, USA

Matthew S. Lucas, Ph.D., M.B.E., R.N. Department of Women, Children, and Family Health Science, College of Nursing, University of Illinois at Chicago, Chicago, IL, USA

Jamela M. Martin, Ph.D., R.N., C.P.N.P.-B.C. Old Dominion University, School of Nursing, Norfolk, VA, USA

Marcus L. Martin, M.D. University of Virginia, Charlottesville, VA, USA

Gabrielle Marzani, M.D. University of Virginia School of Medicine, Charlottesville, VA, USA

Gwyneth Milbrath, Ph.D., R.N., M.P.H. College of Nursing, University of Illinois at Chicago, Chicago, IL, USA

Joel Moll, M.D. Department of Emergency Medicine, Virginia Commonwealth University, Richmond, VA, USA

Denee Moore, M.D. Central Virginia Health Services, Charlottesville, VA, USA

Lisa Moreno-Walton, M.D., M.S., M.S.C.R., F.A.A.E.M. Department of Medicine, Section of Emergency Medicine, Louisiana State University Health Sciences Center- New Orleans, New Orleans, LA, USA

Tiffany Murano, M.D., F.A.C.E.P., R.D.M.S. Department of Emergency Medicine, Rutgers New Jersey Medical School, Newark, NJ, USA

Steven Nazario, M.D., F.A.A.E.M., F.A.C.E.P. Emergency Medicine Residency Program, Florida Hospital, Orlando, FL, USA

Emergency Medicine, Florida State University College of Medicine, Tallahassee, FL, USA

Rachel Nelson, M.D. University of Rochester Medical Center, Rochester, NY, USA

Robert E. O'Connor, M.D., M.P.H. University of Virginia, Charlottesville, VA, USA

Brenda Oiyemhonlan, M.D., M.H.S.A., M.P.H. University of California, San Francisco, Department of Emergency Medicine, Zuckerberg San Francisco General Hospital, San Francisco, CA, USA

Anthonia Ojo, M.D. Eastern Virginia Medical School, Norfolk, VA, USA

Aasim I. Padela, M.D., M.Sc., F.A.C.E.P. MacLean Center for Clinical Medical Ethics, The University of Chicago, Chicago, IL, USA

Munzareen Padela, M.D., M.PP. The University of Chicago, Chicago, IL, USA

Marcia Perry, M.D. University of Michigan Medical School, Ann Arbor, MI, USA

Ava Pierce, M.D. UT Southwestern Medical Center, Dallas, TX, USA

Vivian W. Pinn, M.D. National Institutes of Health, Washington, DC, USA

Gwendolyn Poles, D.O., F.A.C.P. PinnacleHealth System, Faculty, Internal Medicine Residency Program, Medical Director Kline Health Center, Harrisburg, PA, USA

Norma Iris Poll-Hunter, Ph.D. Human Capital Initiatives, SHPEP, Diversity Policy and Programs, Association of American Medical Colleges, Washington, DC, USA

Heather Prendergast, M.D., M.S., M.P.H. University of Illinois, Chicago, IL, USA

P. Preston Reynolds, M.D., Ph.D., M.A.C.P. University of Virginia, Charlottesville, VA, USA

Cynthia Price, M.D. Hartford Hospital, Hartford, CT, USA

Kenyon Railey, M.D. Department of Community and Family Medicine, Office of Diversity and Inclusion, Duke University School of Medicine, Durham, NC, USA

Michael Railey, M.D. Family and Community Medicine, Student Affairs and Diversity, Saint Louis University School of Medicine, St. Louis, MO, USA

Benjamin Ramalanjaona, M.S. State University of New York Downstate Medical Center, Brooklyn, NY, USA

Georges Ramalanjaona, M.D., D.Sc. Essen Medical Associate, Bronx, NY, USA

Lynne D. Richardson, M.D., F.A.C.E.P. Department of Emergency Medicine, Department of Population Health Science and Policy, Icahn School of Medicine at Mount Sinai, New York, NY, USA

Jason M. Rotoli, M.D. University of Rochester Medical Center, Rochester, NY, USA

John S. Rozel, M.D., M.S.L. University of Pittsburgh, Pittsburgh, PA, USA

Altaf Saadi, M.D. University of California Los Angeles National Clinical Scholars Program, Los Angeles, CA, USA

Bisan A. Salhi, M.D., M.A. Departments of Anthropology and Emergency Medicine, Emory University, Atlanta, GA, USA

Swami Sarvaananda, Ph.D., B.C.C. Clinical Pastoral Education Programs, University of Virginia Health System, Charlottesville, VA, USA

Susan Sawning, M.S.S.W. University of Louisville School of Medicine, Louisville, KY, USA

Sarah Sewaralthahab, M.B.B.S., M.P.H. Department of Internal Medicine, University of Maryland Medical Center, Baltimore, MD, USA

Internal Medicine Department, King Saud University, Riyadh, Saudi Arabia

Teresa Y. Smith, M.D., M.S.Ed., F.A.C.E.P. SUNY Downstate/Kings County Hospital, Department of Emergency Medicine, Brooklyn, NY, USA

Audrey Snyder, Ph.D., A.C.N.P., R.N. University of Northern Colorado, Greeley, CO, USA

Michelle Strickland, M.P.A. University of Virginia, Charlottesville, VA, USA

Edward Strickler, M.A., M.A., M.P.H., C.H.E.S. Institute of Law, Psychiatry and Public Policy, University of Virginia, Charlottesville, VA, USA

Katherine Sullivan, Ph.D., R.N., C.T.N.-A., C.E.N. University of Northern Colorado, Greeley, CO, USA

Yoshiya Takahashi, M.Div., B.C.C. Chaplaincy Services and Pastoral Education, University of Virginia Health System, Charlottesville, VA, USA

Taryn R. Taylor, M.D., M.Ed. Emory University School of Medicine, Atlanta, GA, USA

Traci R. Trice, M.D. Office of Diversity and Inclusion Initiatives, Department of Family and Community Medicine, Sidney Kimmel Medical College of Thomas Jefferson University, Philadelphia, PA, USA

Leigh-Ann J. Webb, M.D. University of Virginia, Charlottesville, VA, USA

Marcee Wilder, M.D., M.P.H. Department of Emergency Medicine, Icahn School of Medicine at Mount Sinai, New York, NY, USA

Michael D. Williams, M.D. UVA Center for Health Policy, The Frank Batten School of Leadership and Public Policy and School of Medicine, University of Virginia, Charlottesville, VA, USA

University of Virginia Health System, Charlottesville, VA, USA

Taneisha T. Wilson, M.D. Brown Emergency Medicine, Injury Prevention Center, Rhode Island Hospital, Providence, RI, USA

Alpert School of Medicine, Brown University, Providence, RI, USA

The Miriam and Rhode Island Hospitals, Providence, RI, USA

Gloria Wink, M.S. University of Rochester Medical Center, Rochester, NY, USA

Patricia Workman, A.N.P., M.S.N., C.C.H.P.F. Fluvanna Correctional Center for Women, Troy, VA, USA

Sybil Zachariah, M.D. Stanford University, Stanford, CA, USA

Shanta Zimmer, M.D. University of Colorado School of Medicine, Aurora, CO, USA

Shana Zucker, B.A. Tulane University School of Medicine, New Orleans, LA, USA

Editor Biographies

Marcus L. Martin, M.D. is a professor and past chair of the Department of Emergency Medicine at the University of Virginia (UVA). He held the chair position from July 1996 to December 2006. Dr. Martin's emergency medicine responsibilities included the adult and pediatric emergency departments, chest pain unit, express care, Pegasus air ambulance, the Blue Ridge Poison Center, paramedic training program, emergency medicine residency program, and several emergency medicine fellowship programs. During his tenure at UVA, Dr. Martin served as the assistant dean of the School of Medicine and assistant vice president, associate vice president, and interim vice president and chief officer for diversity and equity. In 2011, he was appointed vice president and chief officer for diversity and equity. Dr. Martin is the principal investigator of the Virginia-North Carolina Alliance, a National Science Foundation-funded Louis Stokes Alliance for Minority Participation (LSAMP) program. He is the founder of Emergency Medicine Center for Education Research and Technology (EMCERT) and initiated the medical simulation program at the University of Virginia School of Medicine.

He earned his Bachelor of Science degrees in Pulp and Paper Technology (1970) and Chemical Engineering (1971) from North Carolina State University and was employed as a production chemical engineer at WESTVACO in Covington, Virginia. A member of the charter class of Eastern Virginia Medical School and the first African-American graduate, he earned his medical degree in 1976.

Dr. Martin was commissioned by the US Public Health Service and later served as a general medical officer at the Gallup Indian Medical Center in New Mexico. He completed his emergency medicine residency training at the University of Cincinnati in 1981 and held a series of staff and administrative/teaching posts at Allegheny General Hospital in Pittsburgh.

He was a board member for 12 years and past president of the Society for Academic Emergency Medicine (SAEM). He is a past president of the Council of Emergency Medicine Residency Directors. He is the recipient of the 2008 SAEM Diversity Interest Group Leadership Award, named the Marcus L. Martin, MD Leadership Award in his honor. Dr. Martin is the lead editor for the books *Diversity and Inclusion in Quality Patient Care* (Springer International Publishing, 2016) and

West Indies Health Care and Disaster Preparedness (Create Space Independent Publishing, 2015). The UVA Board of Visitors established the Marcus L. Martin Distinguished Professorship of Emergency Medicine in December 2016.

Sheryl Heron, M.D., M.P.H. is a professor and vice chair of Administrative Affairs in the Department of Emergency Medicine, the assistant dean for Medical Education and Student Affairs on the Grady Campus, and the associate director of Education and Training for the Injury Prevention Research Center at Emory (IPRCE). Prior to attending medical school, Dr. Heron obtained her Masters in Public Heath degree from Hunter College in New York City in 1989 and focused on community health education. She graduated from Howard University College of Medicine in 1993 and subsequently completed her emergency medicine residency training at the Martin Luther King/Charles Drew Medical Center in 1996. That year, she joined the faculty of Emory University School of Medicine as the first African-American woman in Emergency Medicine. In 2002, she was sworn in by the governor to serve as a commissioner on the Georgia Commission on Family Violence and worked to craft a medical protocol to address family violence in the state of Georgia.

Dr. Heron has lectured extensively on the medical response to intimate partner violence as well as wellness/work-life balance and diversity/disparate care in emergency medicine. She has received several awards including the 2011 Women's Resource Center's Champions for Change, Partnership Against Domestic Violence's HOPE Award, the Woman in Medicine Award from the Council of Concerned Women of the National Medical Association, and the Gender Justice Award from the Commission on Family Violence and was named a hero of Emergency Medicine by the American College of Emergency Physicians. Dr. Heron served as a chair of the National Medical Association's Emergency Medicine section where she mentored several faculty, residents, and students in their career path within emergency medicine. From her efforts, Dr. Heron was selected as the first recipient of the Marcus L. Martin, MD Leadership Award, presented during the SAEM annual meeting in Atlanta in 2009, and served as the inaugural president of the Academy for Diversity and Inclusion in Emergency Medicine (ADIEM) of SAEM. Dr. Heron is also the inaugural recipient of the Emory School of Medicine Excellence in Diversity and Inclusion Award for 2018. She is sought after to be a visiting professor and has lectured extensively on diversity and inclusion in emergency medicine and implicit bias.

Lisa Moreno-Walton, M.D., M.S., M.S.C.R., F.A.A.E.M. is the Nicolas Bazan professor of Emergency Medicine, Department of Medicine, Section of Emergency Medicine, in the School of Medicine at Louisiana State University Health Sciences Center-New Orleans (LSUHSC-NO) and secretary-treasurer of the American Academy of Emergency Medicine.

Dr. Moreno-Walton's academic and professional appointments are numerous. Along with her appointment as a full professor, she serves as the director of the Division of Research, the Division of Diversity, and the Viral Testing Program for the Section of Emergency Medicine at LSUHSC-NO. Dr. Moreno-Walton holds an academic appointment in the Department of Surgery at Tulane University School of Medicine.

Prior to her appointment at LSUHSC-NO, Dr. Moreno served as a faculty physician in emergency medicine at the North Bronx Healthcare Network and at the Lincoln Medical and Mental Health Center, both in the Bronx, New York. She is board certified in emergency medicine and completed her residency training at the Jacobi-Montefiore program in the Bronx.

Dr. Moreno-Walton is the recipient of numerous teaching awards. She has developed graduate and postgraduate curricula for core content and research in emergency medicine and has mentored 300 undergraduates and medical students, residents, and junior faculty to successful career development and research productivity.

Dr. Moreno-Walton earned her Master of Science in Clinical Research from Tulane University in June 2011. Since that time, she has been awarded 20 grants to study trauma, HIV, healthcare disparities, hepatitis C, and syphilis. She has given over 450 abstract presentations and 250 invited presentations and has more than 100 scholarly publications. Dr. Moreno-Walton has won 15 research awards and, in 2013, was named a National Institutes of Health PRIDE Research Scholar. She recently created a curriculum for developing emergency medicine research in resource-poor environments, a course that she teaches internationally. She lectures widely on the topics of cultural competency, healthcare disparities, HIV, and trauma.

Dr. Moreno-Walton wrote the charter to found the Academy for Diversity and Inclusion in Emergency Medicine (ADIEM), Society for Academic Emergency Medicine (SAEM), and continues to serve on its board. In 2013, she was the recipient of the Marcus L. Martin, MD Leadership Award presented during the SAEM meeting in Atlanta, Georgia. In 2014, she was the only physician in the United States to receive the Alpha Omega Alpha Professionalism Award for her work to eliminate healthcare disparities. In 2015, she was designated as a master educator by the Academy for Scholarship, Council of Emergency Medicine Residency Directors.

Michelle Strickland, M.P.A received her Bachelor of Arts in Studio Art from Cedarville University in 2013. In 2016, she received her Master's degree in Public and Nonprofit Administration from the University of Memphis. She began working at the University of Virginia Office for Diversity and Equity in 2016.

Part I
Bias in Health Care

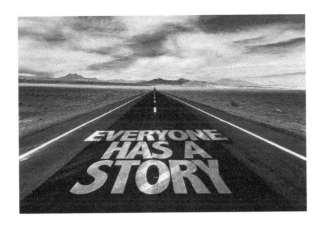

Chapter 1
Introduction

**Marcus L. Martin, Sheryl Heron, Lisa Moreno-Walton,
and Michelle Strickland**

*Diversity and Inclusion in Quality Patient Care, Second Edition: Your Story/Our
Story—A Case-Based Compendium* Part I is a pre-case section containing relevant
chapters addressing bias in health care. The seven chapters that follow are compli-
mentary to those published in our first textbook on *Diversity and Inclusion in Quality
Patient Care* (DIQPC), which emphasizes culturally appropriate care, requiring
healthcare providers to recognize and understand medical education traditions, and
other impeding factors potentially fueling biases. Quality care is created through a
community sensitive to differences in race, culture, sexual orientation, disability,
religion, socioeconomic status, and any other human variations. DIQPC provided a
broad array of chapters and teaching cases to educate the healthcare community
about quality patient care, including the following topics in the pre-case section:

Defining Diversity in Quality Care
Racial/Ethnic Healthcare Disparities and Inequities: Historical Perspectives
*Educating Medical Professionals to Deliver Quality Health Care to Diverse Patient
    Populations*
Culturally Competent Faculty
Culturally Sensitive Care: A Review of Models and Educational Methods

M. L. Martin (✉) · M. Strickland
University of Virginia, Charlottesville, VA, USA
e-mail: mlm8n@virginia.edu; ms2yx@virginia.edu

S. Heron
Emory University School of Medicine, Atlanta, GA, USA
e-mail: sheron@emory.edu

L. Moreno-Walton
Department of Medicine, Section of Emergency Medicine, Louisiana State University Health
Sciences Center-New Orleans, New Orleans, LA, USA

© Springer International Publishing AG, part of Springer Nature 2019
M. L. Martin et al. (eds.), *Diversity and Inclusion in Quality Patient Care*,
https://doi.org/10.1007/978-3-319-92762-6_1

Interpreter Services
The Patient-Physician Clinical Encounter
Spiritual Care Services in Emergency Medicine
Lesbian, Gay, or Bisexual (LGB): Caring with Quality and Compassion
Culturally Competent Care of the Transgender Patient
Looking Past Labels: Effective Care of the Psychiatric Patient
Disability and Access
Racial and Ethnic Disparities in the Emergency Department: A Public Health Perspective
Vulnerable Populations: The Homeless and Incarcerated
Vulnerable Populations: The Elderly
Vulnerable Populations: Children
Religio-cultural Consideration When Providing Healthcare to American Muslims
Disparities and Diversity in Biomedical Research

In Part I of *Diversity and Inclusion in Quality Patient Care, Second Edition: Your Story/Our Story—A Case-Based Compendium*, pre-case topics include unconscious bias, microaggressions, gender and transgender bias, cultural competencies in the deaf patient, and the impact of bias on global health care. In Parts II–VI, teaching cases are presented that address bias in health care related to the experiences of patients, medical and nursing students, residents, nurses, staff, advanced practice providers, and attending physicians.

Chapter 2
The Inconvenient Truth About Unconscious Bias in the Health Professions

Laura Castillo-Page, Norma Iris Poll-Hunter, David A. Acosta, and Malika Fair

"Not everything that is faced can be changed, but nothing can be changed until it is faced." – James Baldwin

Introduction

In 2003, the Institute of Medicine (now the National Academy of Medicine) released two reports that focused widespread attention on the crucial issue of disparities in healthcare access [1, 2]. These pivotal reports documented that Americans' access to quality care was fractured along racial and socioeconomic lines and concluded that "bias, prejudice, and stereotyping on the part of healthcare providers may contribute to differences in care" [1]. The reports included equity of care as one of the six pillars of quality health care and pointed out that, as long as health disparities exist, our health system cannot claim to deliver quality care to all patients [1, 2].

L. Castillo-Page (✉)
Diversity Policy and Programs, Organizational Capacity Building,
Association of American Medical Colleges (AAMC), Washington, DC, USA
e-mail: lcastillopage@aamc.org

N. I. Poll-Hunter
Human Capital Initiatives, SHPEP, Diversity Policy and Programs,
Association of American Medical Colleges, Washington, DC, USA
e-mail: npoll@aamc.org

D. A. Acosta
Association of American Medical Colleges, Washington, DC, USA
e-mail: dacosta@aamc.org

M. Fair
Health Equity Partnerships and Programs, Diversity Policy and Programs,
Association of American Medical Colleges, Washington, DC, USA
e-mail: mfair@aamc.org

© Springer International Publishing AG, part of Springer Nature 2019
M. L. Martin et al. (eds.), *Diversity and Inclusion in Quality Patient Care*,
https://doi.org/10.1007/978-3-319-92762-6_2

More than 15 years later, a multitude of studies demonstrate examples of health disparities and inequities in healthcare delivery. Patients of color—especially black and African-Americans, Hispanics, and Native Americans—have higher overall risks and poorer outcomes than whites with a wide range of conditions, including asthma, diabetes, HIV/AIDS, hypertension, obesity, preterm births, and tuberculosis. Racial and ethnic minority patients have less access to quality care and have lower life expectancies and higher mortality rates [3]. These differences cannot be explained away solely by socioeconomic status, patient preference, lack of health insurance coverage, or other external factors. While health inequity is a multifactorial problem, health professionals must also recognize the role provider attitudes, behavior, and clinical decision-making play in unequal care and disparate health outcomes [3–5].

Despite federal Title VI protections in place against overt discrimination in the workplace or in patient care, incidences of explicit bias—in which individuals are aware of their prejudices toward certain groups—persist [6]. There is also a subtler form of prejudice that can be more difficult to address. This is called unconscious— or implicit—bias, meaning the prejudices we are not aware of.

With today's intense focus on the population's health, healthcare organizations and healthcare professionals of all types are looking at ways to improve the delivery of quality health care. It is clear that meeting the goals of the Triple Aim—to improve the healthcare experience, improve the health of populations, and reduce the costs of care [7]—requires that we confront the unconscious biases that influence quality care [4].

Discussion

Unconscious Bias in Health Care

Healthcare professionals pledge to "do no harm," adhere to ethical standards, and support the rights of patients to receive equal care. Many clinicians would deny that they treat patients differently based on characteristics such as race, gender, weight, age, sexual orientation, or disability [4]. However, reports of discrimination and inequitable care remain common [3–5, 8–11]. This disconnect is likely a direct result of unconscious bias.

Unconscious bias affects everything from the admissions processes at health science schools to the hiring and promotion of healthcare professionals, the administration of healthcare organizations, and—ultimately—the delivery of care to patients [5, 8, 12, 13].

What Is Unconscious Bias?

Based on research into unconscious bias, our brains operate on associations—automatic responses or shortcuts that allow us to quickly interpret and respond to our environment. In the blink of an eye, the brain takes in bits of data, interprets them, and leads us to conclusions—all without us realizing it is happening. By quickly categorizing situations, people, images, and sounds, we recognize friends, family members, symbols, and letters on the page, for example. This sorting is involuntary and happens in a millisecond, without conscious thought. Our capacity to sort helps us learn, keeps us safe, and allows us to build on previous knowledge [14, 15].

While this process is normal, and very human, it also has unintended consequences—especially in health care—where quick thinking can make the difference in a patient's diagnosis and treatment. Sometimes these split-second judgments provide us with accurate, useful, and even lifesaving information. But some may also be inaccurate and unintentionally obstruct our decision-making and relationships with patients and even inflict unintentional harm [5, 9, 10, 14–17]. This is unconscious bias.

None of us are immune to unconscious bias; it permeates all aspects of society. Scholars have detected and documented unconscious bias in education, criminal justice, and employment practices [17]. A recent review of the literature found that the prevalence of unconscious bias in the health professions is as high as it is in the general population. The same review determined that 20 out of 25 studies found at least some evidence of bias in clinicians' diagnosis, treatment, or interaction with patients based on characteristics such as race, ethnicity, sexual orientation, gender, weight, mental illness, substance abuse, disability, and social circumstances [18]. Moreover, the high-stress environment of health care may increase the incidence of unconscious bias [17, 19]. Researchers found that cognitive stressors such as time pressure, competing demands, overcrowding, stress, and fatigue were associated with an increase in implicit bias among emergency room physicians [20].

In 2016, the Joint Commission issued a Quick Safety bulletin on implicit or unconscious bias. The authors wrote:

> The ability to distinguish friend from foe helped early humans survive, and the ability to quickly and automatically categorize people is a fundamental quality of the human mind. Categories give order to life, and every day, we group other people into categories based on social and other characteristics. This is the foundation of stereotypes, prejudice and, ultimately, discrimination…. Studies show people can be consciously committed to egalitarianism, and deliberately work to behave without prejudice, yet still possess hidden negative prejudices or stereotypes [21].

What the Research Shows

In their 2017 literature review, FitzGerald and Hurst found that despite advanced training in a profession that strives for objectivity, clinicians are just as likely as anyone else to harbor unconscious bias. They reviewed 42 peer-reviewed journal articles that examined unconscious bias in different aspects of health care over the course of a decade and noted that there is a complex relationship between clinical decision-making and a clinician's unconscious bias. While this may not always translate into negative treatment outcomes, a trusting relationship between a health-care professional and her patient is essential to providing good treatment. Thus, it seems likely that the more negative the clinical interaction, the worse the eventual treatment outcome. Over time, negative clinical interactions may leave patients less likely to seek medical attention for future worries or problems [18].

Patients can sustain harm, sometimes in subtle forms, even when they are receiving care that appears equivalent. For example, a 2015 study in the *Journal of Pain Symptom Management* examined differences in physicians' verbal and nonverbal communication with black and white patients who were at the end of life [22]. The study looked at how 30 hospital physicians interacted with black and white patients in mock end-of-life scenarios. Verbal communication was consistent across the races: physicians provided accurate and thorough information to all the mock patients. Nonverbal communication, however, differed by the race of the patient. Findings with black patients indicated that physicians were more likely to stand farther away, make less eye contact, and cross their arms when speaking and listening. This study demonstrates that clinician assumptions based on misinformation or biases based on patient characteristics can affect delivery of appropriate care.

Research also has shown that racial and ethnic minority patients tend to be undertreated for pain, compared with white patients [19, 23–26]. In a study published in 2016, researchers at the University of Virginia uncovered perceptions among clinicians that might contribute to these discrepancies in care [27]. The team surveyed more than 400 medical students and residents. The study participants were asked to indicate whether the following false statements had any truth behind them:

- Blacks age more slowly than whites.
- Blacks' nerve endings are less sensitive than whites' nerve endings.
- Black people's blood coagulates more quickly than white people's.
- Whites have larger brains than blacks.
- Blacks' skin is thicker than whites' skin.
- Whites have a more efficient respiratory system than blacks.
- Black couples are significantly more fertile than white couples.
- Blacks have stronger immune systems than whites.

Study findings indicated that half of the students and residents endorsed one or more of these false statements.

In 2014, the AAMC had the opportunity to put unconscious bias in academic medicine under the microscope when it partnered with the Ohio State University Kirwan Institute for the Study of Race and Ethnicity to convene a daylong gathering that included unconscious bias researchers and administrative leaders charged with developing unconscious bias interventions at their institutions. Attendees spoke candidly about instances of unconscious bias they have experienced and observed.

The proceedings from this meeting led to the AAMC-Kirwan Institute publication, *Unconscious Bias in Academic Medicine: How the Prejudices We Don't Know We Have Affect Medical Education, Medical Careers, and Patient Health* [8]. The report details instances of unconscious bias experienced by leaders and also offers appropriate interventions to make academic medicine more inclusive at all levels, ultimately improving patient care and quality outcomes. While the publication focused specifically on physicians and the culture at medical schools and academic medical centers, unconscious bias affects all health professions, and the suggested interventions are equally relevant [28].

Successful Strategies for Mitigating Unconscious Bias

Recent studies demonstrate that becoming more aware of unconscious biases and resolving to overcome them can help shift attitudes and lead to active strategies to mitigate the effects of bias [29, 30]. The AAMC report highlights several of these strategies, including engaging leadership to create a culture of inclusion, encouraging exploration and mitigation of bias through education and training, and using data strategically to identify bias in all aspects of health care from the hiring and promotion of clinicians to the diagnosis, treatment, and delivery of care to patients [8].

Howard J. Ross, a leading expert trainer on unconscious bias and the author of the groundbreaking 2014 book *Everyday Bias: Identifying and Navigating Unconscious Judgments in Our Daily Lives* [15], recommends that we all take the following steps:

- Recognize and accept that we have biases and that if we don't act on our biases, they will act on us.
- Develop the capacity for honest self-assessment. Once we accept that we have biases, we are more capable of recognizing them as they emerge and before they become entrenched.
- Practice "constructive uncertainty." Question assumptions. Are the "gut feelings" we are experiencing actually our own unconscious biases at work?
- Explore awkwardness and discomfort. Realize that specific people, locations, and situations may seem uncomfortable only because we are not familiar with them.
- Engage with people who might be considered "others" and seek out positive role models in those groups.
- Solicit candid feedback from friends and colleagues, or use self-assessment tools such as the Implicit Association Test to analyze progress [15].

We can explore our own biases by taking the Implicit Association Test developed by researchers at Harvard University in 1998 [31]. The test measures the strength of associations between concepts through a matching exercise. The IAT, which has been validated repeatedly, is based on the idea that matching two highly associated concepts is easier and faster than pairing disparate ideas. Taking the test can reveal biases of which we were previously unaware [28, 32–38].

Ultimately, ensuring a more diverse workforce can help address these disparities in care. Research has shown that diverse work teams are more capable of solving complex problems than homogenous teams [39, 40]. Other studies have also shown that diversity in the healthcare workforce leads to improved access and satisfaction with care [2, 41, 42]. Thus, building a diverse health professions workforce is a key component in improving our ability to deliver quality care to all [43, 44].

Unfortunately, diversifying the healthcare workforce remains a challenge. Although some racial and ethnic minorities have made headway in certain healthcare professions, specialties, or regions of the country, others still lag behind their majority counterparts. Women, people of color, and members of other underrepresented groups are still less likely to hold leadership or decision-making positions in healthcare organizations [12, 13, 43].

In recent years, an increasing number of healthcare institutions have been taking steps to mitigate unconscious bias in training, employment, and patient care [8, 45, 46]. Although many healthcare institution leaders have shared the results of these efforts at professional conferences as case studies, relatively few have yet been subjected to the scholarly peer-reviewed process. One peer-reviewed case study looked at medical school admissions at Ohio State University College of Medicine (OSUCOM) and appeared in *Academic Medicine* in 2017 [47].

Capers et al. reported that all 140 members of the OSUCOM admissions committee were required to take the black–white IAT prior to the 2012–2013 admissions cycle to measure implicit racial bias. They collated the results by gender and student versus faculty status. Individual results were visible only to the test taker and only at the time of the test. All other annual admissions cycle activities proceeded normally. At the end of the admissions cycle, committee members took a survey that recorded their impressions of the impact of the IAT on the admissions process. Capers et al. concluded that all groups (men, women, students, and faculty) displayed significant levels of implicit white preference. Men and faculty members had the largest bias measures. Two-thirds of survey respondents thought the IAT might be helpful in reducing bias, and nearly half (48%) were conscious of their individual results when interviewing candidates in the next cycle. Just over one in five (21%) reported that their knowledge of their IAT results influenced their admissions decisions in the subsequent cycle. The class that matriculated following the IAT exercise was the most diverse in OSUCOM's history at that time. This case study indicates that widespread change is possible at both the individual and institutional levels and that purposeful effort can help overcome unconscious biases.

Conclusion

Unconscious bias, while part of the normal human process, can negatively impact the delivery of quality care. However, when we recognize our own biases and how they influence interactions, we can more consciously consider the best steps toward health equity and achieving the Triple Aim. This recognition must happen at all levels of the healthcare system—from the C-suite to support services—to create real and lasting improvement.

As you read the following chapters, which delve into more specifics about different kinds of unconscious bias in the clinical setting, think about what you can do individually and collectively at your healthcare organization to effect meaningful change. The many clinical scenarios that follow should give you much food for thought. Take the initiative to transform thought into deed. The next generation of health professionals and patients will thank you for it.

NOTE: The AAMC publication is available for free download at www.aamc.org/publications

References

1. Smedley BD, Stith AY, Nelson AR, editors. Unequal treatment: confronting ethnic and racial disparities in health care. Washington: National Academies Press; 2003. 780 p.
2. Smedley BD, Butler AS, Bristow LR, editors. In the nation's compelling interest: ensuring diversity in the health-care workforce. Washington: National Academies Press; 2004. 429 p.
3. Hall WJ, Chapman MV, Lee KM. Implicit racial/ethnic bias among health care professionals and its influence on health care outcomes: a systematic review. Am J Public Health. 2015;105(12):e60–76.
4. Matthew DB. Just medicine: a cure for racial inequality in American health care. New York: New York University Press; 2015.
5. White AA. Diagnosis and treatment: the subconscious at work. In: Seeing patients: unconscious bias in health care. Cambridge: Harvard University Press; 2011. p. 199–210.
6. United States Department of Justice. Understanding bias: a resource guide [Internet]. Washington: U.S. Department of Justice; 2016. (Cited Nov 29 2017). Available from: https://www.justice.gov/crs/file/836431/download
7. Berwick DM, Nolan TW, Whittington J. The triple aim: care, health, and cost. Health Aff. 2008;27(3):759–69.
8. Lewis D, Paulsen E, editors. Proceedings of the diversity and inclusion innovation forum: unconscious bias in academic medicine. How the prejudices we don't know we have affect medical education, medical careers, and patient health. Washington: Association of American Medical Colleges; 2017. 105 p.
9. Schulman KA, et al. The effect of race and sex on physicians' recommendations for cardiac catheterization. N Engl J Med. 1999;340(8):618–26.
10. Schulman KA, et al. The roles of race and socioeconomic factors in health services research. Health Serv Res. 1995;30(1.2):179–95.
11. Green AR, et al. Implicit bias among physicians and its prediction of thrombolysis decisions for black and white patients. J Gen Intern Med. 2007;22(9):1231–8.
12. Pololi LH, et al. The experience of minority faculty who are underrepresented in medicine at 26 representative U.S. medical schools. Acad Med. 2013;88(9):1–7.
13. Palepu A, et al. Minority faculty and academic rank in medicine. JAMA. 1998;280(9):767–71.
14. Banaji MR, Greenwald AG. Blindspot: hidden biases of good people. New York: Delacorte Press; 2013. 272 p.
15. Ross HJ. Everyday bias. Lanham: Rowman & Littlefield; 2014. 207 p.
16. Dovidio JF, et al. Disparities and distrust: the implications of psychological processes for understanding racial disparities in health and health care. Soc Sci Med. 2008;67(3):478–86.

17. Staat C. State of the science: implicit bias review 2014. Columbus: Kirwan Institute for the Study of Race and Ethnicity; 2014.
18. FitzGerald C, Hurst S. Implicit bias in healthcare professionals: a systematic review. BMC Med Ethics. 2017;18(19):1–18. https://doi.org/10.1186/s12910-017-0179-8.
19. Burgess DJ, et al. Understanding the provider contribution to race/ethnicity disparities in pain treatment: insights from dual process models of stereotyping. Pain Med. 2006;7(2):119–34.
20. Johnson TJ, et al. The impact of cognitive stressors in the emergency department on physician implicit racial Bias. Acad Emerg Med. 2016;23:297–305.
21. The Joint Commission. Implicit bias in health care. Quick Safety. 2016;23:1–4.
22. Match communication code of conduct [Internet]. Washington, DC: National Residency Matching Program; c2017 (Cited 21 Dec 2017). Avail from: http://www.nrmp.org/communication-code-of-conduct/
23. Elliott AM, Alexander SC, Mescher CA, Mohan D, Barnato AE. Differences in physicians' verbal and nonverbal communication with black and white patients at the end of life. J Pain Symptom Manage. 2016;51(1):1–8. https://doi.org/10.1016/j.jpainsymman.2015.07.008.
24. Epps CD, Ware LJ, Packard A. Ethnic wait time differences in analgesic administration in the emergency department. Pain Manag Nurs. 2008;9(1):26–32.
25. Heins A, et al. Physician race/ethnicity predicts successful emergency department analgesia. J Pain. 2010;11(7):692–7.
26. Telfer P, et al. Management of the acute painful crisis in sickle cell disease—a re-evaluation of the use of opioids in adult patients. Br J Haematol. 2014;166(2):157–64.
27. Todd KH, Samaroo N, Hoffman JR. Ethnicity as a risk factor for inadequate emergency department analgesia. JAMA. 1993;269(12):1537–9.
28. Hoffman KM, Trawalter S, Axt JR, Oliver MN. Racial bias in pain assessment and treatment recommendations, and false beliefs about biological differences between blacks and whites. Proc Natl Acad Sci U S A. 2016;113(16):4296–301. https://doi.org/10.1073/pnas.1516047113.
29. Schaa KL, et al. Genetic counselors' implicit racial attitudes and their relationship to communication. Health Psychol. 2015;34(2):111–9.
30. Teal CR, Gill AC, Green AR, Crandall S. Helping medical learners recognise and manage unconscious bias toward certain patient groups. Med Educ. 2012;46(1):80–8. https://doi.org/10.1111/j.1365-2923.2011.04101.x.
31. Teal CR, Shada RE, Gill AC, Thompson BM, Fruge E, Villarreal GB, Haidet P. When best intentions aren't enough: helping medical students develop strategies for managing bias about patients. J Gen Intern Med. 2010;25(Suppl 2):S115–8. https://doi.org/10.1007/s11606-009-1243-y.
32. Greenwald AG, McGhee DE, Schwartz JLK. Measuring individual differences in implicit cognition: the implicit association test. J Pers Soc Psychol. 1998;74(6):1464–80.
33. Blair IV, et al. Assessment of biases against Latinos and African Americans among primary care providers and community members. Am J Public Health. 2013;103(1):92–8.
34. Cooper LA, et al. The associations of clinicians' implicit attitudes about race with medical visit communication and patient ratings of interpersonal care. Am J Public Health. 2012;102(5):979–87.
35. Oliver MN, et al. Do physicians' implicit views of African Americans affect clinical decision making? J Am Board Fam Med. 2014;27(2):177–88.
36. Phelan SM, et al. Implicit and explicit weight bias in a national sample of 4,732 medical students: the medical student CHANGES study. Obesity. 2014;22(4):1201–8.
37. Sabin JA, et al. Physicians' implicit and explicit attitudes about race by MD race, ethnicity, and gender. J Health Care Poor Underserved. 2009;20(3):896–913.
38. Sabin JA, Rivara F, Greenwald AG. Physician implicit attitudes and stereotypes about race and quality of medical care. Med Care. 2008;46(7):678–85.
39. Sabin JA, Marini M, Nosek BA. Implicit and explicit anti-fat bias among a large sample of medical doctors by BMI, race/ethnicity and gender. PLoS One. 2012;7(11):e48448.

40. Hoever IJ, van Knippenberg D, van Ginke WP, Barkema H. Fostering team creativity: perspective taking as key to unlocking diversity's potential. J Appl Psychol. 2012;97(5):982–6.

41. Page SE. The difference: how the power of diversity creates better groups, firms, schools, and societies. Princeton: Princeton University Press; 2007.

42. Cohen JJ, Gabriel BA, Terrell C. The case for diversity in the health care workforce. Health Aff. 2002;21(5):90–102.

43. Komaromy M, et al. The role of black and Hispanic physicians in providing health care for underserved populations. N Engl J Med. 1996;334(20):1305–10.

44. Sullivan LW. Missing persons: minorities in the health professions. Durham: Sullivan Commission on Diversity in the Healthcare Workforce; 2004. p. 201.

45. Sullivan LW, Suez Mittman I. The state of diversity in the health professions a century after Flexner. Acad Med. 2010;85(2):246–53.

46. Glicksman E. Unconscious bias in academic medicine: overcoming the prejudices we don't know we have [Internet]. Washington, DC: AAMC; 2016 Jan (Cited 21 Dec 2017). Available from: https://www.aamc.org/newsroom/reporter/january2016/453944/unconscious-bias.html

47. Capers Q IV, Clinchot D, McDougle L, Greenwald AG. Implicit racial bias in medical school admissions. Acad Med. 2017;92(3):365–9.

Chapter 3
Microaggressions

Jeffrey Druck, Marcia Perry, Sheryl Heron, and Marcus L. Martin

Introduction

The term "microaggression" was used in the 1970s by Dr. Chester Pierce to describe insults, dismissals, and casual degradation of marginalized groups. More recently, professor of psychology Dr. Derald Wing Sue defined microaggression as "the everyday verbal, nonverbal, and environmental slights, snubs, or insults, whether intentional or unintentional, which communicate hostile, derogatory, or negative messages to target persons based solely upon their marginalized group membership" [1]. A component of the increase in microaggressions may be a result of the societal unacceptability of overt racism. The end of the American Civil War marked an era of change where we saw a decrease in acts of bigotry and overt racism. This also marked the creation of affirmative action and welfare reform. Affirmative action policies were created to help members of minority groups access employment equal to the majority group. Affirmative action in higher education has been marked by bitter debate and has been challenged in the courts, and the focus on racial membership has not lessened. However, racism has changed from overt acts to subtle and covert acts that form the basis of microaggression.

J. Druck, MD (✉)
University of Colorado School of Medicine, Aurora, CO, USA
e-mail: Jeffrey.Druck@UCDenver.edu

M. Perry, MD
University of Michigan Medical School, Ann Arbor, MI, USA
e-mail: marciap@umich.edu

S. Heron, MD, MPH
Emory University School of Medicine, Atlanta, GA, USA
e-mail: sheron@emory.edu

M. L. Martin, MD
University of Virginia, Charlottesville, VA, USA
e-mail: mlm8n@virginia.edu

© Springer International Publishing AG, part of Springer Nature 2019
M. L. Martin et al. (eds.), *Diversity and Inclusion in Quality Patient Care*,
https://doi.org/10.1007/978-3-319-92762-6_3

The Institute of Medicine, now known as the Health and Medicine Division (HMD) of the National Academies, compels us to focus on climate "as it relates to the perceptions, attitudes and expectation that define the institution, particularly as seen from the perspective of individuals of different racial and ethnic backgrounds" [2]. Addressing the barriers that lead to negative stereotypes and low expectations is of paramount importance to creating an environment that addresses healthcare workers' well-being, health disparities, and access to safe and equitable care. "If we live in an environment in which we are bombarded with stereotypical images in the media, are frequently exposed to ethnic jokes of friends and family members, and are rarely informed of the accomplishments of oppressed groups, we will develop the negative categorizations of those groups that form the basis of prejudice" [3]. This idea that the environment creates and perpetuates prejudice is important to understand; prejudice and unconscious biases are the roots of microaggression. A climate where microaggression is ignored fosters a hostile work environment with professionals who provide substandard patient care.

Discussion

Microaggressions include inappropriate humor, stereotyping, and questions of belonging that occur in three forms: microinsults, microassaults, and microinvalidations [4].

Microinsults are characterized by interpersonal or environmental communications that convey stereotypes, rudeness, and insensitivity and that demean a person's racial, gender, sexual orientation, heritage, or identity. These are subtle unconscious snubs that convey a hidden message. The message is intended to threaten, intimidate, and make individuals or groups feel unwanted or unsafe. Microassaults are explicit racial denigrations characterized by verbal (name-calling) or nonverbal (avoidance behavior) attacks that are intended to hurt their victim. These are usually conscious behaviors. Microinvalidations are characterized by communications and environmental cues that exclude, negate, or nullify the psychological thoughts, feelings, or experiential reality of certain groups such as people of color, women, and LGBTs [4].

Figures 3.1 and 3.2 outline general themes of microaggressions and the messages sent to the recipient.

Microaggression in academic medicine and its impact on those caring for patients are increasingly being identified. The 9/11 bombing of the World Trade Center resulted in an increase in the incidence of religious microaggressions. This presented as religious stereotyping of Muslims as terrorists, leading to increased discrimination against Arab-Americans, furthering their isolation in our society. Microaggressions toward persons of sexual minority groups are commonplace in clinical medicine. These are often in the form of microassaults when medical professionals refuse to use preferred pronouns for transgendered patients or use derogatory language when referring to LGBT persons. Studies have shown that racial

Theme	Microaggression	Message
Alien in own land When Asian Americans and Latino Americans are assumed to be foreign-bom	"Where are you from?" "Where are you born?" "You speak good English." A person asking an Asian American to teach them words in their native language.	You are not American You are a foreigner
Ascription of Intelligence Assigning intelligence to a person of color on the basis of their race.	"You are a credit to your race." "You are so articulate." Asking an Asian person to help with a Math or Science Problem.	People of color are generally not as intelligent as whites. It is unusual for someone for your race to be intelligent. All Asians are intelligent and good at Math/Sciences.
Color Blindness Statements that indicate that a White person does not want to acknowledge race	"When I look at you, I don't see color." "America is a melting pot." "There is only one race, the human race."	Denying a person of color's racial/ethnic experiences. Assimilate/acculturate to the dominant culture. Denying the individual as a racial/cultural being.
Criminality - assumption of criminal status A person of color is presumed to be dangerous, criminal, or deviant on the basis of their race.	A white man or woman clutching their purse or checking their wallet as a black or Latino approaches or passes. A store owner following a customer of color around the store. A whiter person waits to ride the next elevator when a person of color is on it.	You are a criminal. You are going to steal/You are poor/You do not belong/You are dangerous.
Denial of individual racism A statement made when whites deny their racial biases	"I'm not a racist. I have several black friends." "As a woman, I know what you go through as a racial minority."	I am immune to races because I have friends of color. Your racial oppression is no different than my gender oppression. I can't be a racist. I'm like you.
Myth of meritocracy Statements which assert that race does not play a role in life successes	"I believe the most qualified person should get the job." "Everyone can succeed in this society, if they work hard enough."	People of color are given extra unfair benefits because of their race. People of color are lazy and/or incompetent and need to work harder.
Pathologizing cultural values/communication styles The notion that the values and communication styles of the dominant / white culture are ideal	Asking a black person: "Why do you have to be so loud/animated? Just calm down." To an Asian or Latino person: "Why are you so quiet? We want to know what you think. Be more verbal. Speak up more." Dismissing an individual who brings up race/culture in work/school setting.	Assimilate to dominant culture. Leave your cultural baggage outside.

Fig. 3.1 Categories and relationships among racial microaggressions [4]

microaggressions and discrimination have a significant negative impact on both mental and physical health and well-being and are likely major contributors to depression, anxiety, and burnout among physician trainees and other employees [5–7]. Changing culture, decreasing the incidence of microaggressions, and coping with microaggressions continue to be the challenges.

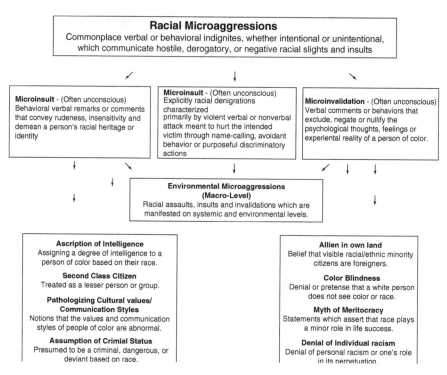

Fig. 3.2 Examples of racial microaggressions [4]

Coping with Microaggression

Microaggressions are often invisible and differ from other stressful events that might elicit a sympathetic response. For example, stressors such as illness or family difficulties are more obvious stressors, where colleagues will be more understanding; in contrast, the invisibility of microaggressions garners no sympathy or emotional support and is often looked upon as people being overly sensitive. Many who experience acts of microaggression post the incident on social media, which often gets them verbal support from allies. In his guide to responding to microaggressions, Kevin Nadal proposes five questions to ponder when making the decision to respond [8]:

1. If I respond, could my physical safety be in danger?
2. If I respond, will the person become defensive and will it lead to an argument?
3. If I respond, how will this affect my relationship to the person (e.g., coworker, family member, etc.)?
4. If I don't respond, will I regret not saying something?
5. If I don't respond, does that mean that I accept the behavior or statement?

Nadal suggests someone responds to microaggression by asking him- or herself the following questions: (1) Did the microaggression really occur? (2) Should I respond to this microaggression? and (3) How should I respond to this microaggression [8]?

An exploratory study of adaptive responses by Hernandez et al. identified eight coping themes that can be used by medical professionals when they experience microaggression [10].

1. Identifying Key Issues in Deciding How to Respond to a Racial Microaggression:
   The decision to respond to a microaggression is very complex. While the response to overt racism might include demonstrations, marches, and media outcry, the response to microaggression tends to require introspection. This often starts with self-reflection: "Did an act of racism truly occur?" Microaggressions are often quick, subtle, and unintentional acts—so people may wonder, "Am I overreacting?" "Am I being too sensitive?" or "Are there other ways to interpret this other than racism? If I choose to respond, it will likely lead to defensive behavior, anger, broken relationships, and increased stress. If I don't respond, I will feel guilty for allowing myself to be treated so poorly." Other reasons for not responding include racial fatigue and fear of retribution or even harm. To minimize the defensive behavior, it is best to address the behavior in a calm manner and avoid personal attacks such as calling someone a racist. It is also helpful to reflect on the situation with others.

2. Self-Care:
   We know from research and our own observations that microaggressions affect the mental and physical health of their victims. It is very important to engage in wellness activities that can help detoxify and maintain positive thoughts in these situations. Mindful behaviors such as meditation, exercise, and acupuncture are often helpful in coping with the stress of microaggression. Taking pride in one's ethnic heritage is also a helpful coping strategy.

3. Spirituality:
   Faith can play a major role in coping with stress. Prayers and other rituals can help one switch focus from oneself to a higher power. One's belief that a higher power can handle the stress can lead to some personal stress relief.

4. Confronting the Aggressor:
   After pondering the potential risk of responding to a microaggression, and ultimately finding one's voice to confront an aggressor, there are still many considerations. One may need to first evaluate the relationship one has with the aggressor. The decision to confront and how to do it will be different if the aggressor is a friend, a family member, or a colleague. Some authors [8, 9] suggest that one uses this as a teachable moment and offers a brief lesson on diversity education. Of course, one will need to decide if that is a battle one chooses to pick as not every microaggression is amenable to a teachable moment. One must balance taking care of their own psychological well-being against providing education to others. Challenging what was said and offering clarity is another option.

5. Seeking Support from Majority Allies:
   There is no question that majority allies are hugely helpful in advancing the cause of equity, diversity, and inclusion. Although it is unfortunate, the same elements of discrimination and racism allow majority allies to make statements that might not be as easily accepted coming from minority populations. People in the

majority may have the financial resources and influential contacts that could be used to address microaggressions. In the case of microaggressions, allies can address microaggressions without seeming defensive. For example, microinvalidation statements such as "It's not a big deal," when offensive statements are made, are harmful, and support from a majority ally can allow others to recognize the underlying fallacy of similar statements. Having allies recognize the importance of microaggressions allows them to call out microaggressions as they happen, as well as be receptive to feedback in case of unintentional statements.

How do you identify allies? From pre-existing organizations, some allies are obvious. Groups with similar aims, such as other minority groups with similar goals, may be helpful. Institutional officials such as chief diversity officers may be able to identify others within a network who are willing to be supportive.

Once allies have been identified, have closed door conversations around overall inclusion; a discussion specifically about microaggressions will allow both public support and a clarification about elements of microaggressions, as well as the opportunity to prep allies with appropriate responses and identification tactics.

6. Keeping Records and Documenting Experiences of Microaggressions:

The documentation of experiences has multiple benefits. From a legal perspective, it can assist with proof of an intolerant work environment. When talking with allies, it helps to have examples, and without documentation, remembering individual experiences is often difficult. With appropriate documentation, a fruitful discussion with employment leadership about microaggressions can open eyes, and possibly change culture. Documenting the frequency of occurrences is also beneficial. When the volume of issues is obvious, microaggressions become apparent. If consistent attempts at success for culture change and administrative support are unsuccessful, legal action and involving the press are alternate options.

7. Mentoring:

Issues regarding microaggressions are difficult to process alone. Having a mentor who one can talk to and receive feedback from is beneficial. A mentor can help frame scenarios, as well as serve as a sounding board for future actions. A mentor can also assist in describing cases in terminology that makes the issues around discrimination more clear.

8. Organizing Public Responses:

Change requires group and public awareness. By utilizing allies, mentors, and documentation, the hope is that the opportunity to speak in a larger venue about discrimination in all forms, and microaggressions in particular, becomes available. From overall lectures and discussion groups about microaggressions, as well as individual conversations about the importance of eliminating microaggressions, communicating the message of inclusion on a larger stage is critical. However, individual events serve as touchpoints for success, and long-term support strategies, such as campus groups and alliances, serve to constantly move the needle forward. Utilizing these groups to develop uniform responses serves two purposes: It provides members with a prepared, measured, vetted method to reply to key issues, and it allows others in the group to understand that their issues are not theirs alone. This solidarity cannot be understated. Along similar lines, research on microaggressions and how they affect self-image, self-worth, career opportunities, and career success is critical to future planning and addressing these issues on a larger scale [11]. When presented with data, majority deniers will have trouble stating these issues do not exist. Further data, examples, and multiple avenues of support will lead to long-term changes in culture and policy [12–14].

Conclusion and Recommendations

Microaggressions occur in everyday life and are not immediately or easily visible to their victims. Even the aggressors of microaggressions may not be immediately aware of their bias. While the impact of microaggression on the well-being of marginalized groups requires more rigorous research, it is clear from the current literature that it has significant impact on the biological, emotional, cognitive, and behavioral well-being of marginalized groups. It is important for educators to teach everyone—not just the marginalized groups—how to recognize and, more importantly, how to cope with microaggressions, as well as to characterize microaggressions for what they are—a form of racism [15].

References

1. Nadal KL, Davidoff KC, Davis LS, Wong Y, Marshall D, McKenzie V. A qualitative approach to intersectional microaggressions: understanding influences of race, ethnicity, gender, sexuality, and religion. Qual Psychol. 2015;2(2):147–63. https://doi.org/10.1037/qup0000026.
2. Smedley BD, Butler AS, Bristow LR, editors. In the nation's compelling interest: ensuring diversity in the health care workforce. Washington, DC: National Academies Press; 2004. 409 p.
3. Tatum BD. Why are all the black kids sitting together in the cafeteria: and other conversations about race. 5th anniversary rev. ed. New York: Basic Books; 2003. 294 p.
4. Sue DW, Capodilupo CM, Torino GC, Bucceri JM, Holder AMB, Nadal KL, Esquilin M. Racial microaggressions in everyday life: implications for clinical practice. Am Psychol. 2007;62(4):271–86. https://doi.org/10.1037/0003-066X.62.4.271.
5. Hammond WP, Gillen M, Yen IH. Workplace discrimination and depressive symptoms: a study of multi-ethnic hospital employees. Race Soc Probl. 2010;2(1):19–30.
6. Hardeman RR, Przedworski JM, Burke S, Burgess DJ, Perry S, Phelan S, Dovidio JF, van Ryn M. Association between perceived medical school diversity climate and change in depressive symptoms among medical students: a report from the medical student CHANGE study. J Natl Med Assoc. 2016;108(4):225–35.
7. Przedworski JM, Dovidio JF, Hardeman RR, Phelan SM, Burke SE, Ruben MA, Perry SP, Burgess DJ, Nelson DB, Yeazel MW, Knudsen JM, van Ryn M. A comparison of the mental health and well-being of sexual minority and heterosexual first-year medical students: a report from medical student CHANGES. Acad Med. 2015;90(5):652–9.

8. Nadal KL. Preventing racial, ethnic, gender, sexual minority, disability, and religious micro-aggressions: recommendations for promoting positive mental health. Prev Couns Psychol. 2008;2(1):22–7.

9. Sue DW. Microaggressions and marginality manifestation, dynamics, and impact. Hoboken: Wiley; 2010. 384 p.

10. Hernandez P, Carranza M, Almeida R. Mental health professionals' adaptive responses to racial microaggressions: an exploratory study. Prof Psychol Res Pr. 2010;41(3):202–9.

11. Embrick DG, Dominguez S, Karsak B. More than just insults: rethinking sociology's contribution to scholarship on racial microaggressions. Sociol Inq. 2017;87(2):193–206. https://doi.org/10.1111/soin.12184.

12. Husain A, Howard S. Religious microaggressions: a case study of Muslim Americans. J Ethn Cult Divers Soc Work. 2017;26(1–2):139–52. https://doi.org/10.1080/15313204.2016.1269710.

13. Platt LF, Lenzen AL. Sexual orientation microaggressions and the experience of sexual minorities. J Homosex. 2013;60(7):1011–34. https://doi.org/10.1080/00918369.2013.774878.

14. DeSouza ER, Wesselmann ED, Ispas D. Workplace discrimination against sexual minorities: subtle and not-so-subtle. Can J Adm Sci. 2017;34(2):121–32. https://doi.org/10.1002/CJAS.1438.

15. Fleras A. Theorizing micro-aggressions as racism 3.0: shifting the discourse. Can Ethn Stud. 2016;48(2):1–19. https://doi.org/10.1353/ces.2016.0011.

Chapter 4
Gender Bias: An Undesirable Challenge in Health Professions and Health Care

Vivian W. Pinn

Introduction

Over the past 25 years, targeted grassroots advocacy and biomedical and government efforts have focused on overcoming and eliminating the historical effects of gender bias on health, health care, and health-related careers. While gender bias may affect to a lesser degree men's health and men's careers in health care, the major effects of gender bias have been challenges to the approach to women's health and challenges for women physicians and health professionals. Recent increased attention to gender bias has helped to identify existing stereotypical impressions about how women's health is perceived, how their health care is delivered, how the science and research that determines standards and practices of health care are designed, and how women's careers in science and health-related careers have been affected. Integral to these is also the role of racial/ethnic bias as it affects women of color and their health and careers. Recognizing and overcoming historical and traditional stereotypical attitudes, overt and subtle, unconscious or intentional, is a challenge that still exists for sex and gender equity in health and in health careers. These lingering stereotypical attitudes may manifest as what is usually referred to as "gender bias" and can impact both interpersonal relationships between health professionals and/or between health professionals and their patients and how the approach to a patient's health complaints may be interpreted.

While "sex" is defined as being male or female according to reproductive organs and functions assigned by one's chromosomal complement, and the term "gender" refers to a person's self-representation in response to or by social institutions but based on biological characteristics shaped by one's environment and life experi-

V. W. Pinn
Former Director (Retired), Office of Research on Women's Health, National Institutes of Health, Washington, DC, USA

ences, the term "gender" is truly more applicable when considerations of bias in health professions are discussed [1].

Further considerations must be given to identities beyond the traditional binary sex/gender categorization, classifications, and identification and require scientific and social thought for clarification and implementation. This discussion of gender bias will focus on two aspects: women as physicians and leaders in healthcare professions, and understanding women's health through the lens of sex and gender and how historical gender bias in research may have an effect on patient care.

Discussion

Women Physicians No Longer Exceptions in the Medical Profession

In an article by Richard C. Cabot published in the Journal of the American Medical Association on September 11, 1915, titled "Women in Medicine," he writes:

> "…Women certainly *can* make good in any department of medicine. But do they *wish* to? Do they like all branches of medicine equally? Do they feel the same natural zest and aptitude for all them all? I think not. One branch–the practice of medicine–is hard for all of us. It is doubly hard for women because it involved competition, not on equal terms, but with an irrational handicap against them. I mean the handicap of a foolish popular prejudice. Quite unreasonable, the majority of people (of both sexes) still prefer a mediocre man doctor to a first rate woman doctor. As long as this is so–and I see no improvement in the last twenty years– women will not have a fair chance to get the broadest experience or to give their best service in medical practice…." [2]

It is now more than 100 years since Dr. Cabot published his comments on women in medicine, recognizing what he called a "handicap of foolish popular prejudice," and yet challenges to women as physicians still exist today in what we generally refer to as gender bias. Yes, much progress has been made regarding the respect for women in medicine over the past 100 years after the publication of his observations, but even now women occasionally have encounters that remind us that there are still some who perhaps "prefer a mediocre man doctor to a first rate woman doctor."

It is unseemly that gender bias exists today for women as physicians, as the numbers of women who are entering and successfully practicing medicine or scientific research have grown expansively over the past 30 years. The first woman to graduate from an American medical school was Dr. Elizabeth Blackwell, who received her medical degree in 1849 from what was then the Geneva Medical College (Hobart College), graduating first in her class [3]. Being the first and only woman American medical school graduate, she obviously experienced extremes of what we would today refer to as gender bias. She was not allowed to participate in some of her medical school's classroom demonstrations, as they were considered inappropriate for women, and she was unable to find employment as a physician. She established her own dispensary, which also provided training for women doctors.

By 1900, approximately 6% of American physicians were women, and although there was increased recruitment of women into medicine during World War II, that effort did not last, and by 1960, only 7% of physicians were women [4]. The trend toward the current increase in women physicians in the United States received impetus from a gender discrimination suit brought by the Women's Equity Action League in 1960. The numbers have risen since then, and the percent of women in medical school entering classes has approached but never exceeded 50%. The entering class of 2016, for example, recorded the largest increase in women over the prior 10 years with 49.5% women and 50.2% men comprising new enrollees, and women represented 49.5% (10,474) of total matriculants compared to 50.2% (10,551) men in that year [5].

However, gender bias for women physicians becomes more evident when identifying challenges to their career advancement, especially in academic medicine. There were times in the not-so-distant past when women were not welcomed into some medical specialties, especially surgical, and that bias was most evident at the time of application for medical internships and postgraduate training. Most of these instances were known through anecdotal experiences, but the differences in the number of women in various specialties reflect these past biases [6]. Over the past 20 years, opportunities for women to enter and practice in every medical specialty have emerged. According to the Association of American Medical Colleges (AAMC), the top ten specialties for women in residency programs (by numbers) in 2013–2014 and 2015–2016 were, in rank order, internal medicine, pediatrics, family medicine, obstetrics and gynecology (OBGYN), internal medicine subspecialties, psychiatry, surgery, emergency medicine, anesthesiology, and pathology; in percentages, OBGYN led with 83% women and pediatrics at 71%. In emergency medicine, 37–38% of residents were women [7, 8]. But this represents quite a change from when women were rare in surgical specialty and other residency programs, perhaps best represented in the relative lack of women in leadership positions in some academic disciplines.

Looking beyond the pipeline and at women in academic medical positions of leadership, the findings are not as encouraging. The increase in women entering medicine has not yet been reflected by parity in academic faculty positions and especially in leadership or decision-making positions such as associate or full professors, department chairs, and other high-ranking academic administrative positions. Only 22% of full professors are women, and the highest numbers of women department chairs in 2014 and 2015 were in OBGYN, radiology, family practice, and pediatrics, although the highest percentages in clinical departments were OBGYN (22%), pediatrics (20%), and family practice and dermatology (19%) [9]. There were ten chairs of emergency medicine, representing 10%. While many still blame this lack of parity in academic representation of women in leadership to "leakage" from the pipeline, that theory is less applicable today than when fewer women were entering medicine and with increased numbers of experienced and accomplished women moving forward for many years in their careers. This observation also holds true for underrepresented minority women. The disparity of women in academic medical leadership has been characterized by Lautenberger, Raezer, and Bunton of the AAMC as "a national issue because it has implications for talent entering the healthcare workforce and our ability to strengthen the broader health system" [10].

There are a number of factors that may contribute to the disparities in the progression of women in academic careers. At a workshop convened by the Office of Research on Women's Health (ORWH) at the National Institutes of Health (NIH) in 1994, the major barriers to advancement of women in biomedical careers that were identified included lack of female role models and mentoring, differences in "rewards" of the profession such as salary differentials and promotion rates, family responsibilities and dual professional and personal roles, need for reentry programs for those who interrupt their careers for family matters, sex discrimination (gender bias) and sexual harassment, lack of sensitivity to gender-specific concerns, and racial bias, especially for women of color [11]. In the years since that report, some progress has been made in responding to these barriers and others, yet even today, many of these same barriers still exist for the advancement of women. A classic article by Handelsman and her co-authors in 2005 emphasized barriers to women in science and medicine such as pipeline issues, the academic and scientific environment, unconscious bias, and balancing family and work [12].

Another landmark report from the National Academies, *Beyond Bias and Barriers*, specifically examined barriers to women in science (including medicine) and engineering and proposed strategies for putting the talents of women to the best use [13]. The committee that prepared this report was charged:

- "To review and assess the research on gender issues in science and engineering, including innate differences in cognition, implicit bias, and faculty diversity.
- To examine institutional culture and the practices in academic institutions that contribute to and discourage talented individuals from realizing their full potential as scientists and engineers.
- To determine effective practices to ensure that women who receive their doctorates in science and engineering have access to a wide array of career opportunities in the academy and in other research settings.
- To determine effective practices for recruiting women scientists and engineers to faculty positions and retaining them in these positions.
- To develop findings and provide recommendations based on these data and other information to guide faculty, deans, and department chairs.
- To develop findings and provide recommendations based on these data and other information to guide faculty, deans, department chairs, and other university leaders; scientific and professional societies; funding organizations; and government agencies in maximizing the potential of women in science and engineering careers" [13].

This comprehensive study reiterated many of the same barriers, providing data to confirm many major points leading to the statement that "it is not lack of talent, but unintentional biases and outmoded institutional structures that are hindering the access and advancement of women." One of the conclusions of this report was that "eliminating gender bias in universities requires immediate, overarching reform and decisive action by university administrators, professional societies, government agencies, and Congress."

In many situations, what is now generally referred to as "work-life balance" or making "work-life compromises" may have an impact on the advancement of women in their medical careers in many ways that can be difficult to quantify. The dual role that many women and even some men face in being successful in their professional responsibilities as well as often having the principal family responsibilities for childcare, family care, or other demands of family or personal life may determine specialty and practice choices, considerations for promotion and time constraints for meeting requirements for promotional advancement, demands of clinical or administrative duties, or undertaking research roles in academia. The competing demands of these dual roles still present major obstacles through institutional environments, schedules, and policies that have been designed and often continue without considerations for these demands because of the previous dominance of men in medicine due to inherent gender bias. This is addressed in terms of "outmoded institutional structures" in the National Academies report [13].

There are also instances where flexibility in timelines for promotion, research or fellowship opportunities, or leave for child or family care may be declined by women physicians and scientists because of fear of stigma rooted in gender bias if they deviate from the usual timeline expectations of their male colleagues. When such policies are promoted as "Family-Friendly Policies," and both men and women are encouraged to take advantage of such flexibility when needed, this may lessen the hesitancy of some to benefit from offered opportunities or to request them. As an example, the NIH now refers to adjustments in the implementation of Federal Grant Policies that are responsive to concerns of women physicians and scientists with dual professional demands as "Family-Friendly Initiatives," and institutions and organizations should consider following this same model of terminology [14, 15].

Of course, women make decisions that may determine their career progression. Their choices may be influenced by their perceptions of the likelihood of success, the ability to see potential for advancement, the courage and confidence to undertake new or different responsibilities especially depending on their life circumstances at that moment, and their experiences with unintended or intended gender biases and unconscious- or conscious-stereotypical attitudes in their work environment.

The intricacies of gender bias are related to the current concepts of the complexity of implicit bias, which is discussed in detail in chapter 2, "The Inconvenient Truth About Unconscious Bias in the Health Professions." Regardless, gender bias, or sexism, is considered as a major contributor to the lack of equity in the career advancement of women in medical careers, especially in academia, some examples of which are referred to in the above text. As one author, Economou, stated, "Women have been achieving near parity in MD and MD/PHD training, but their advancement in academic biomedical science is reduced at every career milestone thereafter" [16]. He further comments that "there are implicit biases—often subtle discrimination based on cultural stereotypes that may be outside of conscious awareness (unconscious bias)—that can affect decisions about one's career at every level…Women might be viewed as having more communal and nurturing traits, whereas men might be expected to have more of a self promoting, leadership phenotype."

Many other studies have specifically reported examples of ways that gender bias affects the careers of women in science and medicine. A piece on *Science Friday* brought attention to a report that scientific papers with female lead authors receive fewer citations than those with male lead authors, perpetuating the myth that there may be some "inherent differences in the content or quality of women's work." The report also referred to studies that suggest gender bias in how letters of recommendation are worded [17]. Trix and Psenka also published a study of recommendations for female and male medical faculty and concluded that letters for female faculty applicants differed systematically from those written for male faculty and tended to describe women more often as teachers and students while those for men more often portrayed them as researchers and professionals [18].

One other action that reflects a stereotypical attitude about women, regardless of career, is sexual harassment, often based on the biased concept of women being seen as less empowered and as sexual beings rather than being respected for their intellectual or scientific abilities. That sexual harassment exists in the sciences has long been known, but only in recent years have the scientific literature and the print media begun to give attention to these problems for women in biomedical careers. While sexual harassment may be inflicted on both men and women, by far the majority of reports have been of women students or faculty members. Few studies of harassment of women in medicine exist [19, 20]. The Committee on Women in Science, Engineering, and Medicine of the National Academies has commissioned a committee to study the influence of sexual harassment in academia on the career advancement of women in the scientific, technical, and medical workforce. The committee expects to release this report in the summer of 2018 [21]. It is anticipated that the study will provide a better understanding of the prevalence of sexual harassment for women in biomedical careers, as well as guidance for how to best eliminate the gender bias in scientific and medical settings that facilitate inappropriate sexual advances or assaults on women (and men).

With the increase in the representation of women in medicine over the past 40 years, it is surprising that even today women may not be fully recognized as physicians in spite of their presence in every specialty, in visual media such as television and movies, and in all aspect of the communities in which they live and practice. Yet, women still report instances of being doubted as physicians in public situations and even occasionally by their patients. Media reports have indicated women physicians being doubted as doctors in public settings, and there are many anecdotal accounts of patients who still have a bias against women as their physicians.

While there have been significant improvements in the status of women in medical careers, the fact that gender bias may still reflect the prejudices Dr. Cabot described in 1915 is extremely bothersome. In the practice of medicine, interrelationships with colleagues have improved as women have demonstrated their ability to function in times of stress and that women are not less capable intellectually. However, there remain concerns about the role of peers and others when instances of gender bias affect the ability of women as physicians, educators, or just colleagues when those with less cognizant views of women in their medical roles present problems related to misinformed stereotypical traditional biases. Do their colleagues speak up in the defense of female (or male) colleagues when gender bias is suggested or manifested? Does each individual become a "committee of one" to rectify biases when they are expressed either openly or in subtle attitudes? Do we insist on institutional transparency, fairness, and accountability to ensure gender equity and diversity? Successful career advancement for women physicians may seem peripheral to clinical practice if only superficially considered. However, the mutual respect of peers, colleagues, and patients based on elimination of traditional biases; conscious recognition that women can be and are as capable as their male colleagues in decision-making and leadership positions in medical academia, industry, or practice; and successful examples of women in positions of authority can erode the negative biases and many of the barriers that still confront women in medicine.

Gender Bias in Research and Health Care: From Bias to Affirmation

Over the past 25 years, stereotypical impressions of what constitutes "women's health" have changed greatly, evolving into what some refer to as "Gender-Specific Medicine," but more importantly, reflecting the new and long overdue scientific approach to medicine based on the contributions of sex and gender to clinical care [22]. Whether it was gender bias or naiveté about the contributions of sex chromosomes and gender influences on health, medical care has not traditionally been based on long known or newly recognized sex and gender differences when they exist in diagnostic presentations of diseases or conditions, in responses to interventions, or how these data should be considered when providing the best care to both women or men patients. Many did not realize or even consider that numerous standards of medical practice related to conditions that affect both women and men had been based on research involving only men or a lack of significant numbers of women. Medical textbooks reinforced the lack of sex differences in even normal anatomy, physiology, and basic principles of diagnosis of non-sex-specific diseases. A sex-/gender-appropriate approach to health care has arisen from the synergy of efforts of the grassroots advocacy, medical and scientific, public policy, and legislative communities over the past 25 years [23]. These principles of sex/gender scientific appreciation can help abolish the impact of gender bias in health practices. Prejudices based on lack of knowledge about sex differences in health or on personal biases about the veracity or needs of patients based on their sex and gender cannot, and should not, be tolerated in our healthcare system.

It has been well documented that until the latter years of the twentieth century, women's health was traditionally considered as that of the reproductive system during the reproductive years, reflecting a gender bias in considerations of health and medical issues. Few studies actually examined how to prevent the major health contributors to mortality or morbidity in postmenopausal women or even how to consider menopause itself as part of the life transition and not as a disease needing treatment. More importantly, for a number of reasons, most research on conditions and diseases beyond the reproductive system were studied predominantly in male populations, although the results were considered to be applicable to women. Demands for defining the role of sex and gender in health through research most often referred to the example of cardiovascular disease in women as understudied and therefore often misdiagnosed. While heart disease was long recognized through statistics as the leading overall cause of death in women, neither most women or physicians seemed truly cognizant of this reality, and what was taught about clinical approaches to cardiovascular disease (CVD) had been based on research studies in which women were often not included. It was not unusual for groups of women or even health professionals to incorrectly identify the leading cause of death for women as breast cancer. (Breast cancer was the most common cancer in women but not the leading cause of death or of cancer deaths.)

During many women's health events throughout the 1990s, women often told anecdotes about going to the emergency room with complaints that did not fit the standard description of an acute myocardial infarction (MI) in men and being sent home with a diagnosis of anxiety or reflux only to return with a later diagnosis of MI becoming evident [24–26]. Later evidence reviews of the scientific literature published in 2003 documented that although coronary heart disease resulted in more than a quarter million deaths per year of women, much of the research of the prior 20 years either excluded women entirely or included limited numbers of women and minorities [27]. These studies further concluded that the published research rarely included findings specific to women. Therefore, it seemed given that research is needed to also include women in studies of CVD – and other conditions and diseases that affect both women and men – which would contribute to what was taught and practiced.

In 1990, the NIH ORWH was established to ensure the inclusion of women in biomedical research, as well as to set a research agenda for gaps in knowledge that needed to be studied. Integral to this focus on women's health was the expansion of the understanding of women's health beyond the reproductive system and reproductive years across the life span and to include conditions that may affect both sexes. Public Law in 1993 required the inclusion of women and minorities in clinical research studies with the additional requirement for analyses of research outcomes by gender, thus resulting in a shift in the design of biomedical research to allow the determination of sex and gender differences [28, 29].

With the strong focus on diseases that had not previously been well defined in women, and the emphasis on sex- and gender-based studies, women's health research and health considerations in care have evolved into the science of sex and gender factors in human health. It is now expected that variables of sex and gender will be examined across the spectrum of research, not just clinical but in basic, molecular and cellular investigations that form the basis for further clinical and translational studies and ultimately what is taught in health professional education and clinical application. The results of such studies can inform personal and professional approaches to patients and the provision of personalized sex and gender-appropriate health [1, 30, 31].

There are still many areas of human health where sex differences have not been demonstrated or explored, but for those conditions where sex/gender differences have been discovered or documented, it is important that this new knowledge be incorporated into medical education and clinical translation to care. Sex differences have been acknowledged in conditions such as many autoimmune diseases including lupus, rheumatoid arthritis, and multiple sclerosis. Similarly, sex/gender differences have been determined in how to approach addiction disorders, pain syndromes, and even gastrointestinal conditions such as irritable bowel syndrome [32, 33]. Definitions of AIDS were changed once sex differences in manifestations in women were identified. Sex differences in brain disorders have been well documented, such as increased prevalence of Parkinson's disease, Huntington's disease, autism, and schizophrenia in men but increased prevalence of Alzheimer's disease, depression, eating disorders, and anxiety disorders in women [34]. Sex differences are seen in the etiology of stroke, as men have more related to atherosclerosis (68% of men versus 19% of women) while women are more prone to cardioembolic origins, which can be of clinical significance for diagnosis as well as preventive or treatment therapies.

Knowledge of sex differences in pathophysiology, health and wellness, natural history of diseases, responses to interventions, and physiologic metabolism of medications is important in patient care; therefore, it is of importance that information from sex-based studies is incorporated into medical education and physicians' approaches to their patients. Pain syndromes are increasingly receiving attention about sex/gender roles and how gender or other biases in the interaction between the physician and patient, the impact of the physician's same or different sex as the patient, or the physician's knowledge about sex differences in the neuroscience of pain may affect accurate evaluation and effective treatment [35]. Women have been shown to have different responses in the effectiveness of some analgesics than men, are believed by some to have a lower pain threshold, and have been reported in some studies to experience more symptoms of pain than men even with similar underlying causes. The results of further research on the physiology and psychology of pain are needed to assist physicians and lessen the effects of gender bias in evaluating and managing pain.

Another example is, again, cardiovascular disease. A report on this topic by Legato, Johnson, and Manson stresses such points as the differential in metabolism affecting survival of women with heart disease, higher rates of atrial fibrillation and arrhythmias in women, and the uniqueness of women, because of a longer cQT interval, to be at increased risk of torsades de pointes in response to certain medications – which has led to the withdrawal of some of these from routine use – and that women are more likely to not show coronary atherosclerotic disease on imaging studies at the time of a MI because the cause may more likely be related to vascular spasm or small vessel disease [36]. There are also reports that women are not referred for diagnostic or therapeutic procedures as often as men. Increased investigations involving women and evaluation of CVD and heart disease will help in the prevention and management of these conditions in women and to correct the biases and myths that have arisen because of historical perceptions that these are the same regardless of sex [37].

There are many other reports of sex differences in pharmacologic responses, including safety and effectiveness, to various classes of drugs and of the need for more evaluation of sex differences in medical devices that may be prescribed for both men and women. Research is providing information about sex differences that can impact considerations of evaluation and treatment by physicians who must be aware of such differences and their importance in managing patient care.

Gender bias in health care can be described in terms of not recognizing that sex and gender differences exist and can affect human health so that sex-specific approaches to prevention, diagnosis, and management are considered. It can also be described in terms of how physicians and other healthcare providers may proceed with prejudicial patient management decisions based upon their own biases. Many other examples of questionable care based on sex have been reported, and many are summarized in the article by Alspach [38]. In addition to the many described above, they include fewer referrals for women for total joint arthroplasty, management of cases of acute coronary syndrome with less aggressive evidence-based drug therapies for secondary prevention, and other instances of differences in the use of expected procedures or treatments in critical care situations.

The education of physicians and other health professionals should include a responsibility to provide, as part of that educational process, information and data that will prevent gender bias from intruding into the approach to patients, consideration of their complaints, and being familiar with new knowledge related to sex differences in diseases and responses to interventions. This should begin with knowledge of sex differences in normal body anatomy, physiology, and aging. The article by Parker [31] suggests that there is a link between gender bias in medical education and negative attitudes and behaviors when practicing physicians. It also suggests that the predominantly male images and stereotypical information in anatomy textbooks may provide inadequate and unrealistic information about patients that can perpetuate gender bias in medicine.

Risberg and her colleagues, in response to the goal of incorporating a gender perspective in medical education to combat gender bias, surveyed medical educators in a Swedish medical school and concluded that it is necessary that "both male and female teachers participate and embrace gender aspects as important. To facilitate implementation and to convince those who are indifferent, this study indicates that special efforts are needed to motivate men" [39]. (Note: This author strongly agrees that both male and female faculty and colleagues must promote concepts of sex and gender in health and in health careers, and that the newly documented facts related to the importance of sex and gender factors in human health will be motivation for both male and female faculty to embrace the transmission to students.)

Gender biases can and should be transformed into *sex and gender awareness* based on scientific information. Future physicians should consider how their own sex/gender might affect both their reception to patients' complaints and how they proceed with the management of their patients' health. The need for improved attention to non-binary gender identities, such as those who are transgender, remains important for future discussions of sex and gender in human health and collegial attitudes [40].

Conclusion

Bias of any type ideally should not exist in a sophisticated healthcare system such as is found in the United States. With the exceptional and comprehensive standards for the accreditation of medical institutions and centers, and for medical licensing and standards of care expected of physicians, prejudicial actions in the care of patients or in career opportunities based on traditional stereotypical biases should not still exist or be tolerated. Further, biomedical research has demonstrated sex and gender differences across the spectrum of health and disease that should eliminate sex biases in health care approaches for women and for men. These findings are important in decision-making for excellence in health care for both women and men. With the current emphasis on personalized medicine, how can one ignore the effects of sex characteristics and gender influences on the totality of the human body, from cells to behaviors, and resulting responses to evidence-based interventions?

Gender bias, based on traditional stereotypical impressions of sex and gender, be it implicit, unintentional, unconscious, or even conscious and intentional, has consequences for the health, health care, and careers of women and men. Unconscious bias has received much attention in many aspects of our lives, but such bias, including either intentional or unconscious that manifests itself in health care or in health careers, should not be tolerated. There are many reports of unconscious bias in medical decision-making, related to either or both sex or race or other factors [41, 42]. It is vital to recognize that such biases exist and to take all possible steps to eliminate the negativism of such influences. Several suggested actions by the Joint Commission to deter bias such as that associated with gender include the following: avoid stereotyping patients, individuate them, understand and respect the magnitude of unconscious bias, recognize situations that magnify unconscious bias, and assiduously practice evidence-based medicine by making the most objective evaluation and decisions possible [43].

Gender bias can and does result in unnecessary morbidity for patients and lack of fair career opportunities for women in health and academic medical careers. To quote Dr. Shirley Malcom, Head of the Directorate for Education and Human Resources Programs of the American Association for the Advancement of Science:

> "Confronting …bias is always difficult, but women and men should be willing to stand
> up to it…"

We all have a responsibility to ensure that gender bias does not affect healthcare decision-making and that both women and men have fairness and equity in their health care and health career opportunities.

References

1. Wizemann TM, Pardue ML, editors. Exploring the biological contributions to human health: does sex matter? Washington, DC: National Academies Press; 2001. 288 p.
2. Cabot RC. Women in medicine. JAMA. 1915;65(1):947–8.
3. Elizabeth Blackwell [Internet]. [New York]: Bio; c2017 (Cited 19 Dec 2017). Available from: https://www.biography.com/people/elizabeth-blackwell-9214198
4. Office of Women's Health, Department of Health and Human Services. A century of women's health: 1900–2000 [Internet]. Washington (DC): U.S Department of Health and Human Services; 2002 (Cited 19 Dec 2017). Available from: https://www.webharvest.gov/peth04/20041102164114/http://4woman.gov/TimeCapsule/century/century.pdf
5. Number of women enrolling in medical school reaches 10-year high [Internet]. Chicago: Association of American Medical Colleges; 2016 Nov 1 (Cited 19 Dec 2017). Available from: https://news.aamc.org/medical-education/article/women-enrolling-medical-school-10-year-high/
6. Boulis AK, Jacobs JA. The changing face of medicine: women doctors and the evolution of healthcare in America. Ithaca: Cornell University Press; 2008. 280 p.
7. The state of women in academic medicine: the pipeline and pathways to leadership, 2013–2014 [Internet]. Chicago: Association of American Medical Colleges; 2014 (Cited 19 Dec 2017). Available from: https://www.aamc.org/members/gwims/statistics/
8. The state of women in academic medicine: the pipeline and pathways to leadership, 2015–2016 [Internet]. Chicago: Association of American Medical Colleges; 2016. Table 2, Distribution of residents by specialty, 2005 compared to 2015. Available from: https://www.aamc.org/download/481180/data/2015table2.pdf
9. The state of women in academic medicine: the pipeline and pathways to leadership, 2015–2016 [Internet]. Chicago: Association of American Medical Colleges; 2016. Table 11, Distribution of chairs by department, gender, and races/ethnicity. Available from: https://www.aamc.org/download/481206/data/2015table11.pdf
10. Lautenberger D, Raezer C, Bunton SA. The underrepresentation of women in leadership positions at U.S. medical schools. Analysis in Brief, Association of American Medical Colleges. 2015;15(2):1–2.
11. National Institutes of Health. Women in biomedical careers: dynamics of change: strategies for the 21st century. Washington, DC: U.S. Department of Health and Human Services; 1994. 228 p. NIH Publication No. 95-3565.
12. Handelsman J, Cantor N, Carnes M, Denton D, Fine E, Grosz B, Hinshaw V, Marrett C, Rosser S, Shalala D, Sheridan J. More women in science. Science. 2005;309(5738):1190–1. https://doi.org/10.1126/science.1113252.
13. The National Academies. Beyond bias and barriers: fulfilling the potential of women in academic science and engineering. Washington, DC: The National Academies Press; 2007. 346 p.
14. NIH family-friendly initiatives [Internet]. Bethesda, MD: National Institutes of Health; 2011 (Cited 19 Dec 2017). Available from: https://grants.nih.gov/grants/family_friendly.htm
15. Rockey S. Update on NIH's implementation of federal grant policies [Internet]. Bethesda, MD: National Institutes of Health; 2015 (Cited 19 Dec 2017). Available from: https://nexus.od.nih.gov/all/2015/03/02/update-on-nihs-implementation-of-federal-grant-policies/

16. Economou JS. Gender bias in biomedical research. Surg. 2014;156(5):1061–65. doi. org/10.1016/j.surg.2014.07.005.
17. Franz J. The weight of gender bias on women's scientific careers [Internet]. Minneapolis, MN: Public Radio International; 2017 (Cited 19 Dec 2017). Available from: https://www.pri.org/stories/2017-01-01/weight-gender-bias-women-s-scientific-careers
18. Trix F, Psenka C. Exploring the color of glass: letters of recommendation for female and male medical faculty. Discourse & Society. 2003;14(2):191–220.
19. Carr PL, Ash AS, Friedman RH, et al. Faculty perceptions of gender discrimination and sexual harassment in academic medicine. Ann Intern Med. 2000;132(11):889–96.
20. Jagsi R, Griffith KA, Jones R, Permumalswami CR, Ubel P, Stewart A. Sexual harassment and discrimination experiences of academic medical faculty. JAMA. 2016;315(19):2120–1.
21. National Academies of Sciences, Engineering, and Medicine. Sexual harassment of women: climate, culture, and consequences in academic sciences, engineering, and medicine. Washington, DC: The National Academies Press; 2018. https://doi.org/10.17226/24994.
22. Legato MJ. Principles of gender-specific medicine. Gender in the genomic era. 3rd ed. London: Academic Press; 2017. 792 p.
23. Pinn VW. Women's health research: current state of the art. Glob Adv Health Med. 2013;2(5):8–10. https://doi.org/10.7453/gahmj.2013.063.
24. Legato MJ, Colman C. The female heart: the truth about women and coronary artery disease. New York: Simon & Schuster; 1991. 252 p.
25. Rubini Gimenez M, Reiter M, Twerenbold R, et al. Sex-specific chest pain characteristics in the early diagnosis of acute myocardial infarction. JAMA Intern Med. 2014;174(2):241–9. https://doi.org/10.1001/jamainternmed.2013.12199.
26. Pilote L. Chest pain in acute myocardial infarction: are men from Mars and women from Venus? JAMA Intern Med. 2014;174(2):249. https://doi.org/10.1001/jamainternmed.2013.12097.
27. Grady D, Chaput L, Kristof M (University of California, San Francisco-Stanford Evidence-based Practice Center). Diagnosis and treatment of coronary heart disease in women: systematic reviews of evidence on selected topics. Evidence report/technology assessment No. 81. Rockville, MD: Agency for Healthcare Research and Quality: 2003 May. 144 p. AHRQ Publication No. 03-E037. Contract No 290-97-0013.
28. Pinn V. Research on women's health: progress and opportunities. JAMA. 2005;294(11):1407–10. https://doi.org/10.1001/jama.294.11.1407.
29. Kelty M, Bates A, Pinn VW. National Institutes of Health policy on the inclusion of women and minorities as subjects in clinical research. In: Gallin JI, Ognibene FP, editors. Principles and practice of clinical research. 3rd ed. London: Academic Press; 2012. p. 147–59.
30. Clayton JA, Collins FS. NIH to balance sex in cell and animal studies. Nature. 2014;509(7500):282–3.
31. Parker R, Larkin T, Cockburn J. A visual analysis of gender bias in contemporary anatomy textbooks. Soc Sci Med. 2017;180:106–13.
32. Moving into the future with new dimensions and strategies: a vision for 2020 for women's health research. Bethesda, MD: National Institutes of Health; 2010. NIH Publication No. 10-7606. Available from: http://orwh.od.nih.gov/research/strategicplan/ORWH_StrategicPlan2020_Vol1.pdf
33. Kim AM, Tingen CM, Woodruff TK. Sex bias in trials and treatment must end. Nature. 2010;465:688–9.
34. Institute of Medicine. Sex differences and implications for translational neuroscience research: workshop summary. Washington, DC: The National Academies Press; 2011.
35. Becker B, McGregor AJ. Men, women, and pain. Gender and the Genome. 2017;1(1):46–50. https://doi.org/10.1089/gg.2017.0002.
36. Legato MJ, Johnson PA, Manson JE. Consideration of sex differences in medicine to improve health care and patient outcomes. JAMA. 2016;316(18):1865–6. https://doi.org/10.1001/jama.2016.13995.

37. Raeisi-Giglou P, Santos A, Volgman AS, Patel H, Campbell S, Villablanca A, Hsich E. Advances in cardiovascular health in women over the past decade: guideline recommendations for practice. J Women's Health. 2017;27:128. https://doi.org/10.1089/jwh.2016.6316.

38. Alspach JG. Is there gender bias in critical care? Crit Care Nurs. 2012;32:8–14. https://doi.org/10.4037/ccn2012727.

39. Risberg G, Johansson EE, Westman G, Hamberg K. Gender in medicine – an issue for women only? A survey of physician teachers' gender attitudes. Int J Equity Health. 2003;2:10–7.

40. Streed CG, Makadon HJ. Sex and gender reporting in research. JAMA. 2017;317(9):974–5. https://doi.org/10.1001/jama.2017.0145.

41. Hamberg K. Gender bias in healthcare. Womens Health. 2008;4(3):237–43.

42. Byyny RL. Cognitive bias: recognizing and managing our unconscious biases. Pharos Alpha Omega Alpha Honor Med Soc. 2017;80(1):2–6.

43. Implicit bias in health care. Quick Safety. 2016;23:1–4.

Chapter 5
A Global Perspective on Health Care

Lisa Moreno-Walton

Introduction

Most readers of this text (*Your Story/Our Story*) live in First World countries, designated as having high levels of life expectancy at birth and education by age 25, as well as a high Human Development Index, Gross Domestic Product indicator, and Press Freedom Index [1]. When we go to our worksite as healthcare providers, we give little thought to the resources we will use during our shifts. We anticipate that the operating room will be provisioned with sterile equipment, that the ventilators will be powered by electricity, that the cardiac catheterization lab will be able to open within minutes, that there will be incubators for premature newborns, and that well-equipped ambulances will be available to transport even non-emergent patients to the emergency department. Our research endeavors and quality assurance projects focus on increasing the quality, efficacy, and efficiency of the practice of medicine. However, there is a vast difference between the medicine that is practiced in the First World and the health care that is available to most of the earth's inhabitants.[1]

Discussion

Each year, upward of two million Americans participate in short-term medical mission trips, and about half of those participants have no formal medical training [2]. Websites advertise to medical professionals seeking an opportunity for travel: "Are

---

[1] Attributed to Professor Lee Wallis, Immediate Past President of the International Federation of Emergency Medicine and Past President of the African Federation of Emergency Medicine.

L. Moreno-Walton
Department of Medicine, Section of Emergency Medicine, Louisiana State University Health Sciences Center-New Orleans, New Orleans, LA, USA

© Springer International Publishing AG, part of Springer Nature 2019
M. L. Martin et al. (eds.), *Diversity and Inclusion in Quality Patient Care*,
https://doi.org/10.1007/978-3-319-92762-6_5

you frustrated and stressed from medical practice in the United States? Do you enjoy travel or have a yearning to help others? If so, why not try a volunteer vacation?" [3]. Other websites encourage medical students and college students interested in considering medicine as a career to participate in mission trips as a way to advance their medical skills by practicing examinations and procedures that they would not be permitted to do in their home country because of their lack of training and credentials [4]. Medical mission trips are often self-funded by medical professionals or funded by crowdsourcing and organizational donations raised by participants. Multiple ethical issues compromise the reputation of such trips, such as, best use of monetary contributions, ethical care of patients, sustainability, and value of skills taught.

A recent article described a mission trip undertaken by 18 college students who worked at an orphanage in Honduras for their spring break. The students raised $25,000 to pay for the trip, and many of them reported that it was a life-changing event for them. However, the orphanage's yearly budget of $45,000 covers staff salaries, building maintenance, and food and clothes for the children. One of the permanent missionaries commented that she knew that the trip benefited the students far more than it benefited the orphans, and the orphanage administrator stated, "We could have done so much with that money" [5]. We exist in a global economy that annually spends the equivalent of US$400 billion on recreational narcotics, where Japanese businessmen spend US$35 billion for business-related entertainment, and where American and European Union consumers spend US$12 billion on perfume. In comparison, only US$13 billion is spent on basic health and nutrition and only US$9 billion is spent on water sanitation [6]. Clearly, the advantage of having a healthy population of global citizens is not obvious to many governments or many individuals in control of organizational budgets, or other needs are deemed more pressing. In a world where the average annual salary in purchasing power parity dollars is $1,480 per month [7], over 3 billion people live on less than $2.50 per day, and 80% of the world's people live on less than $10 per day [6], it is shocking that Americans spend $250 million dollars annually to send themselves on medical mission trips that are of questionable value to anyone but themselves [8, 9].

The ethical issues that are most compelling arise around the actual provision of medical care. Multiple blog sites exist on which medical, dental, premedical, nursing, and pharmacy students discuss their experiences. The oft quoted and variably attributed statement that "the only care that they get is the care that you give them" is a concept that the students themselves often echo [10]. But, it begs the question: Does care rendered by a student actually qualify as medical care? Or more bluntly stated: Does being poor and brown mean that you do not deserve the same level of expertise and consideration for patient safety as someone who is rich and white? There is adequate literature to support the fact that "those in training may lack experience in recognizing serious or unfamiliar conditions and skills in performing particular procedures. In resource-constrained health care settings, trainees from resource-replete environments may have inflated ideas about the value of their skills and yet may be unfamiliar with syndromic approaches to patient treatment that are common in settings with limited laboratory capacity. These challenges may be compounded by…lack of mutual understanding of training and experience, and the possibility that inexperienced or ill-equipped short-term trainees are given responsibilities beyond their capability" [11]. Further challenges to patients' ability to receive adequate medical care are often compounded by the visiting trainee or professional healthcare provider's inability to speak the language of the country where he has chosen to do short-term medical work or his failure to understand the culture [12]. Some American medical colleges and residency training programs propose that work abroad helps meet the Accreditation Council for Graduate Medical Education cultural competency requirements [13], and there is indeed value in exposing students and residents to cultures that are not their own as part of cultural competency training. When inadequately supervised, however, these experiences can again be far more valuable to the trainees than to the patients. Those faculty members with expertise can find opportunities to teach cultural competency to students and residents during the day-to-day, well-supervised patient encounters that are part of their home hospital training. In-country training also ensures that patient outcomes are closely monitored, as opposed to international training experiences, where 74% of missions either fail to document outcomes, or follow patients for only a few days [8].

The issue of sustainability is a major consideration in global health. The translation of skills from physicians in resource- and training-rich nations to physicians in resource- and training-poor nations is far more efficient, both monetarily and in patient access and outcomes, than medical missions conducted by physicians from resource-rich nations. Clearly, an indigenous physician can operate on more patients in a year than a visiting physician can operate on in a month. However, such skills translation is extremely work-intensive. Documented relationships leading to independent practice generally take 10 years or more [14, 15]. One of the most successful programs involves teaching renal transplantation to indigenous surgeons in northern Iraq. Dr. Gazi Zibari, an Iraqi Kurdish physician, returned to his native country in 1992 to lay the groundwork for the program. American physicians work side by side with Kurdish physicians to prepare patients, perform surgery, and manage postoperative routine and critical care [16, 17]. Preliminary analysis of the independent work of the Kurdish surgeons over a 5-year period documents renal transplant outcomes comparable to those achieved in the United States, but the program has a decade-long history of a few in-country visits a year by a stable team of physicians as well as telemedicine and phone contact as needed. The Americas Hepato-Pancreato-Biliary Association, Operation Hope, and the Kurdistan Regional Government Prime Minister Foundation have supplied consistent funding to ensure that all of the necessary resources are consistently available in the local hospital. Additionally, the program is led by a linguistically and culturally competent, resource-sensitive physician who maintains constant contact with government, military, and health ministry officials so that there are no interruptions in supplies or barriers to patient care, communication, or physician training. Perhaps most importantly, Dr. Zibari performed a needs assessment and a feasibility study prior to initiating the program. He was cognizant of the fact that much of what we in the First World seek to teach physicians and other healthcare providers in the Third World is meaningless in the context in which they practice medicine. We all hear of programs, costly in dollars, time, and energy, designed to teach bystander cardiopulmonary resuscitation or put automated external defibrillators in public venues in nations where tuk-tuks and auto rickshaws are used to transport patients to hospitals or where the nearest hospital is 4 h away by the local transport method. Might it be more sensible to train an indigenous healthcare worker, someone who speaks the language, knows the culture, is trusted by the community, and is going to continue to live and work among them, to deliver a breech baby, or to set a fracture? Many global health professionals, this author among them, contend that this is the most cost-effective, culturally competent method of bringing sustainable health care to the majority of the world's population. In countries like Afghanistan or Bangladesh, where there are only 0.3 physicians per 1000 people, or Malawi, Niger, and Sierra Leone, where there are only 0.02, what good would it do to teach renal transplantation or defibrillation? [18]. With UNICEF estimating that 2.2 million children died last year due to lack of immunization [19], providing cheap resources and minimal training to community health workers seems an obvious cure.

One of the most devastating areas of disparities is found among the ever-expanding population of displaced persons and refugees. According to reports issued in June 2017 by the United Nations High Commission on Refugees, 65.6 million people are currently living as forcibly displaced persons, of which 22.5 million are refugees and 10 million are currently stateless people. Of these 65.6 million displaced persons, fully one half of them are under the age of 18. During the year under analysis, only 189,300 of these people had been resettled, with the remainder living in camps or ad hoc communities [20]. Individuals living in such conditions, as well maintained as some of them may be, are subject to infections that are transmitted in environments lacking modern sanitation (cholera, trachoma, schistosomiasis), infections common in crowded environments (tuberculosis, hepatitis, mononucleosis), and diseases that are caused by social stressors (domestic violence, hypertension, low birth weight and premature delivery, sexual harassment and assault, child abuse, human trafficking, prostitution).

Another area of health disparity is research. Eighty percent of the world's scientific literature is produced by only 20 countries. None of these countries is in Africa or the Middle East, and only one (Brazil) is in Latin America. One of the limiting factors is that most of the major indexes, such as Scopus (the largest abstract and citation database of peer-reviewed literature), require that articles be printed in English in order to qualify for listing [21]. The recently published English language study, "Mortality after Fluid Bolus in African Children with Severe Infection," [22] called into serious question the concept that evidence-based medicine can be universally applied to all patients when not all patients share the same resources or genetics as the study population on which the evidence was established. If every patient is to have the benefit of evidence-based practice, then all patient populations must have the opportunity to be studied and have best practices established for their race, ethnicity, culture, and resource environment.

Research is further impacted by who is doing the research. Drug companies are increasingly conducting studies in nations whose ethical review boards are less complex to negotiate than those in Western cultures. Recent studies question "whether the research being conducted is of value to public health in these countries or whether economically disadvantaged populations are being exploited for the benefit of patients in rich countries" [23]. Even non-pharmaceutical studies in Third World countries are most often conducted by Northern investigators. Witness the multiple papers published about the Haitian earthquake experience written by North American authors who traveled to Haiti to do medical mission relief work, but chose not to involve Haitian physicians as co-investigators. Perhaps part of the Fluid Expansion as Supportive Therapy (FEAST) study's success can be attributed to the involvement of local doctors. In a presentation about their work, the investigators stressed the importance of the relationships between the local pediatric staff and the community, both in enrolling patients and in the treatment of the children during the trial. Other studies have documented that the well-established phenomenon of concordance in clinical practice also has a powerful influence in research trials [24].

More recently, the social diseases of human trafficking and orphan tourism have been on the rise. Currently, 20.9 million persons are victims of human trafficking. Each year, 2 million children are forced into sexual slavery. More than half of children trafficked for sex tourism are under the age of 12 and serve about 1,500 customers per year. Ninety percent of children rescued from Southeast Asian brothels are infected with HIV. Two-thirds of victims of child sex trafficking undergo forced abortions, often outside of safe medical environments [25]. Trafficking of girls is sometimes sanctioned by their families, who must sacrifice one child to feed the others or who feel that a female child must contribute to the family. The amelioration of global poverty and the elimination of the gender disparities that prohibit the education of females and their employment in professions and trades will serve to remove one of the root causes of trafficking. Enforcement of the international laws prohibiting trafficking and criminalization of procurement of persons for engagement in sexual activity in exchange for money will help to eliminate the other contributing factors [26].

A recent Al-Jazeera documentary highlighted the facts about the emerging orphanage tourism trade and popularized the slogan, "Children are not tourist attractions." According to their report, two-thirds of children living in orphanages have at least one living parent but are kept out of school and employed as professional orphans. Western tourists are lured into the orphanage and asked to play with the children and to make contributions to social and educational programs to improve life for the orphans. The money is kept by the proprietor of the orphanage. Visitors can enter the children's bedrooms at will, unsupervised, and can "check out" a child for the day to take them to a zoo, an amusement park, or for a meal. There have been numerous incidents of kidnappings and child molestations associated with these activities [27].

Conclusion

While modern health care has made remarkable advances in recent decades, not every citizen of the world can benefit from these advancements. Resource-rich nations should take care to invest money and skills in resource-poor nations in a culturally competent and resource-sensitive manner. Needs assessments, feasibility studies, impact studies, and appropriate governmental permissions and collaborations must be undertaken to ensure the success of any intervention. Local healthcare providers must be involved in the planning, execution, analysis, and publication of any endeavor that takes place in their country and involves their patients if exploitation is to be avoided. Proper supervision of trainees, protection of patient safety, and quality assurance monitoring of complications and outcome measures must be done in the field with the same rigor as it is done in the home hospital environment. Empowerment of local healthcare providers will ensure that sustainable and meaningful assistance is provided in a way that is culturally competent and resource sensitive. Visiting physicians and other providers must be aware that they are guests in the host country. They should provide for their own lodging and food so they do not use resources that could have been made available to patients. They should make every effort to learn the culture and the language of the country where they plan to visit so they can maximize their positive impact and minimize the risk of misdiagnosis or harmful interactions. Visitors must be aware of the high risk of diseases linked to poverty (abuse, trafficking, certain infectious diseases, low birth weight) that may be far more prevalent in the nations that they visit. Everywhere we go, we should be cognizant of the privilege we have as healthcare providers and be certain to honor the patients who trust us with their care. Eventually, every patient will have access to culturally competent, evidence-based, best practices for whatever medical condition presents. We can each be a link in the chain that eliminates poverty and disparity for every patient whose life we touch, regardless of color, race, religion, ethnicity, age, gender identity, or socioeconomic status.

References

1. One world—the nations online project: get in touch with your neighbors [Internet]. [place unknown]: The Nations Online Project; c1998–2017 (Cited 8 Jan 2018). Available from: www.nationsonline.org
2. ShortTermMissions.org. Research and statistics: where can I find data and statistics about short-term missions and their impact? [Internet]. St. Louis (MO): Mission Data International; c2000–2018 (Cited 8 Jan 2018). Available from: http://www.shorttermmissions.com/articles/research
3. Smith JD. What to expect from a medical mission [Internet]. Alexandria (VA): American Academy of Otolaryngology; c2018 (Cited 8 Jan 2018). Available from: http://www.entnet.org/content/what-expect-medical-mission
4. Raymond R. Mission possible: a brief how-to guide on medical missions [Internet]. [Chicago]: American Osteopathic Association; 2014 (Cited 8 Jan 2018). Available from: https://thedo.osteopathic.org/2014/04/mission-possible-a-brief-how-to-guide-on-medical-missions/

5. Van Engen JA. Short term missions: are they worth the cost? The Other Side [Internet]. 2000 (Cited 8 Jan 2018). Available from: http://www.bostoncollege.org/content/dam/files/centers/boisi/pdf/s091/VanEngenShortTermMissionsarticle.pdf

6. Shah A. Poverty facts and stats [Internet]. [place unknown]: Anup Shah; 2013 (Cited 7 Jan 2018). Available from: http://www.globalissues.org/article/26/poverty-facts-and-stats

7. Alexander R. Where are you on the global pay scale? [Internet]. London: BBC; 2012 (Cited 8 Jan 2018). Available from: www.bbc.com/news/magazine-17512040

8. Sykes KJ. Short term medical service trips: a systematic review of the evidence. Am J Public Health. 2014;104(7):e38–48.

9. Statton ML. 7 Reasons why your two week trip to Haiti doesn't matter: calling bull on "service trips" and voluntourism [Internet]. New York: The Almost Doctor's Channel; 2015 (Cited 8 Jan 2018). Available from: http://almost.thedoctorschannel.com/14323-2/

10. About28. The medical mission trip question. In: Pre-Medical-MD [Internet]. [Houston (TX)]: CRG; 2014 (Cited 8 Jan 2018). [about 17 screens]. Available from: https://forums.studentdoctor.net/threads/the-medical-mission-trip-question.1052640/

11. Crump JA, Sugarman J. Ethical considerations for short-term experiences by trainees in global health. JAMA. 2008;300(12):1456–8.

12. Harris JJ, Shao J, Sugarman J. Disclosure of cancer diagnosis and prognosis in northern Tanzania. Soc Sci Med. 2003;56(5):905–13.

13. Campbell A, Sullivan M, Sherman R, Magee WP. The medical mission and modern cultural competency training. J Am Coll Surg. 2011;212(1):124–9.

14. Novick WM, Stidham GL, Karl TR, et al. Paediatric cardiac assistance in developing and transitional countries: the impact of a fourteen year effort. Cardiol Young. 2008;18(3):316–23.

15. Uetani M, Jimba M, Niimi T, et al. Effects of a long-term volunteer surgical program in a developing country: the case in Vietnam from 1993 to 2003. Cleft Palate Craniofac J. 2006;43(5):616–9.

16. Moreno-Walton L. Iraq: field report. Emerg Physicians Int. 2016;19:12–3.

17. Moreno-Walton L. Return, rebuild: one Kurdish surgeon brings healing to northern Iraq. Emerg Physicians Int. 2016;20:20–2.

18. The world factbook [Internet]. Washington: CIA; (Cited 8 Jan 2018). Available from: https://www.cia.gov/library/publications/the-world-factbook/docs/guidetowfbook.html

19. Why are children dying? [Internet]. New York: UNICEF; (Cited 8 Jan 2018). Available from: https://www.unicef.org/immunization/index_why.html

20. Figures at a glance [Internet]. Geneva: UNHCR; c2001–2018 (Cited 8 Jan 2018). Available from: www.unhcr.org/en-us.figures-at-a-glance.html

21. Huttner-Koros A. The hidden bias of science's universal language [Internet]. Washington: The Atlantic Monthly Group; 2015 (Cited 8 Jan 2018). Available from: https://www.theatlantic.com/science/archive/2015/08/english-universal-language-science-research/400919/

22. Maitland K, Kiguli S, Opoka RO, et al. Mortality after fluid bolus in African children with severe infection. N Engl J Med. 2011;364:2483–95. doi:full/https://doi.org/10.1056/NEJMoa1101549.

23. Weigman K. The ethics of global clinical trials. EMBO Rep. 2015;16(5):566–70.

24. Campbell C, Nair Y, et al. Hearing community voices: grassroots perceptions of an intervention to support health volunteers in South Africa. SAHARA J. 2008;5(4):162–77

25. Sex trafficking fact sheet [Internet]. New York: Equality Now; (Cited 8 Jan 2018). Available from: https://www.equalitynow.org/sex-trafficking-fact-sheet

26. Polaris [Internet]. Washington: Polaris; c2018 (Cited 8 Jan 2018). Available from: www.polarisproject.org

27. Papi D. Why you should say no to orphanage tourism (and tell all tour companies to do the same) [Internet]. New York: Oath Inc; 2012 Nov 20 (Updated 2017 Dec 6; cited 2018 Jan 8). Available from: www.huffingtonpost.com/daniela-papi/cambodia-orphanages-_b_2164385.html

Chapter 6
Cultural Competence and the Deaf Patient

Jason M. Rotoli, Paolo Grenga, Trevor Halle, Rachel Nelson, and Gloria Wink

Introduction

People with disabilities or those who require accommodations to access health care and medical information are subjected to increased healthcare disparities. They experience disproportionately reduced appointment availability, lack of accessible and timely transportation, increased cost and insurance barriers, poor physician-patient communication, negative attitudes, lack of respect, and discrimination [1]. This includes people with cognitive disorders, physical limitations, visual impairment, and hearing deficits. In comparison to the general population, obesity, oral disease, diabetes, depression/anxiety, and interpersonal violence are higher among people with disabilities. Within this underrepresented group, those with multiple disabilities tend to have worse overall health outcomes and more prevalent comorbidities. Patients who self-identify as having a disability are also more likely to rate their own health as poor [2, 3].

The term disability is often defined as a physical or mental condition that limits a person's movements, senses, or functional ability leading to an inability to engage in any substantial gainful activity [4]. However, despite having a hearing deficiency, the culturally deaf population does not identify with this definition. The culturally deaf, or capital "D" [Deaf], are a group who use American Sign Language (ASL) as the primary language and have no sense of loss or perceived inability. In fact, there is quite the opposite attitude among its community members. This is a group of people who define their deafness culturally and ethnically, not medically. Unlike most other people with a disability, Deaf people often prefer their children

J. M. Rotoli (✉) · P. Grenga · T. Halle · R. Nelson · G. Wink
University of Rochester Medical Center, Rochester, NY, USA
e-mail: Jason_rotoli@urmc.rochester.edu; Paolo_grenga@urmc.rochester.edu;
Trevor_halle@urmc.rochester.edu; Rachel_nelson@urmc.rochester.edu;
Gloria_wink@urmc.rochester.edu

© Springer International Publishing AG, part of Springer Nature 2019
M. L. Martin et al. (eds.), *Diversity and Inclusion in Quality Patient Care*,
https://doi.org/10.1007/978-3-319-92762-6_6

to be born Deaf in hopes of sharing the same life experiences. In addition, they share a common language, visual art, poetry, and customs. This is in contrast to lower case "d" [deaf], which indicates the medical condition of deafness and incorporates people who were born hearing, use spoken language, and identify with their own race, culture, or ethnicity [5].

For the Deaf ASL user, there are several important statutes, laws, and organizations established to reduce healthcare disparities and facilitate accessible and equitable health care. Established in 1880, the National Association of the Deaf (NAD) is a civil rights organization advocating in the areas of early intervention, education, employment, health care, technology, and telecommunications. Within the NAD, the Law and Advocacy Office advocates for equal access to mental and physical health care across the USA [6]. In 1990, the Americans with Disabilities Act afforded protection against discrimination in employment, transportation, public accommodation, and communications. This empowered people with disabilities by requiring access to appropriate communication accommodations in all public places, including the healthcare setting. For the Deaf ASL user, it requires healthcare professionals to provide a qualified ASL interpreter to facilitate clear communication [7]. In 2004, recognition of American Sign Language as an official foreign language allowed for the application of prior congressional statutes (Bilingual Education Act 1965 and Civil Right Statutes 1974) to deaf students, thereby providing funding for language barrier removal in schools, where there is the first exposure to basic health information [8]. The Joint Commission, a national US hospital accreditation organization in patient quality and safety, is also committed to the reduction of healthcare disparities through supporting education in cultural competence and encouraging hospitals to provide equal access to care for underrepresented groups [9]. Despite these protective agencies and laws, there are still shortcomings leading to educational, socioeconomic, and health disparities. For example, the ADA mandates the cost of accommodations to be placed on the local provider or employer. This creates a sense of hesitation for employers to hire Deaf ASL users, thereby reducing the chance of successful employment and perpetuating a lower socioeconomic status. It may also cause healthcare providers to shy away from caring for Deaf ASL users, which can translate to lower access to care, lower health literacy, and persistent healthcare disparities [10].

While exposed to the same barriers to care as other people with disabilities, the Deaf ASL user is also a linguistic minority, which contributes to a language discordance further resulting in a low health literacy level. Nearly all emergency department/hospital paperwork, medical pamphlets, television commercials (with or without closed captioning), and news channels communicate using written or spoken English. This severely limits access for those whose primary language is American Sign Language, among whom the average English literacy level is between third and fourth grade [5, 11]. As a result of low health literacy and limited English proficiency (LEP), there is a reduced utilization of primary care resulting in increased emergency department visits, limited health surveillance, and poor representation in healthcare literature and research [12–14]. It has also been shown that linguistic minorities rate themselves as having poorer general and emotional health than the general population [13]. The culmination of these factors results in poor overall healthcare access and worse outcomes for the Deaf ASL user [1, 5, 13, 14].

Discussion

Early access to language provides the foundation for normal development and is strongly associated with future literacy, academic achievement, and health [15]. There is often a lack of communication in a Deaf person's early childhood. This void is deeply rooted and, in time, branches into the challenges that permeate all aspects of the culturally deaf adult's life. Inadequate communication leads to delayed social development and social isolation, low English literacy and subsequent low socioeconomic status, poor health and health literacy, inadequate access to health care, and healthcare misconceptions [5].

Social Development and Isolation

Deaf children experience significant obstacles to their social development, often resulting in social isolation. Many are born to hearing parents and share unique challenges to their developmental experiences such as early childhood communication deprivation, family stressors related to their deafness, limited educational opportunities compared to their hearing peers, and social stigma within the hearing world. Together, these challenges shape the ways that Deaf persons learn to interact with the hearing world and set the stage for their ability to function as independent adults [16–19].

Deaf children often demonstrate delays in learning normative social behaviors. For most hearing children, these behaviors are learned from parents who share a common language; however, the majority of Deaf children are born to hearing parents who have little knowledge of ASL or Deaf culture [5, 18, 19]. This creates two challenges for Deaf children. First, their inability to communicate with hearing adults and hearing peers causes them to struggle in learning social customs such as interpreting body language, how to make friends, how to play with others, and how to communicate their needs to others who have a discordant language [5]. Most hearing parents do not know ASL and, consequently, cannot communicate effectively with their children. Subsequently, the stress and frustration of communicating with their child can actually lead to a paradoxical decrease in language exposure and nonverbal communication. This perpetuates the delay in social and emotional development of Deaf children [5, 19, 20]. Secondly, hearing parents are usually unfamiliar with Deaf culture, resulting in delayed or minimal exposure to the social norms specific to Deaf culture. Early in life, this limits a Deaf child's opportunity to learn social norms unique to the Deaf community, also delaying appropriate social development. Rather than learning social norms from their parents, many Deaf children learn basic social skills and Deaf customs only after exposure to and interaction with Deaf peers [19]. It is important for parents of Deaf children to utilize available resources to learn to communicate with their Deaf children and to foster their development through facilitating early interactions with peers, both hearing and deaf.

Incidental learning is the information learned through informal interactions (visual, audio, or kinesthetic) in public settings. Despite being constantly surrounded by information and opportunities for this type of learning, Deaf children do not necessarily have access to it due to a language barrier [21]. For example, many young hearing women learn about aspects of child rearing and pregnancy by overhearing conversations of older women. Due to language discordance, Deaf women are not exposed to those incidental topics of conversation and can be caught off guard by information that is ostensibly common in the hearing world [22]. From childhood playground interaction to understanding basic hygiene, Deaf children are at a disadvantage because of the lack of incidental learning. Additionally, Deaf people may miss out on news affecting their communities. Because most news is communicated verbally or in written English, it is common for Deaf people to be out of the loop regarding current events. Moreover, family news shared around the dinner table, if not signed, can make Deaf persons feel excluded or isolated from family life and limit their knowledge of familial medical histories [20].

Ultimately, it is important for healthcare providers to recognize that Deaf patients may not have the same working knowledge of appropriate social interaction, family history, or community news and events that may be seen in hearing patients.

Limited Education and English Literacy

Part of the aforementioned social isolation stems from language discordance with the surrounding hearing community and low English literacy skills. English proficiency has been shown to be a necessary component of successful acculturation, which is the acceptance or absorption of another culture. It is also an enabling characteristic within the Andersen Behavioral Model of Health Care Access, a model aimed at demonstrating the driving factors behind the use of health services [23, 24]. In the USA, if someone lacks this English proficiency, they may find it difficult to interact effectively within the healthcare system. In patients with limited English proficiency, it has also been reported that language barriers are a deterrent for attempting to access medical care [15]. Although the Deaf community carries with it a strong sense of cultural identity, this portion of the population must cope with gaps in understanding verbal and written English.

The difficulties associated with attaining adequate English education and fluency for the Deaf are believed to be multifactorial. One challenge is the lack of language acquisition at an early age. This is an issue rooted in early neurodevelopment and brain plasticity or the ability to reorganize through the formation of new connections in the brain. Age of acquisition (AoA) of any language occurs within a critical developmental period. In a 2012 study of Deaf British Sign Language (BSL) users, research subjects were evaluated on grammatical accuracy in comparison to their AoA, and it was reported that grammatical accuracy decreased as the AoA increased [25]. In short, younger children acquire linguistic skills better at an earlier age. This is a concept well known among linguists and many instructors of second languages. Another study highlights a similar perspective:

> Children acquire language without instruction as long as they are regularly and meaningfully engaged with an accessible human language...however, because of brain plasticity changes during early childhood, children who have not acquired a first language in the early years might never be completely fluent in any language [26].

If the child is exposed early and often, he or she can acquire the language relatively easily. Unfortunately, many families with Deaf children may only utilize speech-exclusive approaches to language education. Consequently, they feel caught between language exposure through speech and the use of devices such as cochlear implants or sign-only approaches [26]. Sadly, resource and geographical limitations, such as the locations of Deaf schools and affordable housing, also make this type of choice very challenging. Hearing or speech-exclusive schools do not always have readily available interpreters or other auxiliary aids for Deaf students. What is more, a review of historical perspectives on Deaf education and language highlights that most leading educators felt that a combination of reading and oral education was best for Deaf learners. Some previous teaching styles and schools went so far as to disallow the use of signs for communication [27]. These approaches directly contradict the current popular views held by Deaf learners and families, which is to incorporate sign into English-proficiency education in order to optimize the learning environment. Consequently, many Deaf children suffer due to limitations in the current available educational resources and potentially outdated historical perspectives on learning, resulting in delayed or limited communicative abilities.

Another literature-supported challenge to English proficiency suggests that the barrier is due primarily to an inability to hear the complexities of English morphology and grammar (e.g., pronouns, conjunctions, bound morphemes) [28]. In the hearing world, many of these complexities are learned in early childhood solely by hearing the spoken language. Without hearing these innumerable word combinations and their appropriate grammatical syntax, the Deaf person may often find it difficult to understand when exposed to them in written English [28].

The third barrier to English fluency may be related to application of English vocabulary in unfamiliar contexts. Despite efforts to make accommodations to improve English literacy in the Deaf community, many of which have been incorporated from other English as a Second Language (ESL) programs, there have not been substantial improvements over the past 10 years. Some schools are attempting to incorporate a blended approach of online and traditional learning, deviating from some of the more traditionally held perspectives that were discussed previously

[27, 29]. One study demonstrated improvements in English vocabulary between cohorts compared 10 years apart but did not reveal any significant improvement in phonological awareness and reading ability [30]. Therefore, while Deaf patients may be familiar with more traditional English terms, their ability to read in the context of their health (e.g., physician reports, handouts, and other salient information) still appears to be generally low. If one accepts the proposition that language proficiency is critical for optimal development of executive functioning skills, as was suggested in a study published in the *Child Development Journal*, then the Deaf find themselves at a significant disadvantage when confronted with health literature [31]. As it pertains to their health, Deaf people with poor understanding of their own well-being have a higher risk for negative long-term consequences of poor health [5, 11–13]. Furthermore, with weaker executive functioning skills, some of the potential for higher educational pursuits and associated future earnings is lost.

Low Socioeconomic Status

Low English literacy contributes to decreased levels of educational achievement within the Deaf community, which may negatively impact socioeconomic status. In a comparison of median income levels since graduation from college between hearing and Deaf cohorts, Schroedel et al. reported that Deaf males achieved lower levels of education than their hearing counterparts [32]. The authors also noted a disproportionately high percentage of Deaf males in vocational careers or with an associate's degree (55% vs 22%, respectively) and a disproportionately low percentage obtaining doctoral degrees in comparison to the general population (1% vs 5%, respectively). Interestingly, this study found no substantial differences in salary or earnings between hearing and Deaf people at any given level of education. However, a substantial percentage of male and female Deaf people fall into the lower income bracket due to lower levels of educational achievement. Despite having equivalent pay per educational level, the overall result is that a larger portion of the Deaf population remains in a lower income bracket in comparison to the hearing community [32]. The National Deaf Center on Postsecondary Outcomes (NDC) showed that a major contributing factor to the earnings discrepancy is related to employment. In addition to the previously observed differences in education level, the NDC found that a greater percentage of the Deaf population is not in the labor force, resulting in lower cumulative earnings [33]. It is believed that lower education levels likely contribute to the absence from the labor force, emphasizing the need to improve education in order to narrow the earnings gap.

One study further broke down the earnings gap into contributing components, finding that 40% of the gap could be attributed to a combination of education level and potential experience, while the other 60% was explained by differences in communication skills and unobservable characteristics (including occupational segregation and stigma) [34]. Improvements in social awareness and cultural advancement of equality may help decrease the segregation and stigma, but improvements in educational resources and availability may ultimately lie at the core of narrowing the earnings discrepancy.

The implications of lower educational levels and subsequent earnings on health status are well known across the general population. Access to insurance, primary care resources, and day-to-day health factors (exercise, diet, adequate sleep, etc.) is substantially poorer across all lower socioeconomic classes, regardless of ability to hear [35–37]. Lower socioeconomic status, environmental exposures, and limited access to resources remain problematic, negatively influencing Deaf ASL users' lifestyles, life stressors, and more. This can have important implications in chronic diseases (renal failure, heart disease, etc.) as well as care in the acute setting [36, 37]. The full extent of health disparities as they relate to socioeconomics is likely unknown due to limited participation of linguistic and cultural minorities in research; however, one can begin to see why the Deaf population, which often finds itself at a financial and educational disadvantage, may face greater challenges in the healthcare setting [12].

Poor Health Literacy

As previously mentioned, one of the major barriers to adequate health care experienced by many in the Deaf community is poor health literacy, which is associated with poor health outcomes [12]. The problem is multifactorial, due to internal and external forces, often as a result of isolation from health resources and the healthcare system.

As discussed earlier, this isolation often begins early in the lives of many Deaf Americans. Some describe a "kitchen table" phenomenon experienced during childhood, where the Deaf child sits at a table observing family or friends conversing but is not able to participate or understand what is being said. This leads to minimal understanding or awareness of familial medical histories.

While not directly causative, isolation from family can be frustrating and potentially lead to depression in later years. For example, in a survey by Li et al., there was a strong association between patients with any level of self-reported hearing impairment and self-reported depression [38]. While the study actually reported a lower percentage of self-reported depression among deaf people, it failed to include a significant percentage of deaf participants (<0.2% of the total sample size) or any culturally Deaf patients, limiting its generalization to the Deaf ASL user.

Unfortunately, isolation extends beyond the home and immediate network of the Deaf ASL user, spilling over into the area of mass media. Radio and television without accompanying closed captioning undoubtedly make up a significant portion of this media. Health education programs, research studies, public health endeavors or threats, available treatments and advancements, or other important health-related topics are disseminated in written or spoken English, leaving Deaf Americans poorly misinformed in comparison to their hearing peers [12, 39]. Lack of exposure to these resources leaves little opportunity to correct misinformation received from relatively small social circles [12]. Lack of exposure to medical information and limited health literacy leaves Deaf Americans unable to list symptoms of acute myocardial infarction or stroke, which are often second nature to many hearing people simply due to repeat exposure through informal education [40].

Poor health literacy is also sometimes the result of avoidance of healthcare systems by Deaf ASL users. The language barrier imposed on them, particularly by healthcare providers who are not equipped to effectively communicate with Deaf patients (i.e., practices without access to ASL interpreters), directly influences impressions of healthcare encounters. Procedures performed in childhood can be viewed as terrifying or confusing when anticipatory guidance cannot be delivered. In adulthood, Deaf patients can leave encounters misunderstanding a provider's recommendations. Thus, both in early and later years, Deaf Americans often avoid interfacing with healthcare systems out of fear, anxiety, frustration, and myriad other reasons [40, 41].

So what can be done to improve health literacy in Deaf populations? One major improvement is to increase the total number of healthcare providers and workers that are fluent in ASL, thereby providing care in a concordant manner [40]. Similarly, another opportunity for improvement is to increase the availability of technologies (like visual telemedicine) to facilitate meaningful dialogue between Deaf patients and healthcare workers [42]. It has also been shown that providers with previous cultural competency training in the life experiences of Deaf patients create interactions that result in higher satisfaction rates and more effective communication. Increased collaboration between patients with limited English skills and health literacy researchers may expedite novel solutions [12]. Perhaps most importantly, educating hearing parents of Deaf children about the importance of learning ASL could facilitate early language acquisition, improve social development, and develop more meaningful and fulfilling interactions in early childhood.

Inadequate Healthcare Access

While exposed to some of the same barriers to care as hearing people or those with disabilities, the Deaf ASL user is also a linguistic minority, which contributes to a language discordance further resulting in a low health literacy level. Nearly all health-related communication, emergency department (ED) and hospital paperwork, and medical pamphlets communicate using written or spoken English. This severely limits access for those whose primary language is ASL. There is also a lack of linguistic and cultural concordance that leads to poor research engagement, inaccessible informed-consent processes, and limited research materials. This propagates a well-known history of fear, mistrust, and frustration with the biomedical research community [13, 14, 43–46].

What is more, even when Deaf ASL users do interact with healthcare systems, this access is often incomplete for multiple reasons. In addition to the aforementioned language barrier, cost is another obvious obstacle to care. Although not imparted directly on the patient, implementation of telephone relay systems, hiring interpreters, and installing telemedicine interfaces is cumbersome because it is expensive and time consuming. It may also be inconvenient for patients if interpreter resources are limited and the wait times are long.

Even if the patient is able to navigate through multiple obstacles to accessing health care, there is no guarantee that this care will be complete. The language discordance between Deaf patients and their providers mandates accommodation, as it is well known that attempts to communicate in the absence of interpreter services or fluency in ASL are associated with dissatisfaction and, perhaps more importantly, difficulty in understanding complex medical decision-making [39]. Again, cost can be prohibitive, and the initial stages of setup can be labor intensive. To complicate matters, many primary care providers already have little time to spend on a per patient basis, leading to a departure from the typical doctor-patient relationship. Trying to create more time to have conversations that require additional parties and resources does not always seem feasible and may not be possible in the smallest practices. In emergent settings like the emergency department, this is especially difficult, as high acuity situations often require rapid intervention and informed consent before the necessary interpreter services are available.

While there are educational resources such as health-related websites available to Deaf Americans [12], it is evident that this is not sufficient access. Increasing the number of ASL-fluent physicians will help provide improved, language-concordant information to those in the Deaf community, creating a situation where these patients are more likely to seek and comply with preventive efforts [40]. The cost and time expenditures to do this at the local and regional levels are well defined and are paltry in comparison to the long-term detriments of delivering poor and inequitable health care to a vulnerable population.

Healthcare Misconception

Incorrect or minimal understanding of Deaf culture can lead to poor relationship development between providers and Deaf patients. There can be inaccurate communication and poor comprehension on both sides, leading to provider and patient misconceptions [5, 47].

In general, providers often have feelings of discomfort or angst when they encounter a foreign language or culture that may result in culturally insensitive or inappropriate actions. There are a few common mistakes made by providers while caring for Deaf patients. For example, upon initially meeting a Deaf patient, providers inappropriately rely on the patient's ability to lip-read as a sole mode of communication. One challenge with this technique is that not all individuals with a hearing deficiency are able to read lips. Another problem with relying solely on lip-reading is that only approximately 30% of English can be lip read, ultimately creating a high likelihood of inaccuracy. Despite this, the Deaf patient may not advocate against this poor communication method for fear of ridicule or creating a negative perception of Deaf patients [5]. Working with a certified ASL interpreter is typically the best method to have an accurate and successful discussion between providers and Deaf patients. Communicating in simple written English is another alternative for communication, in comparison to lip-reading, when an ASL interpreter is unavailable. Ideally, the provider would ask for their preferred communication method before starting the patient encounter [47].

Another common area for mistakes is while working with an ASL interpreter to mediate a discussion. This stems from a lack of knowledge, training, and experience working with interpreters. Often, providers mistakenly direct their attention toward the interpreter instead of directing their questions or comments to the patient. ASL interpreters are, indeed, part of the healthcare team but should be thought of as a means to convey information. Despite acting as a conduit of information, interpreters are invaluable members of the team, and it is important to refer to them respectfully. For example, providers and staff should avoid using phrases like "using the interpreter." Instead, using language such as "working with an interpreter" or "communicated with the help of an interpreter" creates a welcoming and respectful team atmosphere.

Additionally, medical terminology is commonly used when communicating with Deaf patients. In doing so, the provider is unable to meet the health literacy level of the patient resulting in poor exchange of information [5]. It is imperative that providers figure out and match the literacy of their patients in order to ensure adequate understanding of the medical information.

These misconceptions and mistakes do not originate only from providers but from the Deaf ASL user as well. There are a few common behaviors that Deaf patients exhibit of which providers should be aware. Deaf patients typically have the fear of appearing uneducated, so they often will nod in agreement to anything the provider says regardless of the limited understanding of the medical information being discussed. Unfortunately, some patients cannot, or will not, advocate for themselves by asking questions or questioning the decision-making. This silence can lead to miscommunication, which may result in mistrust of the provider due to the fear of inaccuracy [47]. In addition to the confusion and provider mistrust issues commonly experienced by Deaf ASL users, an already weak relationship may further become stressed due to providers' common tendency to focus on deafness during a patient encounter. This perpetual focus on deafness demonstrates deaf cultural insensitivity and lack of interest in the true presenting medical complaint, again leading to mistrust of the provider [47–50].

Ultimately, it is important to familiarize yourself with the culture of any patient in order to achieve an acceptable level of cultural competence. Cognizance of Deaf culture, Deaf patient communication preferences, appropriate working relationships with interpreters, and the fears Deaf patients may have may help to obviate some of the misconceptions that can lead to miscommunications and inequitable care [47].

Deaf-Friendly Space

There is no "one-size-fits-all" accommodation for Deaf people, but when communicating with a Deaf ASL user, it is important to create a Deaf-friendly space. A Deaf-friendly space not only includes the physical characteristics and spatial orientation of the care area or work space but also awareness of Deaf culture by colleagues and providers.

The first step to establishing successful communication with Deaf patients is to demonstrate your willingness to provide accommodations. Each deaf person has his or her own specific needs. These accommodations should be elucidated and respected by providers to ensure accurate communication and set the stage for a successful patient-provider relationship. For instance, one patient may need an ASL interpreter, while another will require a Certified Deaf Interpreter (CDI). A CDI can be used when a Deaf patient has a low language level or cognitive impairment. There are other resources that can be used by Deaf patients, such as a signed-English interpreter, cued speech interpreter, captionist, hearing-aid loop system, or the use of simple written English. Like with any other patient with limited English proficiency, providers should avoid asking family members or friends to interpret. They could interpret something incorrectly or become emotionally involved, rendering them unable to convey the patient or provider's actual intentions. Not only will this foster miscommunication, but it is also in direct violation of a patient's right to access healthcare information based on the aforementioned Americans with Disabilities Act [5, 7, 51].

Education plays a big role in creating a Deaf-friendly environment. Medical providers should be educated on how to care for and interact with the culturally deaf community. If the goal is to communicate effectively to provide equitable care, providers must have a heightened cultural awareness and increased patience to recognize and implement the appropriate accommodations. Due to their deafness, the majority of Deaf people have experienced discrimination and impatient attitudes or have been perceived negatively at some point in their lives [1, 13, 47–50]. Therefore, Deaf people tend to be cognizant but intolerant of these behaviors and can easily become frustrated, angry, or uncomfortable, resulting in a poor physician-patient relationship and mistrust. Additionally, straightforward or blunt language is the norm in the Deaf community. While this may be uncommon in hearing communities, providers should avoid ambiguous language and subtleties. Lastly, providers should encourage questions from the Deaf patient in order to improve their engagement and health literacy.

While improving provider cultural competency is essential to create a Deaf-friendly environment, the physical and spatial organization of the office or room is equally important [5]. Deaf people are a visual group, which may result in increased eye sensitivity. Physical characteristics such as lighting, wall color, room size, and seating arrangement all need to be considered. Disorganization of the office can cause fatigue or strain on their eyes that may lead to eye discomfort and lack of concentration. Indirect lighting is recommended as direct lighting can be harsh to Deaf patients' eyes. The color blue is well known as causing the least strain to Deaf patients' eyes. Making these adjustments will take institutional buy-in for true efficacy. For instance, after consulting with the Deaf researchers, coordinators, and collaborators in the National Center for Deaf Health Research within the University of Rochester Medical Center, the university has designed meeting rooms with blue walls and sufficient spacing to create a visually appealing atmosphere that allows for effective communication. As mentioned before, the seating arrangement is another key to successful and comfortable communication. Deaf people require eye contact while communicating, so it is important for providers to look at the Deaf person while talking [5]. A Deaf patient will typically need an interpreter and the interpreter should be positioned adjacent to a provider allowing the Deaf patient to observe the provider's body language and facial expressions while communicating [51]. If there are more than three people, the seating arrangement should be circular. Clear visibility is critical. It is best to ask the Deaf patients if they feel comfortable with the physical setting or if any changes are needed before starting the medical interview.

In reality, there are some limitations to meeting the needs of the Deaf patient. Interpreter availability is a common problem if the provider practices in a place with relatively few Deaf ASL users due to a lack of resources and infrastructure. Even in places with well-established Deaf populations, this may still be a common problem. There are even fewer specialized interpreters (such as CDI, Cued, English-signed, or support service providers for deaf-blind patients) regardless of the location. As mentioned earlier, the emergency department is a place with limited or delayed interpreter availability, may be a place for miscommunication, and has been recognized as a significant problem that Deaf patients encounter in the hospital setting [51]. Lastly, the cost of establishing the infrastructure and resources necessary to communicate effectively is often a barrier.

Ultimately, creating a Deaf-friendly space with a provider who demonstrates willingness to change, open-mindedness, patience, and cultural sensitivity will foster a healthy provider-patient relationship [5]. In addition, adjusting the physical layout of the office or room will create a visually appealing and welcoming area that allows for clear and effective communication. Collectively, these can help reduce healthcare misconceptions and improve the quality of care delivered to Deaf ASL users.

Conclusion

The culturally deaf patient belongs to a community with a rich culture and robust language. Unfortunately, being a linguistic minority and sharing similar qualities with other ethnic/racial minority groups, the Deaf ASL user experiences inequities in health care and access to medical information. Being cognizant of the communication barrier that Deaf ASL users encounter throughout their lives and its associated negative impact on social development, education, income level, health literacy, and access to health care may lead to improved clinical competence. However, simply being aware of the barrier is not enough to reduce health disparities. As individual providers and healthcare organizations, there must be purposeful actions dedicated to improve a provider's cultural competence, improve access to care, and improve access to health information. This includes creating a Deaf-friendly environment, providing qualified ASL interpreters, allowing for direct access to information, increasing the representation of Deaf ASL users in healthcare research, and matching the patient's health literacy level when delivering care. These actions will help bridge the gap of healthcare disparities experienced by the culturally Deaf patient and allow for more accessible and equitable care.

References

1. Peterson-Besse J, et al. Barriers to health care among people with disabilities who are members of underserved racial/ethnic groups. Med Care. 2014;52(10 Suppl 3):S51–63.
2. Horner-Johnson W, et al. Disparities in chronic conditions and health status by type of disability. Disabil Health J. 2013;6:280–6.
3. Young ME, et al. Prevalence of abuse of women with physical disabilities. Arch Phys Med Rehabil. 1997;78:S34–8.
4. Merriam-Webster, Inc. Dictionary by Merriam-Webster [Internet]. Springfield, MA: Merriam-Webster; 2015 (Cited 1 Sep 2017). Available from www.merriam-webster.com
5. Richardson K. Deaf culture: competencies and best practices. Nurse Pract. 2014;39(5):20–8.
6. National Association of the Deaf. National association of the deaf [Internet]. Silver Spring, MD: National Association of the Deaf; 2017 (Cited 1 Sept 2017). Available from www.nad.org
7. U.S. Department of Justice. Information and technical assistance on the Americans with disabilities act [Internet]. Washington, DC: U.S. Department of Justice; (Cited 1 Sept 2017). Available from www.ada.gov
8. Elementary and Secondary Education Act of 1965, Pub. L. 89-10, 79 Stat.58 (Apr. 11, 1965).
9. The Joint Commission. Joint commission: accreditation, health care, certification [Internet]. Oakbrook Terrace, IL: The Joint Commission; 2017 (Cited 1 Sept 2017). Available from www.jointcommission.org
10. Smith S, Chin N. Public health – social and behavioral health. Rijeka, HR: InTech; c2012. Chapter 21, Social determinants of health disparities: deaf communities; p. 449–60.
11. Novic S. Debunking the "fourth grade reading level" statistic [Internet]. [place unknown: publisher unknown]; 2012 [updated 2013 Feb 28; cited 2017 Sep 1]. Available from www.redeafined.com/2012/04/debunking-fourth-grade-reading-level.html
12. McKee M, Paasche-Orlow M. Health literacy and the disenfranchised: the importance of collaboration between limited English proficiency and health literacy researchers. J Health Commun. 2012;17:7–12.
13. Ponce N, et al. Linguistic disparities in health care access and health status among older adults. J Gen Intern Med. 2006;21:786–91.
14. McKee M, et al. Emergency department use and risk factors among deaf American Sign Language users. Disabil Health J. 2015;8(4):573–8.
15. Head, Zauche L, et al. The power of language nutrition for children's brain development, health, and future academic achievement. J Ped Health Care. 2017;31(4):493–503.
16. Mitchell R, Karchmer M. Chasing the mythical ten percent: parental hearing status of deaf and hard of hearing students in the United States. Sign Lang Stud. 2004;4(2):138–63.

17. Barnett S. Clinical and cultural issues in caring for deaf people. Fam Med. 1999;31(1):17–22.
18. Hintermair M. Parental resources, parental stress, and socioemotional development of deaf and hard of hearing children. J Deaf Stud Deaf Educ. 2006;11(4):493–513.
19. Calderon R, Greenberg M. The Oxford handbook of deaf studies, language, and education.Vol 1, 2nd ed. Oxford: Oxford University Press; c2011. Chapter 13, Social and emotional development of deaf children: family, school, and program effects; p. 177–89.
20. Boss E, Niparko J, Gaskin D, Levinson K. Socioeconomic disparities for hearing-impaired children in the United States. Laryngoscope. 2011;121(4):181–6.
21. DeafTEC. Incidental learning [Internet]. Rochester, NY: Rochester Institute of Technology; (Cited 1 Sept 2017). Available from https://www.deaftec.org/classact/challenges/teaching/giving-directions
22. Jackson M. Deafness and antenatal care: understanding issues with access. Br J Midwifery. 2011;19(5):280–4.
23. Andersen RA. Revisiting the behavioral model and access to medical care: does it matter? J Health Soc Behav. 1995;36:1–10.
24. Lara M, Gamboa C, Kahramanian MI, Morales LS, Bautista DE. Acculturation and Latino health in the United States: a review of the literature and its sociopolitical context. Annu Rev Public Health. 2005;26:367–97.
25. Cormier K, Schembri A, Vinson D, Orfanidou E. First language acquisition differs from second language acquisition in prelingually deaf signers: evidence from sensitivity to grammaticality judgment in British Sign Language. Cognition. 2012;124(1):50–65. https://doi.org/10.1016/j.cognition.2012.04.003.
26. Humphries T, Kushalnagar P, Mathur G, Napoli DJ, Padden C, Rathmann C, Smith SR. Language acquisition for deaf children: reducing the harms of zero tolerance to the use of alternative approaches. Harm Reduct J. 2012;9:16. https://doi.org/10.1186/1477-7517-9-16.
27. Power D, Leigh G. Principles and practices of literacy development for deaf learners: a historical overview. J Deaf Stud Deaf Educ. 2000;5:3–8.
28. Nielsen DC, et al. The English-language and reading achievement of a cohort of dear students speaking and signing standard English: a preliminary study. Am Ann Deaf. 2016;161(3):342–68.
29. Long GL, et al. Access to communication for deaf, hard-of-hearing and ESL students in blended learning courses. Int Rev Res Open Distrib Learn. 2007;8(3):1–13.
30. Harris M, Terlektsi E, Kyle FE. Literacy outcomes for primary school children who are deaf and hard of hearing: a cohort comparison study. J Speech Lang Hear Res. 2017;60:701–11.
31. Botting N, Jones A, Marshall C, Denmark T, Atkinson J, Morgan G. Nonverbal executive function is mediated by language: a study of deaf and hearing children. Child Dev. 2016;00(0):1–12.
32. Schroedel JG, Geyer PD. Long-term career attainments of deaf and hard of hearing college graduates: results from a 15-year follow-up survey. Am Ann Deaf. 2000;145:303–14.
33. Garberoglio CL, Cawthon S, Bond M. Deaf people and employment in the United States: 2016. Washington, DC: U.S. Department of Education, Office of Special Education Programs, National Deaf Center on Postsecondary Outcomes; 2016. 12p.
34. Benito SG, Glassman TS, Hiedemann BG. Disability and labor market earnings: hearing earnings gaps in the United States. J Disabil Policy Stud. 2016;27(3):178–88.
35. Adler NE, Newman K. Socioeconomic disparities in health: pathways and policies. Health Aff (Millwood). 2017;21(2):60–76.
36. Plantinga LC, Johansen KL, Schillinger D, Powe NR. Lower socioeconomic status and disability among US adults with chronic kidney disease. Prev Chronic Dis. 2012;9:E12.
37. Dalstra JAA, Kunst AE, Borrell C, et al. Socioeconomic differences in the prevalence of common chronic diseases: an overview of eight European countries. Int J Epidemiol. 2005;34(2):316–26.
38. Chuan-Ming LMD, et al. Hearing impairment associated with depression in US adults, national health and nutrition examination survey 2005–2010. JAMA Otolaryngol Head Neck Surg. 2014;140(4):293–302.

39. McKee MMD, et al. Perceptions of cardiovascular health in an underserved community of deaf adults using American Sign Language. Disabil Health J. 2011;4(3):192–7.
40. McKee MMD, et al. Impact of communication on preventive services among deaf American Sign Language users. Am J Prev Med. 2011;41(1):75–9.
41. Tate RMD. The need for more prehospital research on language barriers: a narrative review. West J Emerg Med. 2015;XVI(7):1094–105.
42. Wilson JA, Wells MG. Telehealth and the deaf: a comparison study. J Deaf Stud Deaf Educ. 2009;14(3):386–402.
43. Novic S. Debunking the "fourth grade reading level" statistic [Internet]. [place unknown: publisher unknown]; 2012 (Updated 2013 Feb 28; cited 2017 Sept 1). Available from www.redeaf-ined.com/2012/04/debunking-fourth-grade-reading-level.html
44. Tate RC, et al. Strategies used by prehospital providers to overcome language barriers. Prehosp Emerg Care. 2016;20(3):404–14.
45. Barnett S, et al. Deaf sign language users, health inequities, and public health: opportunity for social justice. Prev Chronic Dis. 2011;8(2):A45.
46. McKee M, Schlehofer D, Thew D. Ethical issues in conducting research with deaf populations. Am J Public Health. 2013;103(12):2174–8.
47. Sheppard K. Deaf adults and health care: giving voice to their stories. J Am Assoc Nurse Pract. 2014;26(9):504–10.
48. Steinberg AGBS, Meador HE, Wiggins EA, Zazove P. Health care system accessibility: experiences and perceptions of deaf people. J Gen Intern Med. 2006;21(3):260–6.
49. Ralston E, Zazove P, Gorenflo DW. Physicians' attitudes and beliefs about deaf patients. J Am Board Fam Pract. 1996;9(3):167–73.
50. Ebert DA, Heckerling PS. Communication with deaf patients. Knowledge, beliefs, and practices of physicians. JAMA. 1995;273(3):227–9.
51. Hoan L, et al. Assessing deaf cultural competency of physicians and medical students. J Cancer Educ. 2011;26(1):175–82.

Chapter 7
Transgender

Adrian D. Daul

Introduction

Terminology

Gender identity is one's internal sense of being male, female, both, or neither – it is a product of both innate and external influences. *Biological sex*, in contrast, is assigned at birth based on anatomical, gonadal, and genetic elements. Also in contrast to biological sex, gender identity can shift over time. The discourse and language around gender is evolving rapidly in our country. Many people, particularly in the younger generations, now describe their gender identity on a spectrum that defies the historical binary of men/women. These individuals may use words like gender fluid, gender non-binary, gender nonconforming, genderqueer, or gender variant to describe their felt gender [1]. The vast majority of people identify as *cisgender*, which means they have a congruent sex and gender identity (e.g., a male that identifies as a man), whereas transgender individuals have a gender identity that does not match their assigned sex (e.g., a birth-assigned female that identifies as genderqueer or a birth-assigned male that identifies as a woman). *Gender expression* is an outward presentation of gender – for example, the clothes, makeup, piercings, or hairstyle one chooses may be feminine, masculine, or androgynous. For transgender individuals, body modifications as result of gender-affirming hormones and surgeries may be an important part of their gender expression. *Gender transition* is the process of shifting one's outward gender expression, usually to match one's internal sense of gender (e.g., from feminine to masculine). For some individuals, gender transition could mean starting gender-affirming hormones and changing one's name/pronouns; for others, it might be something subtler like a shift to more masculine clothing.

A. D. Daul
Department of Emergency Medicine, Emory University School of Medicine,
Atlanta, GA, USA

© Springer International Publishing AG, part of Springer Nature 2019
M. L. Martin et al. (eds.), *Diversity and Inclusion in Quality Patient Care*,
https://doi.org/10.1007/978-3-319-92762-6_7

Case Study

In 2012, Dr. Elliott Elson took the first step in his gender transition. After decades of suppressing the dissonance between his biological sex and gender identity, he finally accepted that his gender identity was masculine-of-center and made a conscious decision to shift his gender expression by starting to shop in the men's department. Four years later, after continuing to experience gender dysphoria, he decided to transition further – to change his name, adopt masculine pronouns, and start gender-affirming hormone therapy (i.e., testosterone). Three months after that decision, he administered his first hormone injection of testosterone. At that point, only his closest circle of family and friends knew about his plan to transition. For the next few months, he continued to live and work as Allison while his body subtly started to take on a more masculine form. Four months after his first shot of testosterone, he had "top surgery" to remove his breasts. In the weeks following the surgery, he made a broad announcement of his transition to his colleagues, extended family, and friends – at this time, he asked everyone to start calling him by his chosen name, Elliott, with male pronouns. Shortly thereafter, a judge approved his case for legal name change to Elliott.

Case Scenario

Long before Dr. Elliott Elson came out as transgender in professional circles, his gender identity and expression had been masculine-of-center. One challenge Dr. Elson faced in being gender nonconforming in a professional environment – where dress codes have historically been dictated by gender – was finding acceptable professional attire that could comfortably house (and simultaneously hide) his female-bodied self. While vulnerable on many levels, it felt important to present his authentic gender in his professional life. A few years ago, he attended a faculty event dressed head-to-toe in masculine attire (including shirt and tie) and he was greeted by a senior, white male colleague with a hearty, "Hello, young lady!" Dr. Elson was mortified. This colleague's comments demonstrated complete disregard for Dr. Elson's masculine gender expression: he felt undressed and unseen.

Discussion

Gendering: Binary Assumptions

Gendering is one mechanism that perpetuates the historical invisibility of gender diversity. Most of us move through our daily lives making automatic, binary assumptions about people's gender identities – subconsciously categorizing the people around us as "men" or "women." This is called gendering. The way we have gendered an individual subsequently informs the words we use to speak with/about that individual – for example, pronouns (he/she), honorifics (Mr./Ms.), and certain terms of respect (ma'am/sir) all have inherent gender meaning. It is important to recognize that this process of subconscious sorting is a way in which we make assumptions about the people around us and that sometimes our assumptions will be wrong. When our assumption is wrong, it is called *misgendering*. Being misgendered (e.g., when a transman is called "Ma'am" instead of "Sir") is a common and often distressing experience for transgender individuals.

How to Do Better

Pay attention to people's gender expression. Just because you can discern someone's assigned sex at birth does not mean that you know that person's gender identity. Look for cues like clothing, hairstyle, makeup, jewelry, and accessories – these are intentional choices people make in order to present their gender to the world. A simple best practice to avoid misgendering people is to simply ask what name they wish to be called and what pronouns they use, and then use them.

Do not conflate sexual orientation and gender identity. Sexual orientation is an identity that describes to whom/what gender(s) someone feels sexually attracted – this is often simplified to men/women/both, which reinforces a binary gender construct. Transgender people, like their cisgender counterparts, might identify as gay, straight, queer, bisexual, etc. Before his gender transition, people who noticed Dr. Elson's masculine presentation may have assumed he identified as a "butch lesbian"; however, his presentation was an expression of his gender identity and not his sexual orientation.

Case Scenario

A month before Dr. Elson planned to announce his gender transition to his fellow faculty/staff (and 3 months into gender-affirming hormone therapy), about half of his patients were perceiving him as a man, which felt encouraging. On one occasion when a patient referred to him as "Sir," a nurse overheard and became visibly upset because she felt the patient had mistaken Dr. Elson's gender. He told the nurse that it was fine and encouraged her to let it go. Yet, she took it upon herself to correct the patient and let him know that Dr. Elson was a "ma'am."

Despite Dr. Elson's attempts to ask the nurse not to intervene, she did anyway. For the nurse, it was a matter of respect – her behavior was likely motivated by feelings of protectiveness toward Dr. Elson. For him, however, it was more than a matter of feeling affirmed in his felt gender: It was also a matter of safety. He was "passing" as a man, and the nurse "outed" him to this patient.

Discussion

Transition: Trapped Between "He" and "She"

Deciding to gender transition is usually preceded by months or, more likely, years of contemplating the risks, benefits, and alternatives. And once someone makes the decision to transition, there is a thoughtful process for how and when to come out to one's friends, family, and colleagues. Transitioning is often a long and fraught journey. Gender-affirming hormones work slowly to exert their effects over months-to-years [2]. Yet, the person transitioning must decide on discrete moments to change names/pronouns, to announce one's transition to family/friends/colleagues, and to swap bathrooms. One of the most vulnerable times during gender transition is the interval between deciding to transition and the carefully timed announcement of transition to family/friends/colleagues. Agonizing moments inevitably arise when asserting one's authentic gender identity would undermine one's intentional and precisely timed plan for coming out.

How to Do Better

If someone's gender presentation shifts over time, you can ask them again about their name and pronouns. If someone tells you that they have no preference for pronouns, that could be a signal they are in the process of transition or they do not feel safe in the current context to voice their preference. In that case, consider using neutral words (e.g., they/them, sibling, parent, child) when talking with/ about them.

Unless specifically instructed to do so, do not speak to someone else's gender. As in this case, you may inadvertently "out" that individual. Many people in the LGBTQ community are "out" in certain spheres (e.g., with friends) but not in others (e.g., work) – this is obviously a delicate decision when one in six transgender people report having lost a job due to revealing their gender identity at work [1]. Perceived safety is an important part of the equation when deciding to be "out." People who identify as sexual and gender minorities vigilantly scan their environment to determine whether it is safe to be out in any given context. And when safety is uncertain, they may hide their identity by censoring personal life from conversations, avoiding pronouns, and modifying dress/presentation. Every time a person hides their gender/sexual minority identity, however, they add to the problem of invisibility for LGBTQ people. Moreover, that person internalizes a message that it is not safe or okay to be themself – this is internalized self-stigma. Internalized stigma is a major driver of violence and discrimination against gender minorities and contributes to the extremely high prevalence of mental illness, suicide, and addiction among transgender people [1, 3].

Case Scenario

Shortly before Dr. Elson's legal name change, he went to his primary care provider's office for blood work to check for the levels and side effects of his gender-affirming hormones. When he registered with the front desk staff, he told them that his preferred name was "Elliott" with "he/him" pronouns. Nonetheless, he got called from the waiting room by the phlebotomist as "Ms. Elson." As he walked down the hall, he told the phlebotomist that he had a different preferred name and did not use "Ms." The phlebotomist shrugged off Elliott's concern with a quick "OK." As the phlebotomist was drawing Elliott's blood, he tried to broach the topic again by explaining that he was transgender and Elliott was his new name. The phlebotomist replied, "There is nothing I can do until you legally change your name."

After this experience, in correspondence to his primary care provider Elliott detailed the incident and his distress over being outed to the entire waiting room when the phlebotomist called him by the wrong name. The primary care doctor sent back a supportive message and assured Elliott she would let her office manager know.

Discussion

Patient Perspective

Healthcare access is challenging for gender minorities. Electronic health records (EHRs) have historically not included fields for gender identity [4]. Many transgender people have had outright negative experiences when they try to access the health system, such as being refused care or misgendered by healthcare staff. Fear of a negative experience causes many transgender people to delay seeking care when they need it [1].

From a broader perspective, the lack of intentional data collection about sexual and gender minorities in EHRs and on major institutional/national surveys has contributed to the ongoing invisibility of this population and the health disparities they experience. The current US government administration intends to roll back recent gains by removing/failing to add sexual orientation and gender identity questions on several important national surveys. This is certain to reinforce the status quo of invisibility [5].

How to Do Better

Make a change to your professional environment that promotes safety and inclusivity. Insist that your EHRs collect both sex and gender identity. Consider hanging LGBTQ inclusive posters, wearing a supportive pin, or offering LGBTQ-geared reading material. Assure access to an all-gender restroom. Every staff member that has patient contact – from registration to phlebotomists to providers – needs to be trained on respectfully interacting with transgender and gender-nonconforming people. Being summoned from a busy waiting room by the wrong name is not only distressing but also presents a safety issue because it "outs" that individual.

If you hear colleagues insisting that a patient's gender identity is irrelevant because they treat all patients the same [4], speak up. Explain how their perspective is skewed by the structural mechanisms that have tried to erase and suppress gender diversity over time [6]. Tell them about the implicit biases that we all have, which drive ongoing health disparities for patients in minority groups [7, 8]. Tell them that we as healthcare providers, with our privilege and our vital impact on vulnerable lives, must fight against these implicit biases every single day.

Conclusion

Gender identity is an underrecognized aspect of diversity in the human species. The preceding case scenarios illustrate a few ways that transgender people are uniquely vulnerable. As we all work to ensure the safety and respect of transgender people, commit yourself to the following imperative actions: Recognize and challenge your own automatic binary gender assumptions both in the clinical setting and in your personal life. Tune in to gender expression. Demonstrate your respect for gender diversity by asking about a person's chosen name and pronouns to avoid misgendering. Examine your clinical environment and cultivate a trans-inclusive atmosphere. If you need training in caring for transgender people, seek out educational opportunities. Insist that data is collected on gender identity because measurability equals visibility. Recognize your role of privilege as a healthcare provider and use it to speak up when you see biases in your clinic, family, and community.

References

1. James SE, Herman JL, Rankin S, Keisling M, Motett L, Anafi M. The report of the 2015 U.S. transgender survey. Washington: National Center for Transgender Equality; 2016.
2. Coleman E, Bockting W, Botzer M, Cohen-Kettenis P, DeCuypere G, Feldman J, et al. Standards of care for the health of transsexual, transgender, and gender-nonconforming people, version 7. Int J Transgend. 2012;13(4):165–232.
3. Herek GM. A nuanced view of stigma for understanding and addressing sexual and gender minority health disparities. LGBT Health. 2016;3(6):397–9.
4. The battle to get gender identity into your health records [Internet]. Boone, IA: WIRED; 2017 (Cited 28 Sept 2017). Available from: https://www.wired.com/story/the-battle-to-get-gender-identity-into-your-health-records/
5. Cahill SR, Makadon HJ. If they don't count us, we don't count: trump administration rolls back sexual orientation and gender identity data collection. LGBT Health. 2017;4(3):171–3.

6. Schuster MA, Reisner SL, Onorato SE. Beyond bathrooms — meeting the health needs of transgender people. N Engl J Med. 2016;375(2):101–3.
7. Hardeman RR, Medina EM, Kozhimannil KB. Structural racism and supporting black lives — the role of health professionals. N Engl J Med. 2016;375(22):2113–5.
8. Sabin JA, Riskind RG, Nosek BA. Health care providers' implicit and explicit attitudes toward lesbian women and gay men. Am J Public Health. 2015;105(9):1831–41.

Chapter 8
Unconscious Bias in Action

Bernard L. Lopez

Introduction

Black patients with acute myocardial infarction (MI) receive percutaneous coronary intervention at a lower rate than white patients. They also wait longer to receive care in the emergency department for their chest pain. A transgender patient gets asked questions about their orientation that have nothing to do with their clinical condition. A Latino woman does not get adequate pain medication because she is being "dramatic." Women have a higher rate of missed MI. Male physicians receive higher pay and achieve leadership positions more often than female physicians. All of these scenarios are commonly cited in the literature and are examples of disparities that exist in health care [1–3]. Generally, these are not intentional – healthcare providers are committed to giving the best care possible to help people get and stay better. Somehow, they continue to happen and are a part of our daily lives. While the causes for these disparities are multifactorial and system-related, unconscious bias plays a major role.

As humans, we receive an overwhelming number of stimuli, and our brains use biases as shortcuts to simplify and understand our surroundings more quickly. Our individual experiences shape these shortcuts (it is an ongoing dynamic process) and create the unique lenses through which we view the world. On an evolutionary basis, bias serves to protect us from harm. Think about it – you are walking on the street at night in an unfamiliar area. Just ahead, you see the shadow of a figure walking toward you and see a glint of light off of a long pointy object in that figure's hand. What do most of us instinctively do? We quickly move away from the figure. Why? Because most of us have developed a strong bias against strange and unknown figures holding presumably sharp objects that may cause us harm. While the figure

B. L. Lopez
Sidney Kimmel Medical College of Thomas Jefferson University, Thomas Jefferson University, Philadelphia, PA, USA
e-mail: Bernard.lopez@jefferson.edu

© Springer International Publishing AG, part of Springer Nature 2019
M. L. Martin et al. (eds.), *Diversity and Inclusion in Quality Patient Care*,
https://doi.org/10.1007/978-3-319-92762-6_8

may not be a true threat, our bias causes us to perform certain actions that serve to protect us. It is unlikely that we would approach the figure, do a careful and detailed assessment, review a long list of potential actions, and choose our best option – we may not be alive if we did so. Our bias works on a subconscious level and allows us to react almost instantaneously. In this scenario (and in reality, in many of our every-day scenarios), the stereotypes that we have work outside of our awareness and affect our decisions.

These automatic responses enable us to make fast decisions. Aside from protect-ing us from harm, bias allows us to function quickly in our busy worlds. Bias can also prompt us to jump to unwarranted conclusions. As humans, we harbor uncon-scious associations – both positive and negative – about other people based on race, ethnicity, gender, age, socioeconomic class, sexual orientation, and appearance. Our biases have been built up over time and are based on the input of our environment. These associations influence our feelings and attitudes, especially under demanding circumstances (which are very common in the healthcare setting). They may result in involuntary discriminatory practices and can negatively affect the care of our patients and the function of our organizations. Additionally, not only do they affect the type and quality of care certain patients receive, they also affect the training and career opportunities available to people identified with certain ethnic, cultural, and other underrepresented groups.

Each of us is a unique individual that has our own individual experiences and education (both formal and informal); these can be described as our "book of rules." Our "schema" is our way of systematically organizing these rules. Together, these form our background – the lens – through which we view the world. We are con-stantly experiencing rules, reshaping our schema, and changing our backgrounds on a minute-by-minute basis throughout our lives. These are our biases. Biases – we all have them. We have biases toward race, sexual orientation, religion, age, hand dom-inance, weight, height, accent, appearance, and more. We cannot help having bias – it is how we are wired as humans.

We view a person, an interaction, and a circumstance through our biased "lens." The impulse travels to the amygdala. A signal is sent to the brain stem and the limbic system, which then stimulates our hippocampus. The cingulate gyrus causes our body to respond – you slam on the brakes with the threat of a collision; you say or do something in response to a statement – all in the blink of an eye. Our cerebral cortex, the thinking portion of our brain, has not been involved, as all of this happens in our unconsciousness. Given the millions of stimuli that we experi-ence in the course of our day, we would not be able to function without these quick reactions. Our biases play an increasing role in demanding and busy situa-tions. Health care has many of these demanding and busy situations, and there is significant evidence that unconscious bias not only plays a role in decisions but it can also have life-altering consequences. It can affect the type and quality of care to those identified with certain racial, ethnic, cultural, and other underrepresented groups.

Discussion

What Effect Does Bias Have on Patient Care?

The lives of our patients are affected by bias, both conscious and unconscious. It is especially important that we consider our own biases, as they affect how we view and treat the most important people we encounter – our patients. Our biases play an unconscious role in how we interpret important clues in the history and physical exam of a patient. If one's unconscious bias is such that one downplays certain aspects, this has the potential to negatively affect patient care – missed MI, reduced analgesic treatment, and longer wait times are a few examples. Unconscious bias also affects the lives of those we work with (our coworkers) and creates a certain patient care environment that may or may not be conducive to optimum care. It is not only the healthcare provider that has bias; patients and their families also harbor biases. A minority patient may not follow the recommendations from a white physician because of their subconscious views that are based on their past experiences.

Consider this scenario: A 52-year-old African-American female presents to a tertiary care, academic emergency department with several hours of intermittent chest pain. The white male emergency medicine physician (whose peers consider him to be one of the most compassionate and knowledgeable physicians around) performs a history and physical examination and elicits a history of waxing and waning anterior chest pain, non-radiating, and slightly worsened with exertion. Her pain at the time was 4 on a scale of 1–10. He orders the typical workup for chest pain. The electrocardiogram shows 1 millimeter ST-segment elevation across the precordial leads. The patient ends up being diagnosed with an acute MI and is admitted for medical therapy. No percutaneous coronary intervention (PCI) is performed. In a day and age where PCI is considered the gold standard for the care of acute coronary syndrome, how does this happen? While treatment decisions are complex and are affected by many factors, studies have demonstrated that women and black patients often do not receive the same care that men and white patients receive.

In 1998, Anthony Greenwald [4] and two colleagues created the implicit association test (IAT). This online tool measures the strength of automatic associations between concepts (e.g., black people, gay people) and evaluations (e.g., good, bad) [5]. It is the most recognized and most commonly used test to measure unconscious bias. The IAT score is based on how long it takes a person, on average, to associate certain evaluative words with the concept being tested. Thus, if one quickly associates "good" words with "white" and "bad" words with black, there may be a preference of white over black (a more detailed description can be found in the "Education" section of the website Implicit.Harvard.Edu). Currently, there are 13 tests on the Project Implicit website: Native Americans, gender science, Asian-Americans, race (black-white), age, disability, weight, presidential popularity, Arab-Muslim, skin tone, sexuality, weapons, and gender career.

Does unconscious bias affect patient care? A study by Green et al. in 2007 [6] used the IAT to test whether physicians show implicit race bias and whether the magnitude of such bias predicts thrombolysis recommendations for black and white patients with acute coronary syndromes (ACS). They presented vignettes of a patient presenting to the emergency department with ACS followed by a question-naire and three IATs. A total of 287 internal medicine and emergency medicine physicians at four academic medical centers in Atlanta and Boston completed the study. Amongst the participants, there was explicit preference for white over black patients on perceived cooperativeness. However, the IATs demonstrated implicit preference for white Americans and implicit stereotypes of black Americans as less cooperative with medical procedures and in general. As the physician's pro-white implicit bias increased, so did their likelihood of treating white patients and not black patients with thrombolysis. The authors conclude that unconscious bias may contribute to racial/ethnic disparities in the use of medical procedures, such as thrombolysis for MI. While the study is a bit dated (many physicians use PCI over thrombolytics for MI), it is the one study linking IAT results to treatment choices. A number of other studies have demonstrated the existence of implicit bias in physi-cians with regard to race [7], obesity, gender, and age [8, 9].

While the IAT has been in existence for many years and is the most widely used test to measure implicit bias, there are differing opinions on what it actually mea-sures and whether it is a measure of racial prejudice. Much research has been done on the IAT since it was first developed. One thought is that the IAT may simply be measuring the association of positive evaluations with the "in" or majority group and negative evaluations with the "out" or minority group. Thus, it may not be a specific attribute effect but rather the manner in which humans behave. Researchers performed a study in which two versions of an IAT were used. In the first, the in-group was "French and me" and the out-group was "North African." An IAT effect was found. In the second version, the two categories were "French" and "North African and me." The IAT effect disappeared. The investigators concluded that in-group/out-group membership, and not nationality, was the important factor [10]. What then is the usefulness of the IAT? Consider it a tool that can be used to stimu-late thought about one's unconscious biases. It should not be used to measure ones "prejudices." Just because one may have a strong preference for a certain group does not mean that one is prejudiced against another – it simply means that one may harbor an implicit bias and must take this into account when dealing with someone from the "other" group.

Consider another scenario: A 43-year-old white male presents to the emergency department with left-sided flank pain that radiates to the left groin. He appears somewhat uncomfortable and is not able to sit still. On interview of the patient, one learns that he had a significant history of heroin addiction, but he states that after 1 year of therapy with buprenorphine/naloxone, he is "cured." On physical exami-nation, he is very thin, has poor dentition, and has multiple tattoos on his body. A workup is positive only for red blood cells in the urine. The patient, who has been given only acetaminophen for pain, is discharged and told to continue with acet-aminophen and to take ibuprofen if this does not work. The patient returns the next day and is ultimately diagnosed with a leaking abdominal aortic aneurysm. How does this happen? Is it possible that the initial-treating physician (again, considered to be a fine caretaker) interpreted the patient as being an opioid-seeker and was unconsciously biased against the possibility of a more serious illness?

Unconscious bias can also work the other way – a patient's bias against the physician – to negatively affect care. In his book, *Black Man in a White Coat – A Doctor's Reflections on Race and Medicine*, Dr. Damon Tweedy describes a scenario of a white patient that he cared for in which the patient was initially resistant to care based purely on the fact that Dr. Tweedy was black [11]. This scenario occurs commonly. Think of the unconscious biases that the patient may have had – "He's black; they must have let him into medical school to fill a quota so he can't be as good" or "He won't really give me good care because I am white" – and how this will affect the patient's ability to accept care. And consider this – black patients may also harbor similar unconscious biases, seeking the "more educated and better" white physician.

What Can We Do?

In chapter 2 "The Inconvenient Truth About Unconscious Bias in the Health Professions", the authors discuss successful strategies for mitigating unconscious bias. Perhaps the most important is the recognition and the acceptance that unconscious bias exists within all of us and that these biases, on both the provider and the patient side, affect the quality of care provided and received. Bias is necessarily a part of who we are as humans. Becoming educated on the effect of unconscious bias on patient care is important and there is an almost unlimited supply of scientific articles that document health disparities that are likely related to bias. Consider how bias works, bring the unconscious bias to the consciousness, and work to change it so one's unconsciousness works in a better way. Remember that our patients have their unconscious biases as well and to consider them in the care that we provide.

Conclusion

Unconscious bias – the attitudes or stereotypes outside of our awareness – affect our understanding, interactions, and decisions and are part of who we are as human beings. They serve as shortcuts to simplify the world and help us to understand our surroundings more quickly. Our individual experiences shape these shortcuts and are continually changing in an ongoing dynamic process. Evidence abounds showing that unconscious bias in medicine can have life-altering consequences. Recognition that these biases exist is the first step in bringing them into our consciousness. This realization allows us to work with our biases, enabling us to challenge our biases to work better with people. This ultimately creates the proper environment in which to work and learn which would allow us to provide optimal, culturally competent patient care.

References

1. Alrwisan A, Eworuke E. Are discrepancies in waiting time for chest pain at emergency departments between African Americans and Whites improving over time? J Emerg Med. 2016;50(2):349–55.
2. Griffith D, Hamilton K, Norrie J, Isles C. Early and late mortality after myocardial infarction in men and women: prospective observational study. Heart. 2005;91(3):305–7.
3. Mosey JM. Defining racial and ethnic disparities in pain management. Clin Orthop Relat Res. 2011;469(7):1859–70.
4. Greenwald AG, McGhee DE, Schwartz JLK. Measuring individual differences in implicit cognition: the implicit association test. J Pers Soc Psychol. 1998;74:1464–80.
5. About the IAT [Internet]. [place unknown]: Project Implicit; 2011(Cited 28 Nov 2017). Available from: https://implicit.harvard.edu/implicit/iatdetails.html
6. Green AR, Carney DR, Palin DJ, Ngo LH, Raymond KL, Iezzoni LI, Banaji MR. Implicit bias among physicians and its prediction of thrombolysis decisions for black and white patients. J Gen Intern Med. 2007;22(9):1231–8.
7. Cooper LA, Roter DL, Carson KA, Beach MC, Sabin JA, Greenwald AG. The associations of clinicians' implicit bias attitudes about race with medical visit communication and patient ratings of interpersonal care. Am J Public Health. 2012;102(5):979–87.
8. Schwartz MB, Chambliss HO, Brownell KD, Blair SN, Billington C. Weight bias among health professionals specializing in obesity. Obes Res. 2003;11(9):1033–9.
9. Uncapher H, Arean PA. Physicians are less willing to treat suicidal ideation in older patients. J Am Geriatr Soc. 2000;48(2):188–92.
10. Popa-Roch M, Delmas F. Prejudice implicit association test effects – the role of self-related heuristics. J Psychol. 2010;218(1):44–50.
11. Tweedy D. Black man in a white coat – a doctor's reflections on race and medicine. New York: Picador; 2015. 302 p.

Part II
Patient Cases

Patient cases on cultural competency in the first book *Diversity and Inclusion in Quality Patient Care* include:

African-American Infant and Family
Cambodian Refugee
Sickle Cell Crisis
Mongolian Spots
Death Disclosure
Coin Rubbing
Toxic Ingestion
Adolescent Indian Male Sikh
Intimate Partner Violence in the Gay Community
West Indian/Caribbean
American Indian
Spiritualism in the Latino Community
Islamic Patient
Pediatric Pain

Part II of *Your Story/Our Story* contains patient experiences with bias in health care covering race, ethnicity, gender, sexual orientation, socioeconomic status (homeless and low-income), deafness, disability, and various other human attributes.

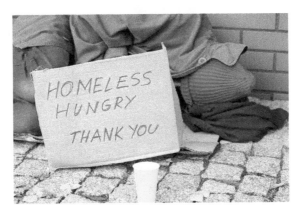

Chapter 9
African-American Patient

Traci R. Trice

Case Scenario

A 21-year-old African-American male presents to the family medicine clinic for a routine physical exam. He was last seen in the clinic approximately 3 years ago. On the day of presentation, he has no acute medical complaints and reports no concerns. The resident, however, asks several times about the patient's general health and health behaviors. When discussing his sexual history, the patient reports that he is sexually active with female partners only. He engages in oral and vaginal penetrative sex with occasional condom use. He has been tested for sexually transmitted infections (STIs) in the past. All tests were negative, but it has been a while since he was last tested. He had eight to nine sexual partners in the last year. The patient occasionally uses marijuana but denies ever engaging in intravenous drug use (IVDU). The resident completes the physical exam and subsequently reviews the presentation with his attending. The resident recommends pre-exposure prophylaxis (PrEP) (a combination of oral medication including tenofovir and emtricitabine to prevent HIV infection in people who do not have HIV but who are at substantial risk of getting it). When the attending asks the resident to explain his rationale, the resident responds that the patient had a high number of sexual partners and that he is black. The patient explains that he is not interested in taking any medications and seems confused by the suggestion.

T. R. Trice
Office of Diversity and Inclusion Initiatives, Department of Family and Community
Medicine, Sidney Kimmel Medical College of Thomas Jefferson University,
Philadelphia, PA, USA
e-mail: Traci.trice@jefferson.edu

© Springer International Publishing AG, part of Springer Nature 2019   77
M. L. Martin et al. (eds.), *Diversity and Inclusion in Quality Patient Care*,
https://doi.org/10.1007/978-3-319-92762-6_9

Review of Symptoms

Positive for penile pain and denies penile discharge or lesions; all other systems are negative.

Past Medical History

Laceration of the face, obesity.

Family History

Hypertension and type 2 diabetes mellitus.

Social History

Drinks alcohol socially, denies cigarette smoking, smokes marijuana on occasion, denies all other recreational drug use.

Physical Exam

Vital signs Temp 97.3 °F (36.3 °C); pulse 67; BP 124/84; respiratory rate 18, SpO_2 98% on room air; height 5′ 9.5″ (1.765 m); weight 223 lb (101 kg); BMI 32.46 kg/m^2.

General Obese African-American male in no distress, well-developed, pleasant.

HEEN Normocephalic and atraumatic.

Eyes Extraocular movements are intact, right eye exhibits no discharge, left eye exhibits no discharge, no scleral icterus.

Neck Normal range of motion, neck supple, no thyromegaly, no lymphadenopathy present.

Cardiovascular Normal rate, regular rhythm, and normal heart sounds, no murmur, no gallop, and no friction rub.

Respiratory Effort normal and breath sounds normal, no respiratory distress, no stridor, no wheezing, no rales.

Abdomen Soft, non-tender, non-distended, obese, normal bowel sounds.

Neuro CN II-XII are grossly intact, alert and oriented to person, place, and time.

Skin Skin is warm and dry, no rash, no diaphoresis.

Psych Mood, affect, and behavior normal.

Questions for Discussion

1. Is being black/African-American a risk factor for contracting HIV? Should race be considered when prescribing PrEP?

Attitudes/Assumptions: The Physician

(a) Black race is a risk factor for HIV.
(b) Black people engage in more risky sexual behavior.
(c) Black men are more sexually potent, having a higher sexual prowess than their other male counterparts.

Attitudes/Assumptions: The Patient

(a) The doctor is trying to use me as a guinea pig by recommending PrEP.
(b) I'm not at risk for HIV. I know I should practice safe sex and wear a condom every time but as long as I'm getting tested and my partner is getting tested then we are good.

Gaps in Provider Knowledge

In simplistic terms, being black is not a risk factor for contracting HIV. On the basis of HIV prevalence data, the United States Preventive Services Task Force (USPSTF) considers men who have sex with men and active injection drug users to be at very high risk for new HIV infection. Behavioral risk factors for HIV infection include having unprotected vaginal or anal intercourse; having sexual partners who are HIV-infected, bisexual, or injection drug users; or exchanging sex for drugs or money. Other persons at high risk include those who have acquired or request testing for other STIs [1].

However, similar to other chronic medical conditions, African-Americans are disproportionately affected by HIV. One cannot ignore the astounding HIV statistics within the African-American community. African-American women and men have the highest rate of new HIV infection in the USA. Although African-Americans represent only 13.2% of the US population, African-American women and men comprised an estimated 61.6% (5,128/8,328) and 40.2% (14,305/35,571) of new HIV infections, respectively [2]. This is not due to biological difference or a higher inclination to risky sexual behavior but to a variety of complex societal factors.

2. Despite the advancements in HIV management, what explains the disparity among African-Americans?

This is a multifactorial problem rooted in the social determinants of health, including but not limited to the lack of a universal adoption of culturally sensitive practices and standards across the US health system, the lack of implicit bias awareness amongst providers, inadequate adoption of prevention strategies including screening and use of PrEP, limited access to health care for patients from lower socioeconomic status (SES), and the mass incarceration of African-Americans [2]. Providers may believe that black patients are more likely to engage in PrEP-associated sexual risk compensation (greater unprotected sex with PrEP) compared to whites, which can lead to reduced willingness to prescribe PrEP [3]. These perceptions are consistent with stereotypes of uncontrolled sexuality and sexual risk that have been documented in association with black men and women and have been pervasive in our society for centuries. Concerns about anticipated patient adherence and perceived risk reduction capacity of PrEP could also influence provider decisions to prescribe this preventative therapy [3].

African-Americans are overrepresented in US correctional facilities. The Bureau of Justice Statistics reports that 38% of state prisoners are black, while they only comprise 13% of the US population [4]. Infectious diseases are highly concentrated in correctional facilities due to lack of condom use with both consensual and non-consensual sex.

The cost of PrEP can also be a barrier. Additionally, there may be fear of associated stigma with initiating PrEP therapy. How one's friends and family members would react to one taking PrEP is a potential barrier. Taking PrEP may be interpreted as an admission that one engages in risky behaviors or lead to a perception that they have HIV [5]. Patients may also find it burdensome to remember to take a daily medication.

3. Which cross-cultural skills could the physician use with this patient?

Cross-Cultural Tools and Skills

HIV still carries a stigma within the African-American community. The physician should respectfully explore the patient's understanding and beliefs about HIV and his sexual behaviors within the context of the patient's culture.

4. What actions should be taken to avoid pathologizing race?

The inclusion of race in documentation of patient histories, oral and written case presentations, and even test questions is a practice that is deeply ingrained in the culture of medicine. The rationale for this tends to center around the perception that race is relevant to one's genetic or biological predisposition for certain disease processes, further influencing treatment/management decisions. Thus, we run the risk of pathologizing race. This type of practice opens the door to inequities in medical care. Race is a sociopolitical construct. Institutions that provide medical education and examination should strongly consider moving away from this practice and instead devote more time to highlighting ethnicity (not to be conflated with race), ancestry, and the social determinants of health that truly impact the health of populations [6].

5. What actions can be taken to eliminate the HIV disparity in the African-American community?

According to the USPSTF, routine screening for HIV is recommended for all adolescents and adults aged 15–65 years, regardless of race. Younger adolescents and older adults who are at increased risk should also be screened [1]. There is insufficient evidence to determine the best time interval for HIV screening. However, the suggested approach is to perform onetime screening of adolescent and adult patients to identify persons who are already HIV-positive. Repeated screenings are suggested for those who are known to be at risk for HIV infection, who are actively engaged in risky behaviors, and who live or receive medical care in a high-prevalence setting [1]. According to the CDC, high-prevalence settings are sexually transmitted disease (STD) clinics, correctional facilities, homeless shelters, tuberculosis clinics, clinics serving men who have sex with men, and adolescent health clinics with a high prevalence of STDs. Furthermore, it is recommended that providers rescreen groups at very high risk for new HIV infection at least annually and individuals at increased risk at somewhat longer intervals (e.g., 3–5 years) [1]. However, this inclusive method of prevention assumes equal access to care for all. Thus, achieving equal access to care is a critical component to eliminating the HIV disparity.

Providers and patients need to be educated about PrEP, its indications for use, as well as its effectiveness as a preventative method. Providers should engage patients in a culturally sensitive manner and be understanding of their cultural norms and practices and how they might influence a patient's decision to accept or decline suggested management. This opens the door for an enhanced dialogue and improved patient-provider relationship and is likely to lead to better outcomes.

6. What components of the ACGME competencies/milestones are addressed in this case?

(a) Patient care – Provide accessible, quality, comprehensive, compassionate, continuous, and coordinated care to patients in the context of family and community, not limited by age, gender, disease process, or clinical setting, and by using the biopsychosocial perspective and patient-centered model of care.

(i) Partner with the patient, family, and community to improve health through disease prevention and health promotion.

(b) Professionalism – Physicians share the belief that health care is best organized and delivered in a patient-centered model, emphasizing patient autonomy, shared responsibility, and responsiveness to the needs of diverse populations. Physicians should place the interests of patients first while setting and maintaining high standards of competence and integrity for themselves and their professional colleagues. Professionalization is the developmental process that requires individuals to accept responsibility for learning and maintaining the standards of the discipline, including self-regulating lapses in ethical standards. Physicians maintain trust by identifying and ethically managing the potential conflicting interests of individual patients, patients' families, society, the medical industry, and their own self-interests.

(ii) Demonstrates humanism and cultural proficiency.

(c) Interpersonal and communication skills – The family physician demonstrates interpersonal and communication skills that foster trust and result in effective exchange of information and collaboration with patients, their families, health professionals, and the public.

(iii) Communicates effectively with patients, families, and the public.

(d) System-based practice – The stewardship of the family physician helps to ensure high value, high quality, and accessibility in the healthcare system. The family physician uses his or her role to anticipate and engage in advocacy for improvements to healthcare systems to maximize patient health.

(iv) Advocates for individual and community health.

Case Outcome

The resident and the attending together returned to the room. They recommended STI testing for HIV, gonorrhea, chlamydia, and syphilis. They educated the patient on what was involved with being treated with PrEP, including follow-up and labs every 3 months and need for medication adherence. They discussed the risks, side effects, and benefits. They asked him what questions/concerns he had regarding PrEP. He had no questions but stated he would give it some thought. The patient was sent home with instructions for STI testing. He tested negative for chlamydia, gonorrhea, and HIV.

References

1. Moyer VA. Screening for HIV: US preventive services task force recommendation statement. Ann Intern Med. 2013;159(1):51–60.
2. McDougle L, Davies SL, Clinchot DM. HIV and African Americans: relationship to cultural competence, implicit bias, social determinants, and US jails and prisons. Spect J Black Men. 2017;5(2):97–111.

3. Calabrese SK, Earnshaw VA, Underhill K, Hansen NB, Dovidio JF. The impact of patient race on clinical decisions related to prescribing HIV pre-exposure prophylaxis (PrEP): assumptions about sexual risk compensation and implications for access. AIDS Behav. 2014;18(2):226–40.

4. Nellis A. The color of justice: racial and ethnic disparity in state prisons [Internet]. Washington: The Sentencing Project; 2016 (Cited 29 Nov 2017). Available from: http://www.sentencing-project.org/wp-content/uploads/2016/06/The-Color-of-Justice-Racial-and-Ethnic-Disparity-in-State-Prisons.pdf

5. Smith DK, Toledo L, Smith DJ, Adams MA, Rothenberg R. Attitudes and program preferences of African-American urban young adults about pre-exposure prophylaxis (PrEP). AIDS Educ Prev. 2012;24(5):408–21.

6. Acquaviva KD, Mintz M. Perspective: are we teaching racial profiling? The dangers of subjective determinations of race and ethnicity in case presentations. Acad Med. 2010;85(4):702–5.

Chapter 10
African-American Patient: Bias in Women's Health

Mekbib Gemeda and Anthonia Ojo

Case Scenario

A 28-year-old gravida six, para five, abortus zero, African-American pregnant female presents to labor and delivery triage with complaints of leg swelling. She is 28 weeks pregnant. The patient reports that she had leg swelling with her previous pregnancies, but this is more than usual. She endorses lower leg edema for the past 2 weeks, with worsening over the past 2 days. She denies headache, contractions, loss of fluids, or vaginal bleeding. She received early prenatal care and has been compliant with her prenatal appointments. Additionally, all of her test results have been unremarkable.

The patient is admitted for evaluation of suspected preeclampsia. The inpatient team consisting of the attending physician, resident physician, and medical student see the patient on rounds the following morning. The medical student is an African-American female who first met the patient in triage. The attending asks the patient more about her history.

Physician: "Hello Mrs. Spencer, I am Dr. Kerry, do you have any questions about your care?"

Patient: "No, thank you for taking good care of me."

Physician: "I see here that you have five previous pregnancies, and this is your first preeclampsia workup. Did all those children have the same…baby daddy?"

Patient: "Yes, they do. I've been married for 10 years to my husband."

(The patient glances at the medical student, with a raised eyebrow. The medical student notices that the patient appears uncomfortable.)

M. Gemeda (✉) · A. Ojo
Eastern Virginia Medical School, Norfolk, VA, USA
e-mail: gemedam@evms.edu

© Springer International Publishing AG, part of Springer Nature 2019
M. L. Martin et al. (eds.), *Diversity and Inclusion in Quality Patient Care*,
https://doi.org/10.1007/978-3-319-92762-6_10

Physician: "Wow, five children, that is a lot. Are you ready for tying those tubes? It's not too early to discuss it."

Patient: "I have thought about it, but my husband and I wouldn't mind having children in the future."

Physician: "Okay, then we can discuss those options after delivery. And do you live close to the hospital in case you have to come back to us for care?"

Patient: "Yes, I actually live very close by."

Physician: "In the projects down the street?"

Patient: "No…we live in the house across the street."

Physician: "Very well. What questions do you have for me?"

Patient: "None."

Review of Symptoms

The patient denies headache, contractions, vaginal bleeding, loss of fluids, blurry vision, and dysuria. She endorses extremity swelling. She denies any fever, rash, malaise, or trauma.

Past Medical History

Five previous vaginal births, term pregnancies, no complications; up to date on immunizations.

Family History

No significant family history.

Social History

The patient denies alcohol, tobacco, or other drug use. She is married and works as a lawyer at her own law firm.

Physical Exam

Vital signs Temp, 97.8; HR, 72; BP, 145/92; RR, 18.

General Well-developed, female, in no acute distress.

Neck No thyromegaly, supple, non-tender.

Cardiovascular Regular rate and rhythm, no murmurs; radial and dorsalis pedis pulses full, 3+ pedal bilateral edema.

Respiratory Clear to auscultation bilaterally, normal respiratory effort.

Abdomen Abdomen is gravid, fundal height 28 cm, bowel sounds present in all four quadrants, non-tender.

Musculoskeletal No cyanosis, no clubbing, full range of motion lower and upper extremities.

Neurologic Cranial nerves II-XII intact, normal sensation to all four extremities, normal gait.

What Was Said?

The physician asks the patient if she has the same "baby daddy" for all of her children. This colloquial phrase is used to describe the biological father of a child. Its use may particularly imply that the relationship between the mother and the father of the child is more casual than that between a married couple. Historically, this choice of language has been predominantly used in African-American culture [1, 2]. In this context, the physician makes an assumption and implies a connotation through his choice of words. The patient replies to the physician's comment by presenting her own term to describe the relationship and paternity of her child's father.

After seeing the patient's obstetrical history of five previous pregnancies, the physician is prompted to ask her about her readiness for a tubal ligation. He poses the question in an assumptive manner, rather than inquiring with open-ended questions. The physician concludes the conversation by introducing another assumption of where the patient lives. Simply by looking at the patient and hearing that she lives very close to the hospital, he suggests the residence down the street that is of lower socioeconomic background, rather than the community much closer and of higher socioeconomic status.

What Was Done?

After the team leaves the room, the medical student is unsure of whether to comment on what she just observed. She later goes to the resident physician to debrief about the pattern of overt assumptions made during the encounter that morning. The resident listens to the medical student's concerns and agrees that the attending's behavior was inappropriate. However, he justifies the attending's actions by saying,

"That is just how he is. He is just straightforward. He is not a racist." The resident physician minimizes the encounter by noting that he has seen that the majority of African-American patients at the hospital refer to the father of the child as "baby daddy." He also explains that for insurance coverage, some women must complete consent far in advance to have a tubal ligation, making it necessary to ask this question early on in a patient's care. The resident then suggests that the medical student focus on learning about medicine-related topics.

Questions for Discussion

1. How can word choice impact the patient's perspective of the care they are receiving?
2. Do you think that the physician would have used this same verbiage of "baby daddy" with a similar patient of Caucasian background?
3. Should physicians try to use colloquial terms specific to the race or culture of their patients?
4. What are neutral phrases that can be used to refer to paternity that do not have negative connotations?
5. What implicit biases exist in women's health for minority patients?
6. How should other providers, regardless of their level of training, address the physician's comment?
7. How should a provider discuss birth control options with a woman without introducing bias?
8. How can providers prevent systematic policies from influencing counseling of options and care to patients?
9. How does a provider survey socioeconomic background without introducing bias?

Attitudes/Assumptions: The Physician

Word choice can reveal the presence of implicit bias and beliefs. In this case, the physician introduced a term that represents a preconceived notion of the patient. More neutral phrases for discussing paternity include "father of the baby" or "the dad." These are terms that do not have a history of implying the same connotation as "baby daddy." It is questionable if the physician would have used this same verbiage with a similar patient of Caucasian background. Unfortunately, by using a colloquial term, he has left room for the patient to interpret his undertone. The patient must correct the provider's choice of words and address the stereotype. Some providers may use colloquial terms to attempt to relate to their patients; however, applying stereotypes of a specific patient population can build barriers to care. As displayed in this situation, the patient's body language communicated that she was disengaging from the physician to identify with another member of the team.

The resident physician comments that there are policies that require consent for sterilization within a certain time frame. He is referring to the consent form and waiting period required for Medicaid-funded sterilizations [3, 4]. This is an example of a systematic policy that may be susceptible to implicit bias and assumptions. Whereas a physician may overemphasize a tubal ligation for the purposes of paperwork anticipation, he or she may subconsciously be placing more emphasis on one form of contraception over another. Furthermore, these conversations may be more biased toward women of certain racial, ethnic, and socioeconomic backgrounds [5].

Understanding a patient's socioeconomic background is important in many aspects of health care in order to provide cost-conscious care and be mindful of access to care. The physician could utilize open-ended questioning and discussion to learn about the socioeconomic background of the patient.

Cross-Cultural Tools and Skills

A core aspect of communication between a provider and a patient should be founded on respect and exploration by the provider of what shape the patient would like the communication to take. The default should be formal communication where the provider addresses the patient with utmost respect and deference, avoiding colloquial, casual communication, which could be achieved by building a relationship and rapport with the patient.

To bridge the gap of communication and relatability, physicians should allow patients to introduce colloquial terms into the conversation. Conversational tools such as echoing the patient's word choice may allow the patient to feel that their provider is following the patient's lead in language and tone. Providers are encouraged to ask for clarification when patients use slang terms so that both parties understand the context of the term in the perspective of the individual patient. Healthcare workers should be cognizant that language, especially if it is slang, may inhibit the ability to build rapport.

Black women in America experience a disproportionately higher rate of infant mortality than their white American counterparts. This has led to investigations into racial disparities experienced by African-American women. Pregnant black women have a compounded source of stress during pregnancy that is influenced by external biases of childbearing, as well as a mistrust of the medical system due to a history of exploitation of black women's bodies [6, 7].

Research has shown that African-American women and women who lack insurance or who utilize public insurance are more likely to undergo sterilization procedures when compared to their white counterparts and women with private insurance [8]. There is little data on birth control counseling and discussion of options preceding sterilization. Providers should be aware of the bias in care that exists for minority women based on their race, ethnicity, socioeconomic status, and number of children. Implicit bias may influence the manner in which patients are counseled on management options [7]. The American College of Obstetricians and Gynecologists recommends that women receive extensive and unbiased counseling for sterilization and all forms of contraception [5].

Open-ended questions are important tools in culturally competent care. They allow the patient to communicate their background, beliefs, and values. When asking very specific questions, it is helpful to identify the reason the question is being asked and the implications to the patient's care.

The core problem in the case is the attending's implicit bias about black women, their socioeconomic space, childbearing, and family structure. His bias surfaced in a comment he made which seemed on the surface to be targeted at creating closer rapport with the patient. The patient looked visibly uncomfortable and made eye contact with the medical student, the only African-American on her care team. At this point, the physician should have recognized the problem, apologized for his word choice, and clarified to the patient why he used it. He should have also made a point to apologize to the students and others in the care team to take advantage of the incident as a learning opportunity.

The medical student made the correct choice in addressing the incident with the resident physician. However, every institution should have policies and procedures in place for how all members of the healthcare team may express concerns about patient care. Institutions should avoid condoning a culture in which specific behaviors and personalities of more senior staff are tolerated. The American College of Obstetricians and Gynecologists has recommended that physicians incorporate issues of bias into teaching of trainees such as medical students, residents, and fellows [7]. This case is an example of a learning opportunity for the entire care team. There is an evident lack of training opportunities for providers to learn how to build rapport with diverse patients in culturally sensitive and respectful ways.

Case Outcome

Diagnosis Gestational hypertension.

Disposition Home.

The workup is negative for preeclampsia. The patient is counseled on preeclampsia signs and symptoms and returns home. At 39 weeks gestation, her water breaks, and she chooses to go to a different hospital for delivery, despite it being a further distance from her home.

References

1. Baby daddy [Internet]. Springfield, MA: Merriam-Webster Inc; c2017 (Cited 6 Dec 2017). Available from: https://www.merriam-webster.com/dictionary/baby%20daddy

2. Nelson LE, Morrison-Beedy D, Kearney MH, Dozier A. Black adolescent mothers' perspectives on sex and parenting in nonmarital relationships with the biological fathers of their children. J Obstet Gynecol Neonatal Nurs. 2012;41(1):82–91. https://doi.org/10.1111/j.1552-6909.2011.01324.x.
3. US Department of Health, Education, and Welfare. 42 Code of Federal Regulations. 441.257; 1976.
4. US Department of Health, Education, and Welfare. 42 Code of Federal Regulations. 441.253; 1978.
5. American College of Obstetricians and Gynecologists. Sterilization of women ethical issues and consideration: committee Opinion No. 695. Obstet Gynecol. 2017;129(4):109–16.
6. Rosenthal L, Lobel M. Explaining racial disparities in adverse birth outcomes: unique sources of stress for Black American women. Soc Sci Med. 2011;72(6):977–83. https://doi.org/10.1016/j.socscimed.2011.01.013.
7. ACOG statement of policy on racial bias [Internet]. Washington: The American College of Obstetricians and Gynecologists; 2017 (Cited 13 Nov 2017). Available from: https://www.acog.org/-/media/Statements-of-Policy/Public/StatementofPolicy93RacialBias2017-2.pdf?dmc=1&ts=20171003T014038341.1
8. Borrero S, Schwarz EB, Reeves MF, Bost JE, Creinin MD, Ibrahim SA. Race, insurance status, and tubal sterilization. Obstet Gynecol. 2007;109(1):94–100.

Chapter 11
Asian Patient

Simiao Li and Michael Gisondi

Case Scenario

An 84-year-old Chinese woman is brought to the emergency department (ED) by ambulance. EMS was called by a friend who found the patient in her kitchen with a large head laceration. By report, a large amount of dried blood was found at the scene, and the patient had applied a poultice to her scalp following the incident.

The patient is sitting calmly in bed, alert, and looking around. She does not speak English but rather a dialect of Cantonese which the ED interpreter assists in translating: "The patient states she was cooking that morning when she slipped on the kitchen floor and fell, hitting her head on the counter. She did not lose consciousness."

Review of Symptoms

Neurologic: Mild headache, denies loss of consciousness.
    All other systems are reported negative.

S. Li (✉)
Department of Emergency Medicine, The Ohio State University Wexner Medical Center, Columbus, OH, USA

M. Gisondi
Department of Emergency Medicine, Stanford University School of Medicine, Stanford, CA, USA
e-mail: mgisondi@stanford.edu

© Springer International Publishing AG, part of Springer Nature 2019
M. L. Martin et al. (eds.), *Diversity and Inclusion in Quality Patient Care*,
https://doi.org/10.1007/978-3-319-92762-6_11

Past Medical History

Non-insulin-dependent diabetes, hypertension.

Family History

Noncontributory.

Social History

The patient is retired and lives alone in senior housing in Chinatown. No family lives nearby. She denies alcohol or recreational drugs.

Physical Exam

Vital signs Temp, 98 °F; pulse, 89; BP, 136/84; respirations, 12, O_2 Sat 99% on room air.

General Thin, petite woman appearing stated age sitting calmly on stretcher with her head in a bandage.

Cardiovascular No murmurs, gallops, or rubs.

Respiratory Clear breath sounds bilaterally.

ENT Edentulous.

Abdomen Non-distended, non-tender with normal bowel sounds.

Extremities No cyanosis, no edema.

Skin 15 cm laceration to scalp at crown with dried brownish powder in wound, shallow abrasion to the anterior forehead.

Neuro Grossly intact, moves all four extremities, no obvious sign of deficit.

Neck Supple, non-tender in posterior midline, no pain on range of motion.

Questions for Discussion

1. Why didn't the patient seek medical attention of her own accord?

Attitudes/Assumptions: The Physician

(a) The poultice the patient applied to her wound will increase odds of wound infection and certainly was not beneficial.
(b) The patient chose to not seek medical attention; therefore, she must not understand the seriousness of her condition and likely won't comply with our recommendations.
(c) The patient doesn't speak English, so she must not be educated.

Attitudes/Assumptions: The Patient

(a) I've treated wounds myself the same way many times in the past, and they all healed fine – Why do I need to go to the emergency room?
(b) None of these doctors or nurses are speaking to me directly – they must not be concerned about me.

Gaps in Provider Knowledge

(a) Lack of knowledge of health beliefs/customs: folk medicine/home remedies.
(b) Lack of knowledge of disparities/discrimination: immigrant communities often lack insurance coverage or access to medical care. If this patient is undocumented, she may defer seeking medical care for fear of deportation [1].

2. What actions can be taken by the doctor to provide the optimal outcome?

Cross-Cultural Tools and Skills

(a) Use a professional interpreter to obtain accurate information within a culturally appropriate context. Use of professional interpreters is associated with improved clinical care with respect to clinical outcomes and patient satisfaction [2, 3].
(b) Acknowledge that the patient acted logically based on her prior knowledge and circumstances.
(c) Understand that the patient may have limited access to medical care for follow-up of her emergency room visit.

3. What medical issues concern you about this case?

(a) The physician should discuss with the patient that she is at greater risk of developing a wound infection, given delay before wound closure.
(b) The physician should determine the patient's ability to obtain follow-up medical care for her wound and blunt head injury.

4. Which components of the Emergency Medicine Milestones of the ACGME competencies [4] are incorporated in the case?

(a) Patient-centered communication: Demonstrates interpersonal and communication skills that result in the effective exchange of information and collaboration with the patient.
(b) Professional values: Demonstrates compassion, integrity, and respect for others, as well as adherence to the ethical principles relevant to the practice of medicine.

Case Outcome

Diagnosis Scalp laceration, blunt head trauma.

Disposition Home with friend.

After a history and physical is obtained, the provider discusses the next steps for her care using the interpreter. The patient undergoes a CT scan of her head, which shows no acute intracranial injury. The wound is thoroughly irrigated and closed using staples. The physician is able to determine that the patient has appropriate follow-up for wound check and staple removal at a sliding-scale community clinic in her neighborhood. Via an interpreter, the patient is given time to ask questions. The patient and provider conclude using shared decision-making to hold antibiotics, and the patient is given strict return precautions for wound infection.

References

1. Beck TL, Le TK, Henry-Okafor Q, Shah MK. Medical care for undocumented immigrants: national and international issues. Prim Care. 2017;44(1):e1–e13.
2. Karliner LS, Jacobs EA, Chen AH, Mutha S. Do professional interpreters improve clinical care for patients with limited English proficiency? A systematic review of the literature. Health Serv Res. 2007;42(2):727–54.
3. Juckett G, Unger K. Appropriate use of medical interpreters. Am Fam Physician. 2014;90(7):476–80.
4. The Emergency Medicine Milestones Project [Internet]. Chicago: Accreditation Council for Graduate Medical Education and The American Board of Emergency Medicine; 2015 (Cited 28 July 2017). Available from: https://www.acgme.org/Portals/0/PDFs/Milestones/EmergencyMedicineMilestones.pdf

Chapter 12
Native-American Patient

Xi Damrell and Kevin Ferguson

Case Scenario

A 63-year-old Native-American woman, accompanied by her son, presents at an emergency room with complaints of dizziness, edema and pain in her extremities, shortness of breath, and a nonproductive cough. She is a practitioner of native traditional religion, is not seen by the Indian Health Service, and claims that she "avoids doctors." Her manner is alternately standoffish and joking. She states to the emergency room physician that she is not averse to Western medicine, however, and sees "traditional medicines" as "complementing white medicine." They both speak English, but, intermittently, the patient and son speak Lakota (their native language) to one another, which makes the physician uncomfortable. Both seem evasive about the patient's history and appear to avoid eye contact. The patient is nonadherent with previously prescribed and unknown diabetic medications, saying that she prefers to treat her condition with "bear root" and other herbs available to her seasonally or from friends. She displays an empty prescription bottle with most of the information worn off. She has tried an unspecified home remedy for cough, but it "won't work until the next moon." She wants the emergency physician to help her decide how to proceed with her cure. At the end of the exam, the son briefly takes the doctor aside to say that his mother is "a highly respected person and not as crazy as she sounds" and that he will make sure she does what she is told.

X. Damrell (✉)
Kaweah Delta Emergency Medicine Residency Program, Visalia, CA, USA
e-mail: xi.damrell@vituity.com

K. Ferguson
Touro University at St. Joseph Medical Center, Stockton, CA, USA
e-mail: kevinferguson@cep.com

© Springer International Publishing AG, part of Springer Nature 2019   97
M. L. Martin et al. (eds.), *Diversity and Inclusion in Quality Patient Care*,
https://doi.org/10.1007/978-3-319-92762-6_12

Review of Symptoms

The patient has increased shortness of breath lately and is unable to lie flat. According to her son, she gets tired easily lately and has been less active.

Past Medical History

The patient says she is diabetic but does not take medication and generally does not follow any dietary restrictions except according to her own beliefs and traditions, preferring wild game and plants to "store-bought" food. Her blood pressure has been high during office visits, but she is not on any blood pressure medication.

Family History

The patient's father died of old age and was diabetic. Her mother died of a heart attack at age 50. Both of her brothers are alcoholics and living, and she is unclear about their medical conditions.

Social History

The patient is a member of a large, multigenerational family group and is considered by them to be an elder and a "medicine woman." She is divorced and lives alone in her small home behind the family farmhouse. There is adequate food in the home, and the patient has children, grandchildren, and neighbors who will "look in on her," although there "may be a problem if medication have to be taken at certain times." The family is seasonally employed by local ranchers and farmers and also farms a small hay plot in addition to maintaining a garden and raising a few horses and chickens. The patient does not use alcohol, illegal drugs, or tobacco.

Physical Exam

Vital signs Temp, 98.3 F; pulse, 110, BP 180/90; respiration, 28, O_2 Sat 93% on room air.

General Obese Native-American woman.

ENT Pupils round, reactive to light, non-icterus sclera, mucous membrane moist, poor dentition.

Neck Jugular venous distention present, no carotid bruits.

Cardiovascular Tachycardia with irregular rhythm, no murmurs, equal palpable distal pulses.

Respiratory Tachypnea, rales in the bilateral lower lung fields.

Abdomen Soft, non-tender, non-distended, no organomegaly.

Extremities 2 plus pitting edema bilateral lower extremities up to the mid-calf.

Skin No rash.

Neuro Awake, alert, and oriented; no focal deficits.

Test Results CBC, normal; metabolic panel, elevated blood glucose of 480; normal bicarb; VBG showed PH is 7.38; BNP, 810; CXR, enlarged heart with bilateral interstitial infiltrates, Kerley B lines, small pleural effusions consistent with pulmonary edema; EKG, atrial fibrillation with V rate of 112, no acute ischemic change; first set of troponin is negative.

Questions for Discussion

1. Why is communication between the physician and the patient difficult?

Attitudes/Assumptions: The Physician

(a) Based on her statements, the patient mistrusts "Western medicine."
(b) She doesn't act educated or well-informed about her condition.
(c) Patient is delusional and has difficulty talking to the physician.

Attitudes/Assumptions: The Patient

(a) I believe in the medicine and the practices of my ancestors. The spirits have answered me in the past and cured my other illnesses.
(b) I know the doctor thinks I am crazy. I saw his facial expression when I told him my medicine will not be ready until the next moon.
(c) White people have always thought we are stupid.

2. What are some cultural issues?

Attitudes/Assumptions: The Physician

(a) Why are they speaking in a Native-American language?
(b) What are they saying that is not translated to me?
(c) What does it mean that the patient considers herself to be a "medicine woman"?

Attitudes/Assumptions: The Patient

(a) I am trying to show the white doctor that I am capable and not uneducated.
(b) I am proud of my native heritage and my bilingual abilities.
(c) The physician may have gone to medical school, but I have learned from the elders during my lifetime.

3. What are some factors related to trust and respect?

Attitudes/Assumptions: The Physician

(a) Even though the patient verbalizes her distrust of medicine, she has communicated that distrust (communication is good).
(b) The patient has offered the doctor an opening by saying that Native American and "white" medicine can complement one another.
(c) Lots of patients are nervous around physicians, and the joking, etc., may simply be this patient's reaction to the situation.

Attitudes/Assumptions: The Patient

(a) I will show this non-Indian doctor that my ways are as valid as his.
(b) I will follow the doctor's advice, so long as it seems to fit with my own beliefs.
(c) When the doctor shows me a little respect and doesn't treat me like I am uneducated, uncultured, or a child, I will reciprocate.

Gaps in Provider Knowledge

(a) The provider may not understand the following: Native-American elders are considered autonomous. They make their own decisions, including medical decisions, although the group (e.g., family and extended family) might weigh in on minute details. Health beliefs are not fixed but are subject to "testing" and "contextualizing" [1]. Western medicines are often sought in addition to native healing (including the use of herbs, ceremonies, sweat lodge rites, and extensive dietary practices) to restore a patient to health. Causes of disease include malevolent spiritual forces and other unknown causes "beyond our understanding" [2].

(b) Owing to her age, the patient has no doubt experienced discrimination by white authorities (including, perhaps, medical providers). She might be using both English and Lakota to "prove" to the doctor that she is competent and capable and also to communicate her autonomy [3, 4].

4. Which components of Emergency Medicine Milestones of the ACGME competencies are incorporated in the case?

(a) *Professional values:* Providers often encounter patients with different cultural beliefs and practices that may conflict with the provider's personal values or beliefs. Respect the different beliefs and establish the therapeutic environment.

(b) *Patient-centered communication:* A professional and nonjudgmental approach is the key when obtaining the history. Understanding the patient's view of her health and likelihood of her compliance will determine her disposition.

(c) *Patient safety:* The provider needs to address psychosocial issues as well as medical emergencies. This patient has no established medical care and will need a primary care physician with cardiology consultation. This could be managed with close follow-up as outpatient.

Case Outcome

Diagnosis Pulmonary edema, new onset atrial fibrillation.

Disposition The patient is admitted to the regular floor with telemetry, and she improved with IV furosemide. Blood glucose improved after 10 units of IV regular insulin in the emergency department. Blood pressure improved with 10 units of IV hydralazine. Serial troponin was negative. A full cardiac workup was done, which included an echocardiogram that showed the patient has a reduced ejection fraction at 40%. The patient's congestive heart failure symptoms improved, and she was discharged home with a multi-medication regiment for heart failure and Coumadin for her atrial fibrillation. There were several long discussions with the patient and her family members. The patient agreed to take her medications as described, and she was given an appointment to follow up with the cardiologist in 2 weeks. The patient also had a primary care appointment scheduled in 2 weeks.

References

1. Treuer A. Everything you wanted to know about Indians but were afraid to ask. St Paul: Minnesota Historical Society; 2012. 184 p.
2. Medicine B. Drinking and sobriety among the Lakota Sioux. Lanham: Alta Mira Press; 2007. 155 p.
3. Weaver H, editor. Social issues in contemporary Native America. New York: Routledge; 2014. 256 p.
4. Trafzer C, Weiner D, editors. Medicine ways: disease, health and survival among Native Americans. Walnut Creek: Alta Mira Press; 2001. 304 p.

Chapter 13
LGB Patient and Mental Health

Charlie Borowicz and John S. Rozel

Case Scenario

A 20-year-old Hispanic male presented alone to the emergency department of a local hospital. He stated that he moved from home to a dormitory before this school year, due to conflict with his family. This was approximately 6 months ago. Since then, he has found it difficult to enjoy things he usually does for fun, has been sleeping excessively (10–11 h per night, with difficulty waking and staying awake), and has been eating one meal per day for the last 2–3 weeks. He reported suicidal thoughts with a plan to drink chemicals obtained from his dormitory's cleaning cart. He stated that his family recently found out he was dating another young man at school, which prompted the conflict. Since then, he has had limited contact with his mother and two brothers and no contact with his father. The doctor conducting the interview asked whether his family has a problem with the patient being gay. The patient immediately said he is not gay and became withdrawn for the rest of the interview, answering with monosyllabic responses.

C. Borowicz (✉) · J. S. Rozel
University of Pittsburgh, Pittsburgh, PA, USA
e-mail: rozeljs@upmc.edu

© Springer International Publishing AG, part of Springer Nature 2019
M. L. Martin et al. (eds.), *Diversity and Inclusion in Quality Patient Care*,
https://doi.org/10.1007/978-3-319-92762-6_13

Review of Symptoms

Psychiatric evaluation is significant for hypersomnia, anhedonia, and lack of appetite. The patient reported suicidal thoughts with a plan to drink chemicals obtained from the housekeeping cart at his dormitory.

Past Medical History

He endorsed one past suicide attempt 2 years ago via hanging himself, in which he tied a belt around a banister in his home but was interrupted by his sister.

Family History

The patient believes his mother has anxiety, but she has never been formally diagnosed. He has one paternal uncle who has been hospitalized for psychiatric reasons, for which the patient does not have details.

Social History

The patient recently moved to a dormitory in his second year of undergraduate education. Prior to this, he was commuting from home.

Physical Exam

No significant findings.

Questions for Discussion

1. Why did the patient become withdrawn?

Attitudes/Assumptions: The Doctor

(a) The patient dating a man means he is gay.
(b) The patient is depressed because his family rejects him for being gay.

(c) His family is a traditional Hispanic family, probably with a strong Catholic background, and therefore will reject him because of his sexuality.

Attitudes/Assumptions: The Patient

(a) The doctor didn't bother to hear my whole story before putting a label on me.
(b) I'm here to talk about my symptoms, not my sexuality.

Gaps in Provider Knowledge

(a) Lack of knowledge about the client's family and variation within religious groups. Some families of many religions can still be accepting of family members on the LGBTQ spectrum.
(b) Lack of knowledge regarding dating/sexual behavior vs. orientation. Dating someone of the same sex does not make that person gay. The person could identify as bisexual or pansexual, for example [1].

This patient possibly identifies as bisexual. However, some men who have sex with men do not identify themselves as gay or bisexual. The doctor labeling him as a gay man invalidates his identity.

2. What actions could have been taken by the doctor to avoid this discomfort during the interview?

Cross-Cultural Tools and Skills

(a) Never assume sexual orientation. Allow the patient to divulge their orientation/identity spontaneously, if they are comfortable doing so.
(b) Allow the patient to discuss their symptoms and triggers and draw parallels between them. Do not assume causation if a set of circumstances exists together.
(c) If sexual history is clinically relevant, the healthcare provider can ask, "How would you describe your sexual orientation?" If the patient chooses to answer, the doctor can proceed with, "I understand that to mean [*describe*]. Can you clarify what it means for you?" Patients have expressed that they feel respected when providers ask questions instead of making assumptions [2, 3].

Case Outcome

Diagnosis DSM-5 296.33 (ICD-10 F33.2) Major depressive disorder, recurrent episode, severe [4].

Disposition   The patient should be referred to inpatient hospitalization for stabilization of suicidal thoughts. Following that, he should be referred to an outpatient therapist for continuing care and a psychiatrist for medication management.

References

1. Alpert AB, CichoskiKelly EM, Fox AD. What lesbian, gay, bisexual, transgender, queer, and intersex patients say doctors should know and do: a qualitative study. J Homosex. 2017; 64(10):1368–89.
2. Rossman K, Salamanca P, Macapagal K. A qualitative study examining young adults' experiences of disclosure and nondisclosure of LGBTQ identity to health care providers. J Homosex. 2017;64(10):1390–410.
3. Rounds KE, McGrath BB, Walsh E. Perspectives on provider behaviors: a qualitative study of sexual and gender minorities regarding quality of care. Contemp Nurse. 2013;44(1):99–110. https://doi.org/10.5172/conu.2013.44.1.99.
4. American Psychiatric Association. Diagnostic and statistical manual of mental disorders. 5th ed. Washington: American Psychiatric Publishing; 2013.

Chapter 14
Transgender Patient and Mental Health

Charlie Borowicz and John S. Rozel

Case Scenario

A 36-year-old African-American female presents to the emergency room of a psychiatric hospital with her sister. On the intake paperwork, she indicates that she is a transgender woman. The doctor makes several errors in calling the patient "him" upon getting report from the nurse. When the nurse reminds the doctor that the patient is transgender, the doctor states that it is difficult because she was "born as a man" and still has "masculine features." This is said within earshot of the patient.

The patient endorses racing thoughts, including intrusive thoughts of self-injury by cutting with a razor. She denies intent to act on these thoughts, labeling them as intrusive, and claims she "just wants them to stop." During the interview, she consistently picks at her hair, ripping out several pieces during the assessment. Her sister gently takes her hands and reminds her to stop several times, but the patient returns to hairpulling in very short intervals. The doctor also observes several adhesive bandages on the patient's fingers. The patient confirms that these are from picking the skin around her fingers. The patient reveals that she has recently separated from her partner of the last 10 years. The doctor asks the patient about hormone usage. The patient confirms that she has been taking them for the last 15 years. The doctor then asks about gender-affirming surgeries, at which the patient gets agitated and asks, "What that has to do with anything?" The doctor asks whether the picking and anxiety started before or after the surgeries. The patient becomes angry and shouts at the doctor, prompting the doctor to call security.

C. Borowicz (✉) · J. S. Rozel
University of Pittsburgh, Pittsburgh, PA, USA
e-mail: rozeljs@upmc.edu

© Springer International Publishing AG, part of Springer Nature 2019   107
M. L. Martin et al. (eds.), *Diversity and Inclusion in Quality Patient Care*,
https://doi.org/10.1007/978-3-319-92762-6_14

Review of Symptoms

Psychiatric evaluation is significant for trichotillomania (compulsive pulling out of the hair) and intrusive thoughts of self-mutilation via cutting. The patient rates anxiety as 9/10 on a 1–10 scale with 10 being the highest and reports that this has been consistent for the past 3 days.

Past Medical History

The patient endorses a history of hypertension, which is usually well managed through medication. She reports a cholecystectomy 5 years prior. Medical records indicate several gender-affirming surgeries performed over a 3-year period, beginning 10 years ago. She denies past psychiatric history.

Family History

The patient denies family history of psychiatric issues.

Social History

The patient is recently separated from a partner of 10 years. She has strong support from her sister, with whom she now lives. Her parents live nearby and are supportive.

Physical Exam

Skin Superficial abrasions to the fingers.

Cardiovascular Mild hypertension, for which the patient takes medications; she reports that she forgot her medication this morning. Mild tachycardia.

Laboratory studies are unremarkable except for a mildly elevated white blood cell count.

Questions for Discussion

1. Why did the patient become agitated?

Attitudes/Assumptions: The Doctor

(a) The patient is experiencing anxiety related to her identity as a transwoman.
(b) Transgender individuals have a higher incidence of mental illness.
(c) Recent onset of symptoms could be a result of identity confusion or social barriers to being trans, as well as surgical regret.

Attitudes/Assumptions: The Patient

(a) The doctor thinks of me as a case study, not as a person.
(b) The doctor is being hostile and invasive.
(c) The doctor doesn't understand transgender issues.

Gaps in Provider Knowledge

(a) Lack of knowledge related to the effects of surgery. Often gender-affirming surgeries will alleviate anxiety and improve mental health [1, 2].
(b) Lack of knowledge related to etiquette in medical examination. Many individuals feel their identity/orientation is not relevant to examinations for non-transition-related care [3].

2. What actions could have been taken by the doctor to avoid this situation?

Cross-Cultural Tools and Skills

(a) Acknowledge that the patient is going through a difficult time. Allow her to tell you what she believes led to the change in her mood and anxiety. Communication and interpersonal skills have been identified as a main component of positive provider-patient interactions [4].
(b) Refrain from discussion of surgery and hormone issues unless prompted to do so by the patient. Assuming a patient's anxiety stems from transition-related issues may cause a person to feel the provider is judging them negatively [4].

Case Outcome

Diagnosis DSM-V V61.10 (ICD-10 Z63.0) Relationship distress with spouse or intimate partner; DSM-V 300.3 (ICD-10 F42) Obsessive-compulsive disorder; DSM-V 312.39 (ICD-10 F63.3) Trichotillomania [5].

Disposition The patient should be referred to intensive outpatient therapy with medication management, followed by individual therapy for maintenance.

References

1. Nahata L, Chelvakumar G, Leibowitz S. Gender-affirming pharmacological interventions for youth with gender dysphoria: when treatment guidelines are not enough. Ann Pharmacother. 2017;5(11):1023–32. https://doi.org/10.1177/1060028017718845.
2. Crall CS, Jackson RK. Should psychiatrists prescribe gender-affirming hormone therapy to transgender adolescents? AMA J Ethics. 2016;18(11):1086.
3. Rossman K, Salamanca P, Macapagal K. A qualitative study examining young adults' experiences of disclosure and nondisclosure of LGBTQ identity to health care providers. J Homosex. 2017;64(10):1390–410.
4. Rounds KE, McGrath BB, Walsh E. Perspectives on provider behaviors: a qualitative study of sexual and gender minorities regarding quality of care. Contemp Nurse. 2013;44(1):99–110. https://doi.org/10.5172/conu.2013.44.1.99.
5. American Psychiatric Association. Diagnostic and statistical manual of mental disorders. 5th ed. Washington: American Psychiatric Publishing; 2013.

Chapter 15
Transgender Patient and Registration

Gabrielle Marzani and Esteban Cubillos-Torres

Case Scenario

A patient has arrived for her routine visit to the clinic. She is well known to the clinic and is greeted by the registration staff. She sits down. Soon, she is called from the busy waiting room by a nurse: "Mr. Rivera?"—no response. "Mr. Cari Rivera?" The patient, a well-attired woman, hesitates and then stands up. She does not know this nurse – the usual nurse is not here. The nurse is confused and then realizes what has happened. It is too late. Flushed with embarrassment, the patient is brought back to the clinic room.

The provider finds her in tears. She feels humiliated and tells the provider that she is not sure she can come back.

The patient is transgender male to female. She defines herself as female but is designated as male because the electronic health record (EHR) system designates sex, not gender. The clinic, working within the restrictions of the system, has created an unofficial work-around and is sensitive to this situation. However, no one remembered to advise the nurse working in the clinic that day, nor was there a formalized gender-neutral way to call the patients back from the waiting room.

This is a woman with panic disorder and post-traumatic stress disorder. Venturing out of her home is an act of courage. She has now been triggered and is at risk of more panic attacks as she now feels vulnerable and exposed, not just here but everywhere. This episode has caused her to question if she should return to the clinic. Of additional significance is that the patient has HIV.

G. Marzani (✉) · E. Cubillos-Torres
University of Virginia School of Medicine, Charlottesville, VA, USA
e-mail: ec4fy@virginia.edu; grm2a@virginia.edu

© Springer International Publishing AG, part of Springer Nature 2019   111
M. L. Martin et al. (eds.), *Diversity and Inclusion in Quality Patient Care*,
https://doi.org/10.1007/978-3-319-92762-6_15

Review of Symptoms

Positive for panic attacks, sleep disturbance, and anxiety.

Negative for loss of interest for the reader, increased feelings of guilt, decreased energy, and suicidal or homicidal ideation.

Past Medical History

HIV and hepatitis C.

Family History

Noncontributory.

Social History

Normal developmental milestones, graduated from high school, works in a service industry.

Physical Exam

Mental Status   The patient appears her stated age. She is neatly groomed in a dress, makeup, and earrings. Her eyes are downcast at times, although other times she maintains good eye contact. At times she becomes tearful when discussing her stressors. Her speech is normal in rate, rhythm, and volume. She describes her mood as "anxious" and this is reflected by some hand wringing. Her affect is anxious and restricted. Her mood is described as "anxious." She denies any suicidal or homicidal ideation. She denies any auditory or visual hallucinations, and she does not appear to be responding to any internal stimuli. She denies any obsession, compulsion, or phobia. Her insight and judgment are intact.

Questions for Discussion

1. What assumptions or gaps in knowledge contributed to this situation?

Attitudes/Assumptions: The Provider

(a) The nurse assumed that the patient name on the EHR was correct and that the name correlated with the patient's sex. A sex-based designation in the registration system was clearly a by-product of a system-level bias and a set of assumptions encoded in the registration system. The registration system mandated a binary selection of male or female. Ms. Rivera was placed as male based on the health system policy that existed at the time. In the existing EHR, gender was not a category, and there was no place to leave blank or provide an alternative choice in the electronic medical record.

(b) The nurse believed that calling out a name in public is appropriate.

(c) The nurse was not aware of the fixed gender assignations of the EHR.

Attitudes/Assumptions: The Patient

(a) The patient assumed that all staff and healthcare providers were sensitive to gender identity issues, especially given that this is a highly specialized HIV clinic that serves many LGBTQ patients.

(b) The patient had developed a sense of security, as she had been seen in this clinic before by staff who were aware of her sexual identity.

Gaps in Provider Knowledge

(a) The provider was not familiar with this patient.

(b) The provider was unaware of the non-binary aspect of the patient's identity.

(c) The provider was not aware of gender-neutral designations that could be used with unfamiliar patients.

2. In what ways does the EHR directly impact a patient's physical health?

Changing her sex from male to female impacted her care in other ways, as many health screenings are triggered by the sex of the patient in the system. Thus, the patient was vulnerable to being forgotten for screenings such as prostate screenings. The system as it existed was going to let her down in one form or another.

3. What actions could have been taken to avoid this situation?

Cross-Cultural Tools and Skills

Calling a Person Back from the Waiting Room

As a matter of respect, calling a patient by Mr., Miss, Ms., or Mrs. was part of the culture of this and many other clinics. This was particularly important for patients who felt invisible or who did not have a voice in the community. Generationally, some patients were offended by the use of a first name without a pronoun in front of it, if called back by a younger staff member. There is also more confidentiality in not using the first and last name. So, Ms. Rivera would be the name the patient would have been called, and preferred to be called, rather than Mr. Cari Rivera. Using a system, such as a numerical system, could be seen as disrespectful. Asking someone how they wish to be addressed is reasonable, although that would have to happen at the point of registration and the information sent back to the clinic staff.

Transgender or gender nonconforming individuals are estimated to make up about three million persons (1%) in the US population. These individuals have the same healthcare necessities as any other patient in terms of healthcare screenings, prevention, and treatment as well as additional needs that are unique to or are worsened by their gender status. For example, these patients are at increased risk of mental health problems, sexually transmitted illnesses, and illnesses related to the effects of hormone therapy [1].

Despite the additional need for care, this population, like other minority populations, tends to suffer adversely from health disparities including access to health care. For example, the levels of uninsured transgender individuals are higher than that of many other groups [2]. Transgender individuals also face many barriers to care, ranging from social stigma that prevents them from seeking care to denial of services because of their transgender status [1]. Given these barriers, it is not surprising that a 2003 survey by Feldman and Bockting found that only 30–40% of transgendered individuals seek routine medical care [3]. The National Gay and Lesbian Task Force and the National Center for Transgender Equality published a report in 2011 after collecting online or paper surveys from 6450 individuals representing all 50 states, the District of Columbia, Puerto Rico, Guam, and the US Virgin Islands. They documented the impact of being transgender or gender nonconforming in multiple areas of their lives. When asked about seeking care, significantly, over a quarter (28%) postponed care when sick or injured because of discrimination. In addition, 28% reported harassment in medical settings, and 2% were victims of violence in a doctor's office. Half reported that they had to teach their medical providers about transgender care. In addition, 24% of transgender women and 20% of transgender men were denied service altogether by physicians and other providers [4].

Thus, there is a clear need to improve access and care for this population. One way to do so, and what the patient in the above case was in need of, is gender affirmation. According to Reisner et al., gender affirmation is a key social determinant of health for transgender individuals. Providing this affirmation to patients increases mental well-being and overall quality of life for this population. On the other hand, lack of this affirmation led to delays in or avoidance of necessary preventative care, health screenings, and medical treatment. Reisner states that the process of gender affirmation is a multidimensional concept, which includes social gender affirmation (i.e., usage of the preferred name and pronoun), psychological affirmation (i.e., feeling that chosen gender is respected and validated), medical affirmation (i.e., hormone therapy, surgical gender confirmation), and legal affirmation (i.e., legal name change and legal gender indicator change) [5].

Against this backdrop enters the electronic health record (EHR). EHRs are used in most major healthcare settings. They were created for many reasons: ease of documentation, access to many pieces of data, communication across providers, and provision of quality care for patients. These systems extract data and use this data to drive clinical decision-making. In doing so, EHRs have sometimes removed subtleties of practice. One such place is in identity, based on a binary model of male/female sex, rather than sex and gender. This structural discrimination occurs when the patient is most vulnerable and has led to a multitude of mishaps for individuals who are transgender or gender nonconforming. EHRs often communicate with other systems, such as billing and coding systems, laboratory systems, and pharmacies. A misidentification can lead to errors in interpreting labs (e.g., kidney function which has normal ranges based on sex), confusion in medications (e.g., hormone replacement), radiographic images, etc. Proper identification, beyond gender affirmation, is critical for the health and well-being of our patients.

The World Professional Association for Transgender Health EMR Working Group notes that a two-step question technique to determine gender identity information is best [6]. The recommendation is to first ask the patient their gender identity and then to ask about the sex assigned at birth. They note that asking the questions in this order respects the priority of gender over the assigned sex. Although this can be asked in person, there is some evidence that it will be more accurately collected if done via patient's self-registration kiosks or patient portals. Practical recommendations by Deutsch and Buchholtz include having the following gender identity data in the electronic health record: gender ID, birth-assigned sex, legal sex, preferred name, and legal name [7]. Other literature has also recommended inclusion of the preferred pronoun. This should be done in the demographic area that would include ethnicity.

It should be recognized that these names and/or pronouns may differ from document to document. The working group reminds us that these name changes may occur at various points in an individual's self-identity or in stages of transition. There may be a significant difference between the identity of a passport, birth certificate, driver's license, health insurance policy, etc. They note that both state and federal regulations may impact how these documents can be created or changed. In addition, the medical record should accurately record the transition and not retroactively change the sex and/or gender.

Deutsch et al. [6] provide the following examples:

1. A patient may have been assigned female at birth and have transitioned to male through the use of testosterone and surgical removal of the breasts; they may also have obtained a court-ordered name and sex or gender change and are registered in the EHR system under a male name and gender. However, since this patient still has a cervix, ovaries, and uterus, healthcare providers will require the ability to enter pelvic exam findings and gynecologic review of systems and to order a cervical pap smear within the EHR system. EHR products that restrict or pre-populate an individual encounter with sex-specific history, exam, or ordering templates will prevent this patient's provider from accurately and efficiently documenting their care.

2. A patient may have been assigned male at birth and have transitioned to female through the use of estrogen; however, this patient has not yet changed her government-issued identity documents and is currently listed with a male name and sex or gender. The patient has an outwardly female appearance and wishes to be referred to using a feminine name and pronouns. The patient also has breasts as a result of their hormone treatment and will require a breast examina-tion and ordering of a mammogram. An EHR system should guide the adminis-trative and clinical staff to use the patient's chosen name and pronoun, which should serve to improve patient engagement and comfort while improving reten-tion in care. An EHR system should also allow the provider to document a breast examination and order a mammogram—even though the patient remains regis-tered as male.

3. A patient with a female birth sex and male gender identity, currently registered as a female, who is taking testosterone, may have a hemoglobin of 17 g/dl flagged as "high" by the interfacing laboratory system. A local flag driven by the patient's birth sex, gender identity, and current testosterone prescription could alert clini-cians to reconsider this "high" flag and review laboratory male reference ranges.

The ideal electronic medical record has the capacity to include non-binary gender-sex identifiers which are uncoupled from traditional sex-oriented demo-graphics, diagnoses, procedures, and reference ranges.

- Sex as a binary identifier should be replaced with a gender/sex model. The patient should be able to select their own identify and be able to state their preferred name and preferred pronoun.
- This needs to be done at the time of the first appointment being made and then routinely (as things change), and a mechanism needs to be in place so that all members of a team are aware. Standard ways of doing this, rather than work-arounds, are the best way to ensure education and communication with perma-nent and transient staff, students, and clinicians.
- Information may be most accurate when requested online or on paper.
- A good place to document this is where the demographic variables are (such as where ethnicity is). It should not be binary.
- It should be recognized that these are not static changes; individuals may change things surgically and/or legally over time, or they may never transition.

- There should be a system in place for everyone who comes in contact with or communicates with patients to see before they have contact with the patient.
- It may be helpful to have a flag/alert if the clinic does not routinely care for these populations, which is triggered at a helpful time in the staff's workflow.
- The electronic medical record needs to be able to accommodate these changes and maintain the integrity of the patient's history; the system should allow for these changes and automatically change anything retroactively.
- These pieces of data should be "uncoupled" from a sex-/gender-coded template (this will uncouple labs, diagnoses, and procedures as well).
- This should include EHR, registration systems, billing and coding systems, laboratories, pharmacies, and anything that would have a label.
- Changing sex for a patient in the electronic medical record can lead to problems in providing quality health care.

Case Outcome

After a series of discussions with the administration, Ms. Rivera was allowed to have her sex changed to female. This was empowering for her and protected her in the clinics. It left her vulnerable to being missed for screenings and also incorrect lab interpretations (with normal values associated with male or female). Workarounds had to then be created for her health screenings. The electronic health record, which includes the registration, laboratory, billing, and coding system, is being patched in conjunction with the vendor to have fields for both sex and gender.

References

1. Redfern JS, Sinclair B. Improving health care encounters and communication with transgender patients. J Commun Healthc. 2014;7(1):25.
2. Johnson CV, Mimiaga MJ, Bradford J. Health care issues among lesbian, gay, bisexual, transgender and intersex (LGBTI) populations in the United States: introduction. J Homosex. 2008;54(3):213–24.
3. Feldman J, Bockting W. Transgender health. Minn Med. 2003;86(7):25–32.
4. Grant JM, Mottet LA, Tanis J, Harrison J, Herman JL, Keisling M. Injustice at every turn: a report of the national transgender discrimination survey. Washington: National Center for Transgender Equality and National Gay and Lesbian Task Force; 2011. 228 p. Available from: http://thetaskforce.org/static_html/downloads/reports/reports/ntds_full.pdf
5. Reisner SL, Radix A, Deutsch MB. Integrated and gender-affirming transgender clinical care and research. J Acquir Immune Defic Syndr. 2016;72(Suppl 3):S235–42.
6. Deutsch MB, Green J, Keatley JA, Mayer J, Hastings J, Hall AM. Electronic medical records and the transgender patient: recommendations from the world professional association of transgender health EMR working group. J Am Med Inform Assoc. 2013;20:700–3.
7. Deutsch MB, Buchholtz D. Electronic health records and transgender patients – practical recommendations for the collection of gender identity data. J Gen Intern Med. 2015;30(6):843–7.

Chapter 16
The Rastafarian Patient

Cynthia Price and Tanya Belle

Case Scenario

A 43-year-old Jamaican woman is brought to the emergency department by her 50-year-old husband. They both have dreadlocks (ropelike braids of hair) and are wearing traditional African robes and turbans. She (the wife) has been having an increasingly severe left-sided headache since the morning of presentation. She denies any head trauma but complains of blurred vision and dizziness. She was reluctant to come to the hospital but presented as her symptoms were worsening and unrelieved with her home treatment. She is found to be hypertensive at triage with a blood pressure of 255/130 mm Hg and is sent to a patient room to be urgently seen. Her physician and nurse are both male and Caucasian-Americans. No other nurse is available at this time. The patient's husband is present and requests female attendants for his wife. He also refuses to allow her to be changed into a hospital gown or "exposed" to be connected to the monitors. The physician explains the urgent need to treat his wife's blood pressure. The patient's husband, however, does not want any "unnatural" substances in his wife's body and refuses to allow the physician to administer any medications until he knows what is in them. The physician believes he is being obstructive and is having difficulty communicating with him due to his "heavy" accent. The physician requests that the husband step outside of the room until the patient can be examined and stabilized. The husband refuses and

C. Price (✉)
Hartford Hospital, Hartford, CT, USA
e-mail: Cynthia.price@hhchealth.org

T. Belle
Emergency Medicine Residency Program, University of Connecticut, Storrs, CT, USA

© Springer International Publishing AG, part of Springer Nature 2019   119
M. L. Martin et al. (eds.), *Diversity and Inclusion in Quality Patient Care*,
https://doi.org/10.1007/978-3-319-92762-6_16

complains loudly about the "system" and the "lack of respect." The patient refuses further care until her husband agrees.

Review of Symptoms

As per the wife, she has been having headaches off and on for the past week. She does endorse nausea after headache became acutely worse; no vomiting noted. She denies any fevers. No mental status changes were reported, as well as no speech changes or weakness. All other systems were reported as negative.

Past Medical History

Diagnosed with high blood pressure years ago, which she treated with herbal remedies.

Family History

Hypertension and diabetes; no cancer or heart disease.

Social History

She lives with her husband and five children, as well as her mother and father-in-law. She does not use alcohol and is strictly vegetarian. She does not reply when asked about "drug" use.

Physical Exam

Vital Signs Temp, 98.2 °F; pulse, 100; BP, 255/130; respirations, 16; O_2 Sat 99% on room air.

General Healthy appearing female, in no respiratory distress; appears in some discomfort; complaining of headache.

Cardiovascular Tachycardic with no murmurs, gallops, or rubs; normal S1 and S2; pulses equal bilaterally and regular.

Respiratory No use of accessory muscles, clear breath sounds.

HEENT No posterior pharyngeal erythema; no cervical adenopathy; pupils equal, round, and reactive; approximately 4 mm bilaterally.

Abdomen Non-distended, non-tender with normal bowel sounds, no masses.

Extremities No cyanosis, no edema.

Skin No rashes or lesions.

Neuro Grossly intact, moving all four extremities, right upper extremity strength slightly reduced; Right nasolabial fold flattening.

Neck Supple, non-tender, no adenopathy, no meningismus.

Questions for Discussion

1. What was the basis for the husband and wife's refusal to accept certain aspects of her care?

Attitudes/Assumptions: The Physician

(a) The husband is being unreasonable with his requests and obstructing his (the physician's) care of the patient.
(b) Likely, the husband is not as educated as him (the physician) and does not understand the repercussions of inappropriate management of the patient's condition.
(c) The department is busy, and this is the only staff available at the moment to assist with the care of the patient.
(d) It is difficult to understand what the husband is saying, and he is becoming unreasonable. I will have him removed and continue my care of the patient.
(e) The husband is being very domineering and not allowing the patient to speak for herself; this may be an indicator of underlying inter-partner violence. I will speak to the wife when her husband is no longer in the room.

Attitudes/Assumptions: The Husband

(a) I am her husband, and my wife's body is sacred and as such should not be exposed or touched by another man.
(b) Western medicine cannot be trusted; I will not allow anything to be given that may contaminate my wife's body.

Attitudes/Assumptions: The Patient

(a) As the head of the household, my husband is my "king" and ultimate decision-maker; therefore, I will defer to him in deciding what treatment is best for me.
(b) This white doctor is rude and likely thinks we are stupid for choosing herbal medications and faith to treat our illnesses.

Gaps in Provider Knowledge

(a) Lack of knowledge of health beliefs/customs by the provider: Rastafarians generally believe their bodies are the temple of God and should be free of anything unclean. They believe in natural remedies and as such are more receptive to alternative methods of healing. They believe strongly in the body's ability to heal itself. They are generally skeptical about western medicine and may refuse procedures that they deem invasive, such as injections, transfusions, and surgery [1].
(b) Lack of knowledge regarding this specific community: Women are generally referred to as "queens" or "empresses" in Rastafarian society. Their bodies are considered sacred and should only be seen by their husbands. In many cases, they may refuse to wear hospital gowns as they are deemed to be inappropriate or immodest [2]. While marriages may not exist in the traditional sense, the male partner is generally considered the head of the household and decision-maker [3].
(c) Lack of knowledge of disparities/discrimination: Patients may fear they may be judged as drug abusers and be reluctant to disclose marijuana use as it is still "illegal" in many places. However, in Rastafarian culture, it is considered a core tenet of religious ceremonies and "herbalism." The overall use of herbal remedies and preparations tends to play a large role in spiritual sessions and healing [3, 4].

2. What actions could have been taken by the doctor to avoid/prevent this negative outcome?

Cross-Cultural Tools and Skills

(a) Assume that the husband cares for his wife's health and safety. His reluctance to treatment is likely not meant to be obstructive but rather comes from a lack of understanding of the current circumstances.
(b) Make the effort to communicate effectively and explain health-related concerns to the husband. Do not assume he lacks the capacity to understand.

(c) Acknowledge the wife's deference to her husband as the decision-maker may be more out of a cultural view of respect rather than submission in the setting of domestic abuse. Attempt to clarify the situation by speaking to the patient in private if possible (e.g., when taking the patient for imaging).

(d) Assume that the patient is concerned about her health, but modesty is important to her and her husband. Attempt to make the situation more accommodating for the patient. There may be alternatives available to the standard hospital gowns, which the patient would be more comfortable wearing.

3. What medical issues are of concern in this case?

(a) Given the patient's symptoms and elevated blood pressure, there is the very high possibility of an evolving stroke. The resident should take the time to explain the correlation between elevated pressures in the setting of a possible stroke and the risk of progression and worsening symptoms if not treated.

(b) The patient will require antihypertensive medication on discharge. Given the patient's preference for herbal remedies, some negotiation will likely be required. The physician should be prepared to have a discussion surrounding the pros and cons of medication usage. Shared decision-making should be employed, incorporating both the patient's and husband's opinions.

4. Which components of the Emergency Medicine Milestones of the ACGME competencies are incorporated in the case?

(a) Professional Values: Demonstrates compassion, integrity, and respect for others as well as adherence to the ethical principles relevant to the practice of medicine.

(b) Patient-Centered Communication: Demonstrates interpersonal and communication skills that result in the effective exchange of information and collaboration with patients and their families [5].

Case Outcome

After an appropriate history and exam are done, the patient is sent for imaging which confirms a small intracerebral hypertensive bleed.

Diagnosis Hypertensive emergency with left intracerebral bleed.

Disposition Admitted.

The physician carefully explains the cause of the patient's illness to both the patient and her husband and addresses his concerns regarding not administering medications. The husband is allowed to ask as many questions as he needs to feel reassured, and he agrees with medical treatment. The physician assigns the next female nurse to care for the patient and assures both the patient and her husband that their beliefs will be respected to the best of his ability while under his care. The patient's blood pressure is treated, and she is admitted to a monitored unit.

References

1. Olmos MFCC, Paravisini-Gebert L. Creole religions of the Caribbean: an introduction from Vodou and Santería to Obeah and Espiritismo. New York: New York University Press; 2011. 262 p.
2. Baxter C. Nursing with dignity part 5: Rastafarianism. Nurs Times. 2002;98(13):42.
3. Religions: Rastafari at a glance [Internet]. London: BBC; (Updated 2009 Oct 2; cited 2017 Aug 1). Available from: http://www.bbc.co.uk/religion/religions/rastafari/ataglance/glance.shtml
4. Hollins S. Religions, culture, and healthcare: a practical handbook for use in healthcare environments. Oxford: Radcliffe Publishing; 2009. 143 p.
5. The Emergency Medicine Milestone Project [Internet]. Chicago: The Accreditation Council for Graduate Medical Education and the American Board for Emergency Medicine; c2012 (Cited 14 Oct 2017). Available from: http://www.acgme.org/acgmeweb/Portals/0/PDFs/Milestones/EmergencyMedicineMileston es.pdf

Chapter 17
Rastafarianism and Western Medicine

Heather Prendergast

Case Scenario

A 42-year-old male presents to the emergency department for evaluation of a non-healing laceration on his lower leg. The patient is accompanied by his girlfriend, who is employed at the hospital as a medical assistant. The doctor learns from the girlfriend that the patient was very reluctant to seek medical attention. He currently lives in Jamaica, is a practicing Rastafarian, and is only visiting the United States. Per the girlfriend, the patient was given a "savve" for the cut, but it has not helped with healing. The patient is a thin, well-groomed male with shoulder-length hair (dreadlocks) who appears older than his stated age.

Engaging the patient in a meaningful conversation is very difficult. Although the patient is pleasant, he appears very suspicious of the questions he is being asked and answers every question with an additional question [1]. Despite the challenges, the doctor is able to obtain a few meaningful pieces of information concerning the laceration from the patient that makes the doctor very concerned for a serious underlying infection and undiagnosed metabolic abnormality. The doctor, believing the patient to be minimizing the potential seriousness of the situation and trying to embarrass him in front of the staff, becomes more impatient with the patient. He assumes that the nonchalant attitude of the patient may be due to his use of "ganja" (also known as marijuana). The doctor, believing that the patient is "impaired," begins to discuss his working differential diagnosis and treatment plan with the girlfriend. He intentionally positions himself between the patient and his companion and turns his shoulder slightly away from the patient. Although the doctor received no confirmation from the patient that he has recently smoked marijuana, his assumption is based on the general appearance of the patient, preconceived ste-

H. Prendergast, MD, MS, MPH
University of Illinois, Chicago, IL, USA

© Springer International Publishing AG, part of Springer Nature 2019
M. L. Martin et al. (eds.), *Diversity and Inclusion in Quality Patient Care*,
https://doi.org/10.1007/978-3-319-92762-6_17

reotypes about "practicing Rastafarians," and the perceived widespread use of marijuana among this group of individuals [2]. The doctor suggests to the girlfriend that the patient's complaints could be limb-threatening and "it may already be too late." Specifically, the dialogue is as follows:

Physician (enters the room and immediately begins with his questioning): "Hello sir, how long has that laceration been present on your leg?"
Patient: "Well, doctor, it has been there for quite a while. Why do you ask?"
Physician: "Well, it doesn't look like it is healing well from here."
Patient: "How can you say that Doc?"
Physician: "I understand that you have been putting an ointment on it. How long have you been using it, and do you know what type of ointment it is?"
Patient: "I'm not sure, but it has been off and on. In my line of work, I always have a cut or scrape here and there. Why does it matter? They typically come and go."
Physician: "Have you had fevers, weight loss, or tingling in your legs?"
Patient: "Whoa Doc, is this a fishing expedition? How does that relate to the cut on my leg, Doc? I only came because my girl insisted. I am very healthy and active."
Physician: "Okay, sir." The physician repositions himself and begins to address the girlfriend more directly. "Based upon the appearance of the laceration, it looks infected. I am concerned that the infection has spread to the bone. This can be very serious and he could lose his leg, especially if he has an underlying problem such as diabetes."
Both the patient and his companion are shocked, evidenced by the puzzled looks on their faces, and are speechless.
The physician, feeling that he has gained control of the situation and effectively "put the patient in his place," continues to speak with the patient's companion. However, now he is entirely using medical jargon. "Yes, if he has osteomyelitis in addition to undiagnosed diabetes that is out of control, then he may be looking at a below the knee amputation in the worst case scenario. This is a very serious situation. We will have to be aggressive if the infection has spread to your bones."
Physician: (feeling superior and victorious, turns to exit the exam room) "I'll have the nurse come in and draw the blood, get the x-rays ordered, and start fluids and antibiotics. Once we get some results, I can answer any additional questions."

Review of Symptoms

Provided by the girlfriend: The patient has experienced increased thirst and has had frequent urination. These symptoms are attributed to his line of work in Jamaica as a roofer where he works long hours under the sun. There is no history of vomiting or documented fevers.

Past Medical History

Unknown; the patient routinely sees a "healer" in Jamaica and has not been formally diagnosed with any illnesses [1, 3–6].

Family History

Strong family history of diabetes on both paternal and maternal sides.

Social History

Smokes marijuana, no tobacco, no alcohol.

Physical Exam

Vital Signs Temp, 99.8 °F; pulse, 121; respirations, 22; BP, 100/72; O_2 Sat 98% on room air.

General Thin male, well-developed, appears generally healthy

Cardiovascular Tachycardia rate and rhythm, S1 and S2 normal

Respiratory Clear to auscultation

ENT Pupils equal and reactive, extraocular movements' intact

Neck Supple, mucous membranes moist

Abdomen Soft, flat, +normal bowel sounds, no rebound, no guarding

Extremities There is a 3 × 2 cm irregularly shaped chronic appearing ulceration with surrounding erythema, warmth, and purulent drainage. There is tenderness to palpation. Pulses are palpable. There is a trace amount of pretibial edema. No clubbing of nails.

Skin Warm, dry, intact, clean

Neuro Alert and oriented × 3, cranial nerves II–XII intact

Questions for Discussion

1. Why did the physician-patient relationship suddenly change to an adversarial one?

Attitudes/Assumptions: The Physician

(a) I am the doctor, and I have a medical degree. You came to me for help. Don't challenge my knowledge or pretend that we are on the same intellectual level.
(b) Based upon the patient's repeated questions as answers to my questions, the patient is trying to embarrass me in front of my staff and thinks I am incompetent.
(c) The patient is a practicing Rastafarian, which means that he smokes marijuana frequently and most likely is always under the influence of marijuana.
(d) The patient's chronic use of marijuana has impaired his ability to understand the seriousness of his illness.

Attitudes/Assumptions: The Patient

(a) The doctor is trying to manipulate me and manufacture illness.
(b) The doctor is arrogant and believes I am inferior to him.
(c) Western medicine practitioners in general are not trustworthy.
(d) The doctor does not understand Rastafarian culture and attitudes [5]. He probably thinks I am under the influence of ganja.

Gaps in Provider Knowledge

(a) Lack of knowledge of health beliefs/customs by the provider: Rastafarians place a high value on maintaining one's health. It is part of the foundation of Rastafarian ideology. Rastafarianism involves a holistic approach to healing, and Rastafarians often seek "remedies" as part of their healing regimen. There is a strong belief in the body's natural ability to heal itself. These "remedies" involve tonics comprised of "herbs, barks, and roots" [1, 6]. Remedies are passed down within families. The usual sequence of managing illness/ailments involves (1) self-diagnosis and self-medication with herb tonics, followed by (2) recommendations from family and friends, (3) a healer visit, and finally (4) seeking professional medical assistance. Western medicine is utilized to treat diseases, whereas "Jamaican folk healers" are utilized primarily for treating "illness problems" [1]. Nonetheless, because of the underlying distrust of western medicine, seeking medical attention is often facilitated by close family and friends and usually not by the individual themselves. In addition, there is often a great deal of suspicion toward plans that involve invasive or aggressive forms of medical treatment because of Rastafarians' strong belief in the body's natural ability to heal itself.

(b) Lack of knowledge of Rastafarian as a religion: Rastafarians see themselves as very spiritual individuals. Ganja is regarded as a herb that aids religious mediation and is a "medical food" not for recreational use. Smoking ganja is optional for Rastafarians, and some Rastafarians choose not to smoke weed at all. Those who smoke do so for the perceived spiritual benefits gained by smoking [2].

(c) Lack of knowledge of disparities/discrimination: There is a misbelief that marijuana or "ganja" use is widespread in Jamaica, especially among Rastafarians. Dreadlocks are stereotypical of affiliation with Rastafarian beliefs [2, 5].

2. What actions could have been taken by the physician to avoid/prevent this negative change?

Cross-Cultural Tools and Skills

(a) Greetings or acknowledgment of an individual's presence is an important cultural value. Absence of the greeting implies a lack of interest in the well-being of the individual.

(b) Listen carefully to understand what is being said. Many Jamaicans may speak with an accent. Simply clarify what has been said in order to prevent any misunderstanding on your part or the part of the patient. Make sure that efforts to achieve clear communication and dialogue are not conveyed in a condescending manner.

(c) Remember that Rastafarians bring with them a cultural history and that "one size does not fit all."

(d) Be understanding of cultural norms and tendencies without imposing judgment.

3. What medical issues concern you about this case?

(a) The patient is concerned about his health and condition and attempts to engage the physician by asking his own questions in response to the physician's questions. However, the engagement is ineffective and interferes with the ability to obtain a good history from the patient.

(b) Most Rastafarians are unsure whether their beliefs will be respected while in the hospital [6]. It is therefore important to create an environment where the patients will feel comfortable to ask questions and engage in dialogue.

(c) Discuss or explain the reasoning behind your questions. This may help improve the quality of the patient's responses. For example, explaining why the type of herbal ointment used by the patient and the duration may be important in establishing what type of treatment exposure has occurred. Many herbal ointments do not contain antibiotics, and many contain barks and roots that may be irritants to the skin.

4. Which components of the Emergency Medicine Milestones of the ACGME competencies [7] are incorporated in the case?

(a) Patient Care: Establishes and implements a comprehensive disposition plan that uses appropriate consultation resources, patient education regarding diagnosis, treatment plan, medications, and time- and location-specific disposition instructions.

(b) Patient-Centered Communication Skills: Demonstrates interpersonal and communication skills that result in the effective exchange of information and collaboration with patients and their families. Taking the time to introduce or greet the patient can serve to set the tone for a good physician-patient relationship and a potentially positive service outcome. For example, by asking the patient specifically if there are any concerns related to his religious practices that the physician should be aware of would go a long way in establishing a trustworthy relationship. Ask when in doubt. Most Rastafarians are proud of their religion and are happy to talk about it [3, 5].

(c) Professional Values: Demonstrates compassion, integrity, and respect for others as well as adherence to the ethical principles relevant to the practice of medicine. Listen carefully to the patient's concerns. Communicate openly in a nonjudgmental manner, and do not minimize the patient's participation in the conversation.

Case Outcome

Diagnosis Infected diabetic ulcer complicated by osteomyelitis of the fibula.

Disposition Admit for hyperglycemia control and intravenous antibiotics.

After an appropriate history and physical examination is obtained utilizing the principles above, screening laboratory studies revealed glucose of 320 mg/dl, urine negative for ketones and evidence of infection, and white blood cell count of 18,000 with no previous baseline. X-ray of the left fibula demonstrates deep soft tissue swelling, a periosteal reaction, cortical irregularity, and demineralization. Based upon the X-ray findings consistent with osteomyelitis, the physician concludes that it is secondary to infected diabetic ulcer from undiagnosed type II diabetes mellitus. The physician explains his concerns to the patient, his companion, and his family and provides the correlation between the patient's symptoms and the physician's findings. The physician provides recommendations for admission to the hospital and discusses in detail the proposed treatment plan and the expected hospitalization time frame. The patient is allowed to ask questions and conference with his family. The patient is concerned about a prolonged hospital stay and agrees to a 24-h observation admission to receive intravenous hydration, glucose management, and intravenous antibiotics while arrangements are made to continue treatment on an outpatient basis.

References

1. Hesler K, McGurrin L, Sanborn M, Gray M. Natural medicine and healing [Internet]. [place unknown]: WordPress; 2012 Apr 23 (Cited 1 Sept 2017). Available from: http://caribbeanreligionuvm.wordpress.com/category/natural-healing-and-medicine

2. Myers G. 10 things to know about Rastafarian beliefs [Internet]. [place unknown]: Listverse; 2014 Jan 6 (Cited 1 Sept 2017). Available from: http://listverse.com/2014/01/06/10-things-to-know-about-rastafari-beliefs/

3. Chevannes B. Rastafari: roots and ideology. 1st ed. Syracuse: Syracuse University Press; 1994. 298 p.

4. Rastafari health care, selassie's utterance & creating the EWF medical units asap [Internet]. [place unknown]: YouTube; 2011 Nov 23 (Cited 10 Nov 2017). Available from: https://www.youtube.com/watch?v=2n6XU121fEQ

5. Kitzinger S. Protest and mysticism: the Rastafari cult in Jamaica. J Sci Study Relig. 1969;8(2) 240–62.

6. Baxter C. Nursing with dignity part 5: Rastafarianism. Nurs Times. 2002;98(13):42.

7. The Emergency Medicine Milestone Project [Internet]. Chicago: The Accreditation Council for Graduate Medical Education and the American Board for Emergency Medicine; c2012 (Cited 12 Nov 2014). Available from: http://www.acgme.org/acgmeweb/Portals/0/PDFs/Milestones/EmergencyMedicineMilestone.pdf

Chapter 18
Elderly Female Appalachian Patient

Edward Strickler and Marcus L. Martin

Case Scenario

An 83-year-old woman presents for a follow-up visit at the office of a pulmonary specialist with primary diagnosis of nonspecific interstitial lung disease also called pulmonary fibrosis. This visit is the first follow-up from a previous hospitalization 3 months ago following an emergency admission for shortness of breath. Bi-level positive airway pressure (BiPAP) was used during her last hospitalization which the patient said was very distressing; the patient signed a declaration that she would not want BiPAP therapy again. The patient was sent home with orders for oxygen therapy with a nasal cannula whenever she feels short of breath.

Review of Symptoms

Her chief complaints are shortness of breath, frequent cough, feeling tired after getting through the morning activities of daily living, and weakness, including legs "feeling wobbly like Jell-O." She also complains of occasional cognitive struggle ("just can't remember the right word and that makes me feel so bad") and leg swelling that makes it difficult to put on compression stockings. The patient refers to her legs "getting bigger" through the course of the day and says that her legs "are little" when arising from sleep overnight. The patient is embarrassed by a discolored scar

E. Strickler (✉)
Institute of Law, Psychiatry, and Public Policy, University of Virginia, Charlottesville, VA, USA
e-mail: els2e@hscmail.mcc.virginia.edu

M. L. Martin
University of Virginia, Charlottesville, VA, USA
e-mail: mlm8n@virginia.edu

© Springer International Publishing AG, part of Springer Nature 2019
M. L. Martin et al. (eds.), *Diversity and Inclusion in Quality Patient Care*,
https://doi.org/10.1007/978-3-319-92762-6_18

on her right leg from a past MRSA infection and tries to keep the stocking pulled high enough to cover the discoloration.

Past Medical History

Two previous hospitalizations within the past 5 years for shortness of breath; hospitalization for fecal impaction; two surgeries for left hip fracture; postpartum depression, more than 60 years ago; rheumatoid arthritis, congestive heart failure, arrhythmia, anxiety, sleep apnea, implanted cardiac pacemaker

Medications Oxygen therapy, metered doses of albuterol and fluticasone, naproxen, lasix, metoprolol, lorazepam

Family History

Husband of 61 years died at age 97 while in hospice care at home with heart failure. Parents are deceased, both from heart attack. She has seven siblings, two living.

She has four children, all living. One, with a recent stroke at age 64 (retired from work early), lives about an hour away but has trouble driving after the stroke. One had a recent intervention to place a stent at age 62, works full time, has "a good job," and lives 2 h away. One, with alcohol abuse, age 60, works occasionally in building trades but cannot legally drive and lives 20 min away. One, age 56, has "a real responsible job at a local plant," working 50–60 h a week.

Social History

The patient lives alone in an unimproved early twentieth-century farmhouse in a mountain valley of western Virginia. The house is heated with portable electrical heaters supplemented by a wood stove. Family, church friends, and neighbors bring cut wood and check in on the patient to see when wood is needed. Running water that is piped from a nineteenth-century hand-dug well is used for bathing, washing, and laundry. Drinking and cooking water is obtained from a local spring. Family, church friends, and neighbors help load a vehicle with gallon jugs of spring water to bring to the patient's house. She stores them underneath a raised back porch in warm weather, and they must be stacked indoors in cold weather. The patient reports, "The works in the back of the commode is gummed up so I have to flush with water from a bucket." When asked to explain, she said she means that the commode has broken components and will not flush automatically. The patient hand-washes her few clothes in a large kitchen sink and hangs them out to dry on a line outdoors, including, as she says, on "sunny airish days" in winter. She also may hang a line of clothes indoors. The patient reports, "Sometimes I do have an accident [meaning occasional incontinence] so I wash them out in the bathtub." When asked if she uses or would use pads, the patient reported that she would use them but that they are "plenty dear" (meaning costly) and that she would "feel like a jasper" (meaning embarrassed) to ask neighbors or church friends to dispose of them. Cooking is done with an electric range top with one working burner. Baking is done with the wood cook stove but the patient says, "Not much baking these days." The patient has a small microwave but says, "The bottom broke so it's chancy." The patient does not have a telephone but does have an old television and a radio. The patient says, "The front porch is sigogglin [out of balance] but everything else is right tight" (meaning that the structure is leaning but still in livable condition). The patient says with a smile, "It's my place, for now, until my mansion above" (referring to religious beliefs about a heavenly home after her death).

The patient completed "most of high school" and is proud when she reports that accomplishment. Other than occasional agricultural work, the patient did not work outside the home. The patient receives Social Security benefits—as her husband's survivor/beneficiary—of about $1,173/month or about $14,078/year. With regular expenses approximating 80–90% of this income, little is left for emergencies of extraordinary expense.

Physical Exam

Vital Signs Temp 98.6, BP 140/90, pulse 90

General Somewhat disheveled appearance

Head Normal

Neck Supple

ENT Poor dentition, mild erythematous pharynx

Cardiovascular Regular rate and rhythm, Grade II systolic murmur

Respiratory Bilateral fine crackles, heard loudest during mid to late inspiration, particularly lower lungs

Abdomen Soft, non-tender

Extremities 2+ pitting edema bilaterally

Skin Warm, moist

Neuro No neurologic deficits

During the visit, the pulmonologist reviewed chest X-rays taken earlier that day and compared them to images obtained during the previous hospitalization.

The patient was informed she has increasing fibrosis in both lungs and an enlarged heart. The specialist asked if the patient had someone to talk with about hospice care or if she would like for someone from the hospital to talk with her about hospice care. The patient was quiet at first and then remarked, "Well, thank you for saying that I have a big heart."

Questions for Discussion

1. How broadly, deeply, or persistently should providers inquire about the patient's understanding of clinical findings, diagnosis, prognosis, and medical care?

   The patient understands what she hears about diagnoses, clinical findings, and prognoses in ways influenced by Appalachian cultural norms [1] and experiences of her rural, Southern, and impoverished life course. For example, the patient relates everything to some illustrative or descriptive story about how she has cared for others in her family or community and stories she had heard about caring for others, including helping her husband to live his last days at home, which is what she wishes for herself. Systems of care that are familiar and available to her have been informal, personal, and low-resource, reflecting Appalachian cultural values of self-reliance, as well as remoteness and isolation of settings with lack of accessible formal systems of care.

2. To what extent should providers engage the patient to understand what she means, or what she expects, regarding the blending of medical knowledge and faith experiences?

   The patient validates religious faith as a primary resource for understanding and describing reality, orienting decision-making for self-care and end-of-life care, and requesting resources and services [1, 2]. For example, the patient talks about faith as a personal, immediate, and powerful relationship with God.

3. How will providers, through the team serving the patient, ensure that stereotyping is minimized, prejudice is challenged, and stigma in any form will not compromise healthcare communications, continuity of care, or best health outcomes possible for the patient?

   Studies report many ways in which Appalachian identity involves stigma, including stereotyping contrary to effective healthcare communications necessary for best outcomes, as well as prejudice that may threaten or destroy trust and therefore may adversely impact current and subsequent healthcare encounters [3].

4. When considering the snapshot of the patient's resources and burdens on her resources, how will providers assure best clinical, social-cultural care?

   Studies suggest that the values of home and family are primary for Appalachians seeking health care and implementing care plans [4]: "Older Appalachian women in this study defined themselves and their health in terms of their homes and as women who care for themselves informally and value independence and privacy." The patient in this case identified many infrastructure and system deficits in her home that may threaten her safety, health, and well-being, but highlighted cultural values and expectations: "The front porch is sigogglin…it's my place, for now, until my mansion above." The patient expresses an expectation of remaining in her home and as independent as possible despite threats to her safety in the home, many challenges in the family system, and her very low income.

Attitudes/Assumptions: The Clinical Team

(a) The clinical team may assume the patient's psychological, emotional, and spiritual self-understanding regarding her illness and health, and planning for death may be lacking.
(b) The clinical team may assume that by her choice of words she is uninformed about her health. For example, if the front porch is "sigogglin," she may not understand that the house is not safe for habitation. She may not understand the possibility for falling and injury when she feels "wobbly like Jell-O."
(c) Considering her description of her facilities, including the "gummed up" commode, is she able to accomplish critical activities of daily living (maintaining continence, personal hygiene)?
(d) The clinical team may assume they will cause embarrassment or shame if they question the patient about this vocabulary that is unfamiliar to them (for instance, when the patient feels "like a jasper").

Attitudes/Assumptions: The Patient

(a) The patient expressed beliefs and expectations about her health and well-being with confidence and clarity, but from within a cultural and social framework, and with values that may be unfamiliar to some providers and that some providers may find disconcerting.
(b) The patient has an attitude of rugged independence. "Many factors make this [Appalachian] culture rich and diverse including the values of rugged independence and a distrust for outsiders; the geographical challenges of mountains and harsh winter weather; the ideals of faith, family, and community; and the confounding variables of educational disadvantage, low socioeconomic status, and poverty" [5].

Gaps in Provider Knowledge

(a) Lack of familiarity with a patient from an Appalachian social and cultural context.

(b) Specific lack of knowledge of Appalachian culture. Mixer, Fornehed, Varney, and Lindley provide a helpful overview to consider the social and cultural contexts of an Appalachian patient: "Appalachian people have a unique geographic, cultural, and economic heritage. They represent a large group of Americans who have been traditionally under-represented in healthcare studies in general, and in cultural care research specifically. As a group, they have been misunderstood, ridiculed, stereotyped, and called 'stupid,' 'rednecks,' and 'hillbillies.' Appalachians' rich cultural values and beliefs include a sense of belonging, love of 'our mountains,' strong family ties, firm faith, appreciation of hard work, fierce independence, self-reliance, and pride. The Appalachian area also is impoverished. For example…the percentage of the population living below the poverty level is 19%, compared to 13.0% in the United States" [5].

Cross-Cultural Tools and Skills

Despite the expanse of the Appalachian region—hundreds of counties in more than a dozen states—few comprehensive, up-to-date resources are available to train health service providers on culturally competent care and services with Appalachian populations. Some research and practice identify themes that should be incorporated in cultural competence training. Perspectives from geriatric social service professionals in a rural Appalachian region revealed several prevalent themes that identify areas of cultural competence with rural Appalachian communities, especially, but not exclusively, regarding aging Appalachian populations [6].

Scarcity of services, resources, and other economic and community development These include scarcity of jobs that propel out-migration of health, social, and community service providers as well as family members who might typically become formal and informal caregivers; these then drive many gaps in services to meet patient needs.

Reliance on neighbors and family Scarcities limit the ability and availability of unpaid family caregivers to provide assistance when chronic illness or disability necessitate the need for care. The so-called fictive kin is an important feature of Appalachian social and cultural norms. "Fictive kin" are neighbors, church members, or occasional contacts in the community who are not "blood kin" but are nevertheless invited to be formal or informal helpers when family are no longer living in the area or are unable to be helpful (because of poverty, incarceration, illness, or disabilities).

Place, impoverished but still home Research on cancer education and treatment in Appalachian populations emphasizes the critical value of establishing trust and trustworthy communications: "There is clearly a distinguishable Appalachian culture, and 'place' is a prominent feature in that culture. Actions and beliefs in

Appalachia are largely based upon discussion among community members about their experiences with disease and health care. Communication and use of care is influenced by skepticism, some distrust of health professionals, and fear of being taken advantage of by 'the system'" [7]. Behringer and Friedell conclude: "Cultural issues undergird one final dilemma…the Appalachian regional population has lower income and poorer educational achievement and is older than the general U.S. population. These characteristics are generally seen as precursors to poorer health status." Knowledge of and sensitivity to the widespread poverty in Appalachian populations is a key tool of cultural competency with Appalachian patients [7].

Case Outcome

The pulmonary specialist reached out to agencies in the Appalachian region in which the patient lives, including a free clinic about 2 h from the patient's home and the area agency on aging serving the county in which the patient lives. The pulmonary specialist also identified several resources and services that could be helpful to the patient, who wanted to live in her home as long as possible. These services were culturally attuned to the patient's values, expectations, and wishes about her quality of life and self-determination, as well as informed about resources that may be affordable and accessible for the patient. The pulmonary specialist's experience with this patient provides the opportunity for continuing education and intervention regarding Appalachian regional health disparities.

References

1. Diddle G, Denham SA. Spirituality and its relationships with the health and illness of Appalachian people. J Transcult Nurs. 2010;21(2):175–82.
2. Lowry LW. Exploring the meaning of spirituality with aging adults in Appalachia. J Holist Nurs. 2002;20(4):388–402.
3. Coyne CA, Demian-Popescu C, Friend D. Social and cultural factors influencing health in southern West Virginia: a qualitative study. Prev Chronic Dis. 2006;3(4):A124.
4. Hayes PA. Home is where their health is: rethinking perspectives of informal and formal care by older rural Appalachian women who live alone. Qual Health Res. 2006;16(2):282–97.
5. Mixer SJ, Fornehed ML, Varney J, Lindley LC. Culturally congruent end-of-life care for rural Appalachian people and their families. J Hosp Palliat Nurs. 2014;16(8):526.
6. Pope ND, Loeffler DN, Ferrell DL. Aging in rural Appalachia: perspectives from geriatric social service professionals. Adv Soc Work. 2014;15(2):522–37.
7. Behringer B, Friedell GH. Appalachia: where place matters in health. Prev Chronic Dis. 2006;3(4):A113.

Chapter 19
Low-Income White Male Appalachian Patient

Xi Damrell and Kevin Ferguson

Case Scenario

A disheveled 78-year-old man in boots, overalls, and a work shirt presents with a severe nonproductive cough, which his accompanying daughter says has become worse over the last few days. The patient quit smoking 5 years ago and drinking 20 years ago but already had mild chronic obstructive pulmonary disease (COPD) and what he calls "hard liver." He does not use inhalers for his COPD. He says that the cough began after he spent time in his woodworking shop where he has been making cabinets. He has not been able to eat and sleep for 2 days due to the cough and complains of dizziness and agitation. His daughter prefers that he go to their church so that the minister and congregation can undertake a healing, but the patient insisted they come to the emergency room first to "get an x-ray picture." Both have strong, Southern regional accents and are somewhat evasive in their answers, especially regarding the patient's history and who is presently caring for the patient. A group of about ten people are waiting outside for the patient and his daughter, who frequently leaves the examining room to relate the goings-on between physician and patient.

X. Damrell (✉)
Kaweah Delta Emergency Medicine Residency Program, Visalia, CA, USA
e-mail: xi.damrell@vituity.com

K. Ferguson
Touro University at St. Joseph Medical Center, Stockton, CA, USA
e-mail: kevinferguson@cep.com

Review of Symptoms

The patient has no fever or night sweats, has lost some weight for the past year, and denies hemoptysis or chest pain.

Past Medical History

Besides his COPD and "hard liver," the patient also had skin cancer that was removed from his face and a clot in his leg for which he took a blood thinner for a while.

Family History

Patient's parents died of old age; his brother and sister both died of cancer, and details are unknown.

Social History

Both the patient and his daughter are members of an evangelical church that limits medical practice because "God comes first," but without detailed prohibitions. Patient quit smoking 5 years ago and drinking 20 years ago.

Physical Exam

Vital Signs Temp, 100.3 F; pulse, 98; BP 160/90; respiration, 22; O_2 Sat 90% on room air

General Elderly thin male with uncombed hair and dirty boots

ENT Pupils round, reactive to light, non-icterus sclera, mucous membrane moist, missing several teeth

Neck No jugular venous distension, no carotid bruits

Cardiovascular Regular rate and rhythm, no murmurs, equal palpable distal pulses

Respiratory Scattered rhonchi, bilateral lower lung fields

Abdomen Soft, non-tender, non-distended, no shifting dullness; liver is not palpable.

Extremities No edema or cyanosis; there is some clubbing of the nails.

Skin No rash; faint surgical scar left forehead

Neuro Awake, alert, and oriented; no focal deficits

Test Results CBC, mild leukocytosis at 12,000; metabolic panel, Na 128, albumin at 3.0, ALT 120, AST 180; VBG showed PH is 7.45; PCO2 48. BNP, 110; EKG, sinus rhythm with right heart strain pattern; CXR, hyperinflated lung without focal infiltration or pleural effusion, heart is normal sized; CT of the chest was ordered after the CXR showed 6 mm peribronchial nodule which is highly suspicious for cancer.

Questions for Discussion

1. What attitudes and assumptions about medicine, health, and identity on the parts of the physician and the patient might result in gaps in knowledge for both?

Attitudes/Assumptions: The Physician

(a) The patient and his daughter have heavy accents and are difficult to understand.
(b) This patient probably had bronchitis.
(c) The patient appears disheveled; no one in the family is caring for him.
(d) I'm busy and the patient is taking a long time getting to the point to give me a history.
(e) The patient is not educated. Will he be able to understand, let alone follow through with his diagnosis and subsequent medical treatment? Will all those people in the waiting room help or hinder his recovery?

Attitudes/Assumptions: The Patient

(a) The doctor assumes I'm "white trash" and therefore doesn't respect me.
(b) The doctor is probably not a churchgoer and doesn't know how we live.
(c) What does the doctor know about how close-knit a family we are? We may look poor but we get along.
(d) Why do I have to do all these tests when the doctor can just give me something for the cough?
(e) The doctor probably thinks we won't be able to pay for this visit.
(f) The doctor doesn't know about woodworking and therefore doesn't realize that sometimes the fumes get too strong, which caused my symptoms.
(g) If the doctor seems to know what he/she is doing, I'll try to do my part and follow his/her orders.

Gaps in Provider Knowledge

(a) Belief in the sanctity of family, region, and religion; core values of personal privacy, integrity, and autonomy; combined with pride in personal skills; a belief in patriarchy and woman's "place"; and fatalism in the face of adversity are found throughout Appalachia. However, the population has become more diverse via influences from the outside such as mass media, travel, military service, college, and tourism, making beliefs more fluid [1].

(b) The Great Smoky Mountains in North Carolina contain numerous small rural communities with distinct traditions and lifestyles that are, apart from common (and often mistaken) stereotypes, unfamiliar to outsiders [2].

(c) Poverty is endemic, and many people cycle in and out of periods of extreme want, relying on family and friends, with occasional support from public assistance. While food stamps and other social services may be available, though far from abundant in some areas, they are sought after with reluctance, as these benefits conflict with the core values of self-sufficiency, self-reliance, community membership, and religion. All may result in people being slow to take a sick or injured person to the emergency room and then being unwilling or unable to follow the recommendations of doctors [3, 4].

Gaps in Patient Knowledge

(a) I know that this cough came after I stayed in the woodshop too long.

(b) Once you get cancer, that's usually a death sentence. My skin cancer was cut off, but other types of cancer will usually kill you eventually.

(c) These tests are going to cost a fortune.

(d) I don't know my list of medications and what they are supposed to do, so I might not take them.

2. What cross-cultural tools and skills can be used by the doctor to avoid unnecessary anxiety during the exam and encourage compliance with treatment?

Cross-Cultural Tools and Skills

(a) Social class standing and regional, ethnic, or national origins, together with race, religion, and comportment, influence how people judge those with whom they interact. The differential power equation between patient and physician sometimes can be exacerbated by the patient exhibiting qualities with which the physician is unfamiliar or else holds in disdain. Demonstrating interest in the patient – including his or her name, where they live, what they enjoy, and what they expect from the physician – can go a long way toward making the encounter fruitful.

(b) Simple courtesies can have a major positive impact. While physicians are pressed for time, especially in an emergency room setting, they can still show their concern and respect by being courteous and mannerly.

(c) Self-deprecating humor, the downplaying of symptoms, and denial of seriousness of the presenting complaint all correspond with the aforementioned values held by "mountain people." Appreciation of this by the physician will help to normalize the interaction.

3. Which components of Emergency Medicine Milestones of the ACGME competencies are incorporated in the case?

Patient-Centered Communication

(a) The patient must be seen as a member of a group in order to get compliance with the medical treatment, etc. By consulting with the patient and family, a consensus can be reached, which will increase the trust everyone has in the physician and the treatment.

(b) Stoicism, quietude, lack of seriousness, and other signs of patient disinterest or disavowal of medical authority should be seen as corresponding with values of personal authority and integrity.

(c) Using a person's name, explaining steps in medical procedures, and listening to both the patient and the accompanying person will decrease the likelihood of a patient dismissing the physician as a bigot or uncaring outsider.

(d) If religion is a factor, encouraging the patient to see medicine and spiritual healing as complementary might promote compliance. Emphasis should be on the patient's well-being.

Systems-Based Management

(a) Arrangements could be made through a social worker for follow-up to make sure that the patient has adequate nutrition, transportation, and prescriptions.

(b) Because of the negative stigma associated with "social welfare," care should be taken to assure the patient that additional "help" is part of medical service and not just for "poor people."

Case Outcome

Diagnosis Lung cancer

Disposition The patient is admitted to the regular floor. Pulmonology is consulted, and biopsy through bronchoscopy confirmed small-cell lung cancer. After discussion with the patient and family, the patient is started on chemo and radiation therapy and discharged with oncology outpatient follow-up.

References

1. Baird S. Stereotypes of Appalachia obscure a diverse picture [Internet]. Washington: NPR; 2014 [cited 2017 Nov 6]. Available from: http://www.npr.org/sections/codeswitch/2014/04/03/298892382/stereotypes-of-appalachia-obscure-a-diverse-picture.
2. Williamson KD. The white ghetto [Internet]. New York: National Review; 2014 [cited 2017 Nov 6]. Available from: http://www.nationalreview.com/article/367903/white-ghetto-kevin-d-williamson.
3. Vance JD. Hillbilly elegy: a memoir of family and culture in crisis. New York: Harper Collins; 2016. 272p.
4. Cavender A. Folk medicine in southern Appalachia. Chapel Hill: University of North Carolina Press; 2003. 282p.

Chapter 20
Rural Patient Experiencing Intimate Partner Violence

Camille Burnett and Loraine Bacchus

Case Scenario

Patricia is a 30-year-old woman who lives in a small rural community. She has been married for 8 years to her college sweetheart, and they are the parents of twin boys aged 5. Her husband Charles is the primary breadwinner and is now retired from the military. He completed two active tours of duty in Afghanistan before being honorably discharged a year ago. Charles has been unable to find work since returning home and is increasingly exhibiting short-fused and aggressive behaviors toward Patricia.

Everyone in town knows Charles and his family. It is the community where he was born and raised and where his family has farmed their land for generations. Patricia was raised in a large metropolitan city where you rarely knew your neighbors, but there was a great variety of things to a do, places to go, and people from all walks of life. If it had been up to her, she would have stayed in the city. She enjoyed city life and all of her family and friends were there. However, once she gave birth to her children, Charles insisted that the boys be raised just as he was, in the country where it was safer and more wholesome. Patricia complied and settled on Charles' family farm at the edge of the small town.

At first, she enjoyed the slower pace and the opportunity to stay home full-time to raise their twins. Gradually, Patricia discovered how isolating and lonely her existence had become. When Charles was home between tours, the stress in

C. Burnett (✉)
University of Virginia School of Nursing, Charlottesville, VA, USA
e-mail: cjb4yw@virginia.edu

L. Bacchus
London School of Hygiene and Tropical Medicine, Faculty of Public Health and Policy,
Department of Global Health and Development, London, UK
e-mail: Loraine.Bacchus@lshtm.ac.uk

© Springer International Publishing AG, part of Springer Nature 2019   147
M. L. Martin et al. (eds.), *Diversity and Inclusion in Quality Patient Care*,
https://doi.org/10.1007/978-3-319-92762-6_20

the home escalated. He was sullen, noncommunicative, and easily angered. Patricia found ways to accommodate his moods by busying herself with chores. However, with no Internet service, poor cell service, and no cable, her options are limited.

Once a week, her in-laws pick her up and take her to the grocery store and to run errands, as there is no public transportation. Charles used to take their only car with him to the base that was 2 h from their home. Now that Charles is at home full-time, Patricia hoped to have more freedom to use the car so that she could venture out, but to her dismay, he continues to keep a tight rein on the vehicle as he does with everything else. Her nearest neighbor, who she rarely sees, lives half a mile down the road. When she does venture into town, she is known as Charles' "city slicker" wife, yet beyond that no one really knows her and people barely speak to her. Her life feels lonely and empty. Even with Charles being home, he really is not there. Not the old Charles anyway.

Whenever Patricia tries to speak to him about her feelings, Charles makes jokes about how easy her life is, how she does not know how good she has it compared to the lives of the women he has seen, and that maybe she needs to go and live in another country if she thinks her life is so tough. If she persists, he quickly shuts down the conversation, with an insult, a broken glass, or a punch in the wall. Recently Charles' behavior has begun to scare Patricia, but because of the children, she does whatever she can to keep the peace. She does not want her boys to grow up thinking that this is how they should behave. The stress and anxiety of living this way is taking its toll on Patricia's health. She has difficulty sleeping, regularly suffers migraines, and has very little interest in anything. Even taking care of the twins is beginning to feel difficult.

Patricia tells Charles that she needs to see their family physician, as lately she has not been feeling well. Charles arranges for his sister to take her to Dr. Carpe's office. It is the only family practice in their small community, and Charles' family has received care from Dr. Carpe for many years. However, Patricia has only visited him for prenatal care.

Dr. Carpe invites Patricia into his office, and her sister-in-law immediately gets up to accompany her. Patricia tells her sister-in-law there is no need to accompany her into the office. Dr. Carpe notices that Patricia looks agitated. He reassures her sister-in-law that they will not be long and that it is practice policy to see patients confidentially. Patricia begins to list her symptoms to Dr. Carpe. He asks her how things are at home, and she tells him that things have not been easy since she had the twins and that her relationship with Charles is under a lot of strain now that he does not work. She tells him that sometimes Charles does things that make her feel uneasy. Dr. Carpe asks her to give an example. She recounts an event where Charles threw the remote control in her direction and how it barely missed her during an argument about money. Dr. Carpe tells Patricia that it is common for men who have served in the military to experience moments of agitation upon returning home. He tells her that he can prescribe her some tablets to help her get some sleep and offers to talk to Charles.

Review of Symptoms

Experiencing stress and anxiety, difficulty sleeping, regular migraines, possible depression (has very little interest in anything), loneliness, isolation and overall feeling unwell.

Past Medical History

Gravida 2, Para 2; no previous surgeries, no major health issues/or diseases; vaccinations up to date; no known food or medication allergies

Family History

Married for 8 years, mother of 5-year-old twins, family history of hypertension (on father's side of the family); spouse is a veteran (possible PTSD). No family history of mental health issues or any major diseases/disorders on either side of the family.

Social History

Stay-at-home mother, limited social supports, and no extracurricular activities; is a member of the local congregation at the local church but attends infrequently; non-smoker, occasional alcohol use, no history of substance use

Physical Exam

Vital Signs   BP 130/90, HR 96, resp 18

Questions for Discussion

1. Identify areas of strengths and weaknesses in Dr. Carpe's consultation with the patient.
2. What could Dr. Carpe have done differently?
3. How could he follow-up at the next appointment?

Attitudes/Assumptions: The Physician

(a) It is a good practice to ensure that Patricia is provided with confidential time.
(b) He asks her how things are at home.
(c) He follows-up on Patricia's comments about Charles' behavior by asking for an example of what he does to make her feel uneasy.
(d) He observes Patricia's irritation when her sister-in-law tries to accompany her into his office for the consultation and defuses the situation by explaining it is routine procedure to see patients alone.
(e) He does not ask Patricia about intimate partner violence (IPV), assess her safety and that of her children, or offer information and referrals to community resources and support.
(f) He treats Patricia's symptoms (i.e., sleeping tablets) without properly exploring the underlying causes of her health issues.
(g) He excuses Charles' behavior by implying that it is acceptable or normal in men who have done active service but in doing so is inadvertently engaging in victim blaming.
(h) He ignores patient confidentiality by offering to talk to Charles. He does not recognize that this may increase Charles' aggression toward Patricia and result in further controlling and isolating behaviors.
(i) The physician is oblivious to the fact that Patricia has been exposed to IPV evidenced by his lack of inquiry along those lines and no implementation of IPV screening or IPV interventions.
(j) The physician focuses on Patricia as the primary source of her health issue without considering the impact that IPV has on health outcomes.
(k) The physician has limited or no training or knowledge of IPV best practices, including identification and intervention, and limited or no training or knowledge of using a trauma-informed care approach.

Attitudes/Assumptions: The Patient

(a) In moving to Charles' rural hometown, Patricia has become socially and geographically isolated.
(b) Patricia does not have her own income as she no longer works and is a full-time mother. In addition, she does not have access to transportation.
(c) Patricia lacks social support (e.g., friends, family, work colleagues, employer) and is socially isolated.
(d) Patricia is experiencing various forms of intimate partner violence. Charles is controlling what Patricia can do day-to-day, for example, by not giving her access to their car and making sure family members accompany her to the grocery store and to run errands. He exhibits threatening and aggressive behavior by throwing objects at her and punching the wall. He verbally abuses Patricia.

(e) The stress of living in an abusive relationship may be linked to Patricia's recent migraines, sleeping disturbance, and low mood. She may be depressed and experiencing anxiety.

(f) Patricia presents as a quiet, yet very attentive young woman. She provides limited amounts of information to inquiries, and responses are very specific to what is asked, with very little elaboration. She tends to be quite temperate in her responses, not overly expressive. She does not appear to be very outgoing; however, she is very polite and able to clearly articulate her thoughts.

Gaps in Provider Knowledge

(a) Lack of training and general knowledge of IPV.

(b) Unable to recognize and identify IPV exposure in a patient.

(c) Does not know best practices in how to respond to IPV exposure in a patient. Providers should follow evidence-based guidelines for an appropriate healthcare response to patients who are exposed to intimate partner violence [1–3].

(d) Not screening for IPV. Screen for intimate partner violence using a recognized tool [1]. For example, "We've started to talk to all our patients about safe and healthy relationships because it can have such a large impact on your health. Before we get started, I want you to know that everything here is confidential, meaning that I won't talk to anyone else about what is said unless you tell me (insert the laws in your state about what is necessary to disclose, i.e. child protection). Has Charles ever threatened you or made you feel afraid? Has he ever threatened to hurt you or your children if you did or did not do something? Has he ever physically hurt you?"

(e) Not assessing safety of patient exposed to IPV. Assess Patricia's immediate safety and that of her children. For example, "Is it safe to you and your children to be in the home today?"

(f) Not referring patient to IPV supports and services. Offer information about community resources, including organizations that support women and children exposed to intimate partner violence (e.g., shelters), and, at the very least, offer the National Domestic Violence Hotline number 1-800-799-SAFE (7233) [1, 2]. Offer to make a warm referral. Remind Patricia that if she feels that her life or those of her children are being endangered by Charles that she should call 911.

(g) Gaps in the use of effective therapeutic communication techniques and trauma-informed care approach.

   (i) Create a nonjudgmental and empathic atmosphere that is conducive to disclosure of intimate partner violence and discussion [4]. For example, "Intimate partner violence is very common and affects 1 in 3 women. Charles' behavior towards you is not acceptable and he is responsible for his actions not you. It's always wrong to physically hurt or threaten another person." This will help Patricia to recognize that Charles' behaviors are abusive, validate her experiences, and destigmatize the issue so that she can talk about it openly.

(ii) Keep the lines of communication open. For example, "I'm glad that you have talked to me about this. I want you to know that you can talk to me again about this."

(h) Did not identify nor discuss potential barriers/challenges to care that patient might be facing. Recognize that providing health care in rural communities presents unique challenges for patient care. This includes lack of transportation, geographical and social isolation, limited community resources and support (e.g., shelters), lack of confidentiality related to physician and community, limited economic opportunities, and greater health disparities [5].

Cross-Cultural Tools and Skills

(a) Use evidence-based screening and brief counselling assessment tools for IPV such as the Abuse Assessment Screen (AAS) [6], Women's Experience with Battering (WEB) scale [7], and Domestic Violence Enhanced Perinatal Home Visits (DOVE) [8].

(b) Use therapeutic interviewing skills and compassionate care techniques. Use trauma-informed care approach to all patients [9].

Case Outcome

Patricia returns home after seeing her physician and continues to experience the same symptoms. Over time, her symptoms progress to include headaches and GI disturbances. Patricia becomes frustrated that she is not improving and that with the additional symptoms she is experiencing, she is finding it increasing difficult to manage day-to-day family responsibilities.

Diagnosis Patricia is an abused woman who has been exposed to intimate partner violence that includes isolation, emotional/psychological abuse (physical threat of violence by punching walls), and financial abuse. As a result, she is suffering from the health effects of this exposure. She schedules another appointment to see Dr. Carpe. Treatment includes addressing the symptoms and reducing or eliminating her exposure to IPV by discussing safety plans and offering referral to community resources, including specialist IPV organizations.

References

1. Committee on Health Care for Underserved Women. Intimate partner violence. Committee opinion no. 518. Obstet Gynecol. 2012;119:412–7.
2. Chamberlain L, Levenson R. Addressing intimate partner violence, reproductive and sexual coercion: a guide for obstetric, gynecologic and reproductive health care settings [Internet]. San Francisco: Futures Without Violence. 2013 [cited 2017 Nov 28]. Available from: https://www.futureswithoutviolence.org/addressing-intimate-partner-violence/.
3. Moyer VA. Screening for intimate partner violence and abuse of elderly and vulnerable adults: U.S. preventive services task force recommendation statement. Ann Intern Med. 2013;158:478–86.
4. Bacchus LJ, Bullock L, Sharps P, Burnett C, Schminkey D, Buller AM, Campbell JC. "Opening the door": a qualitative interpretive study of women's experiences of being asked about intimate partner violence and receiving an intervention during perinatal home visits in rural and urban settings in the USA. J Res Nurs. 2016;21(5–6):345–64.
5. Burnett C, Schminkey D, Milburn J, Kastello J, Bullock L, Campbell J, Sharps P. Negotiating peril: the lived experience of rural, low-income women exposed to IPV during pregnancy and postpartum. Violence Against Women. 2016;22(8):943–65.
6. McFarlane J, Parker B, Soeken K. Physical abuse, smoking and substance use during pregnancy: prevalence, interrelationships and effects of birth weight. J Obstet Gynecol Neonatal Nurs. 1996;25(4):313–20.
7. Smith PH, Earp JA, DeVellis R. Measuring battering: development of the women's experience with battering (WEB) scale. Womens Health. 1995;1(4):273–88.
8. Sharps PW, Bullock LF, Campbell JC, Alhusen JL, Ghazarian SR, Bhandari SS, Schminkey DL. Domestic violence enhanced perinatal home visits: the DOVE randomized clinical trial. J Women's Health. 2016;25(11):1129–38.
9. Elliot B, Bjelajac P, Fallot R, Markoff L, Reed B. Trauma-informed or trauma denied: principles and implementation of trauma-informed services for women. J Community Psychol. 2005;33(4):461–77.

Chapter 21
The Homeless Patient

Bisan A. Salhi

Case Scenario

A 68-year-old man presents to the emergency department (ED) with a complaint of right arm pain. He states that the pain was sudden in onset and started 4 h prior to arrival, while he was walking outside. He reports no prior ED visits for the same complaints. The patient is homeless and is well known to the ED staff, who note that he frequently comes to the ED for frivolous complaints and to seek shelter or food. He has a history of a previous stroke and requires a walker to ambulate. He denies any history of trauma or any changes to his daily routine. The patient appears disheveled, wears multiple layers of clothing, and carries a large garbage bag that contains all of his belongings.

Upon review of the patient's chart, it appears that he has had many past visits to the ED for various complaints. A musculoskeletal exam is documented in his chart, noting no bony deformities and that he is spontaneously ranging all joints in the affected extremity. He is discharged from the ED with a diagnosis of upper extremity sprain and advised to take acetaminophen or ibuprofen as needed for pain. He returns the next day with complaints of continued arm pain. The resident undresses the patient to examine him and discovers a cool, pulseless right upper extremity.

B. A. Salhi
Departments of Anthropology and Emergency Medicine, Emory University,
Atlanta, GA, USA
e-mail: bsalhi@emory.edu

© Springer International Publishing AG, part of Springer Nature 2019
M. L. Martin et al. (eds.), *Diversity and Inclusion in Quality Patient Care*,
https://doi.org/10.1007/978-3-319-92762-6_21

Review of Symptoms

The patient complains of right arm pain. He also complains of low back pain, which he states is chronic and unchanged. He denies trauma, edema, or erythema to the affected extremity. All other systems are reported negative.

Past Medical History

History of stroke, hypertension, and schizophrenia

Family History

Hypertension

Social History

The patient reports drinking heavily for many years but states he has not consumed alcohol in more than a decade. No current history of tobacco or drug use. The patient has been homeless for 6 years and usually stays in shelters or on the street.

Physical Exam

Vital Signs Temp, 37 °C; pulse, 110; BP, 140/80; respirations, 20; O_2 Sat 99% on room air

General Chronically ill-appearing man who appears older than his stated age. The patient is disheveled and requires a walker to ambulate.

Cardiovascular Irregularly irregular rhythm; tachycardia with no murmurs, gallops, or rubs

Respiratory No use of accessory muscles, clear breath sounds

ENT Tympanic membranes clear, throat clear, no erythema uvula midline

Abdomen Non-distended, non-tender with normal bowel sounds, no hepatosplenomegaly

Extremities   The right forearm and hand are cool and mottled. No palpable radial or ulnar pulse in the right upper extremity. The left upper extremity is normal. Motor function is preserved in bilateral extremities.

Skin   No rashes or lesions

Neuro   Grossly intact, moves all four extremities, no obvious sign of deficit

Questions for Discussion

1. Why was this patient dismissed during the first ED visit?

Attitudes/Assumptions: The Physician

(a) The patient is here all the time and misusing the ED for food and shelter.
(b) The patient is malingering to get his social needs met and has no real medical complaints.
(c) This patient is homeless and mentally ill. Therefore, he is less likely to have an emergent complaint, and his history and presenting complaint should not be trusted.

Gaps in Provider Knowledge

(a) Lack of knowledge of health effects/outcomes associated with homelessness, including the fact that homeless persons suffer from mortality rates three to six times those of the general population, with homelessness being found to be an independent risk factor for mortality. Despite the focus on "inappropriate" or "excessive" ED utilization by the homeless, evidence suggests that the homeless are more likely to delay care until they perceive their symptoms to be emergent in nature [1].
(b) Lack of knowledge regarding this specific community: beware of stereotyping. Homeless persons experience higher rates of chronic illness, chronic injury, infectious disease (e.g., tuberculosis, HIV, and hepatitis C), substance use, and mental illness than their low-income, housed counterparts [2]. Although substance use and mental illness are overrepresented among homeless populations, the majority of homeless persons are neither substance users nor mentally ill. Moreover, homeless patients have difficulty storing and taking medications as prescribed due to their housing circumstances, which further contributes to their poor health outcomes [3].
(c) Lack of knowledge of disparities/discrimination: homeless persons have been subject to systematic discrimination and unethical research practices in the

United States. Physicians continue to use stereotypes of poverty and homelessness (e.g., unkempt appearance) to identify homeless patients [4]. Furthermore, it is common to deviate from standard of care when treating these patients. This may further render these patients vulnerable to stigma and discrimination by emergency providers, thereby exacerbating existing health inequalities.

2. What actions could have been taken by the doctor to avoid/prevent this unfortunate outcome?

Cross-Cultural Tools and Skills

(a) Always assume that these patients are sicker than they actually appear.
(b) Resist the temptation to expedite the treatment of these patients and to forego a full history and physical examination.
(c) Assume that if you communicate with patients effectively, you may obtain a reliable history and physical examination.
(d) Acknowledge the difficulties the patient may be having in caring for himself/herself on the streets or in a shelter. Work with the patient to come up with a feasible treatment plan based on their circumstances.

3. What medical issues concern you about this case?

(a) Although the patient's diagnosis was eventually recognized and treated appropriately, his homeless status and preconceived notions by staff led to a delay in diagnosis with potentially catastrophic effects.
(b) Like all other patients, homeless patients should have a full history and physical examination performed with a detailed examination of the affected organ system.

4. Which components of the Emergency Medicine Milestones of the ACGME competencies are incorporated in the case?

(a) Patient-centered communication: demonstrates interpersonal and communication skills that result in the effective exchange of information and collaboration with the patient.
(b) Professional values: demonstrates compassion, integrity, and respect for others as well as adherence to the ethical principles relevant to the practice of medicine.

Case Outcome

Diagnosis Acute brachial artery occlusion secondary to new-onset atrial fibrillation

Disposition Admission

After the physician utilizes the principles above to obtain an appropriate history, heparin is started, and the patient receives an emergency surgical consultation. A discussion occurs between the physician and the patient regarding the next steps of treatment and prognosis. The patient is given the time to ask additional questions and to voice his immediate needs and concerns. Social work is involved to determine the appropriate options for the patient upon discharge.

References

1. Martins DC. Experiences of homeless people in the health care delivery system: a descriptive phenomenological study. Public Health Nurs. 2008;25:420–30.
2. Hwang SW, Dunn JR. Homeless people. In: Galea S, Vlahov D, editors. Handbook of urban health. New York: Springer US; 2005. p. 19–41.
3. Coe AB, Moczygemba LR, Gatewood SB, Osborn RD, Matzke GR, J-VR G. Medication adherence challenges among patients experiencing homelessness in a behavioral health clinic. Res Social Adm Pharm. 2015;11:e110–e20.
4. Wen CK, Hudak PL, Hwang SW. Homeless people's perceptions of welcomeness and unwelcomeness in healthcare encounters. J Gen Intern Med. 2007;22:1011–7.

Chapter 22
Low-Income Patient

Taryn R. Taylor

Case Scenario

An 87-year-old woman has been hospitalized after sustaining a femur fracture sub-sequent to a fall. She has also developed a urinary tract infection. Given her ongoing care needs, she and her children have decided it best that she be transitioned to an assisted living facility. During the discharge planning process, the patient advises the multidisciplinary team that she will be utilizing Social Security and Medicaid benefits to subsidize the cost of the facility. The patient overhears the resident physician, who has been newly assigned to her team, complaining about people "abusing the system" because his parents had to "pay cash" for similar care for a family member. He further went on to express annoyance that "these people get their prescriptions for free," and "she probably won't even know how to take her medications correctly."

History of Present Illness

Per the patient and her daughter, the patient seemed more confused than usual and fell while getting out of the bathtub. Upon presentation to the emergency department, she was noted to be febrile and confused, with left leg pain. All other review of symptoms was negative. X-ray confirmed a left distal femur fracture, as well as a pan-sensitive *E. coli* urinary tract infection. She was hospitalized for IV antibiotics and intramedullary nailing of her femur.

T. R. Taylor
Emory University School of Medicine, Atlanta, GA, USA
e-mail: Taryn.Taylor@emory.edu

© Springer International Publishing AG, part of Springer Nature 2019
M. L. Martin et al. (eds.), *Diversity and Inclusion in Quality Patient Care*,
https://doi.org/10.1007/978-3-319-92762-6_22

Past Medical History

The patient has a past surgical history of a left knee replacement, as well as thyroidectomy and hysterectomy. She currently has hypertension, for which she takes Diuril.

Family History

There is a history of type II diabetes mellitus in two of the patient's siblings, both of whom are now deceased. One of her children has hypertension, and her daughter has been successfully treated for breast cancer.

Social History

The patient is a retired nurse, who recently moved in with her daughter, a real-estate agent, and her son-in-law, an attorney. She has three other children, all of whom are college-educated professionals. She has never been a smoker or drinker and is a vegetarian.

Physical Exam on Discharge Planning Rounds

Vital signs Temp, 99.2 ° F; pulse, 79; BP, 141/96; respirations, 19; oxygen sat 98% on RA

General Slender elderly female who appears to be sleeping comfortably in bed

ENT TMs pearly, moist mucous membranes, nose and throat are clear

Neck Supple, non-tender, no adenopathy

Cardiovascular Regular rate and rhythm with no murmurs, rubs, or gallops

Respiratory Easy work of breathing, lungs are clear with good air exchange bilaterally and no accessory muscle use

Abdomen Well-healed surgical scars, soft and non-distended, non-tender

Extremities Surgical dressing to left leg appears clean, dry, and intact; 2+ popliteal and dorsalis pedis pulses with no clubbing or cyanosis noted to extremities

Skin Bruising noted to left leg, but no additional rashes or lesions

Neuro Will wake, answer questions appropriately, no obvious sign of deficit, appears to fall back asleep quickly

Questions for Discussion

1. Why did the resident get annoyed upon learning that the patient would be utilizing Medicaid benefits?

Attitudes/Assumptions: The Physician

(a) The patient appears to be unaware of the conversation on rounds, so it is acceptable to air his grievances.
(b) This woman (patient) is using government resources that are not afforded to others, and it is not fair.
(c) Because she (the patient) is of lower socioeconomic status, she probably also has poor health literacy and will not understand discharge instructions regarding how to take her medications. Because of this, she will likely return to the hospital.

Gaps in Provider Knowledge

(a) Lack of knowledge of disparities/discrimination: poverty is associated with higher rates of morbidity and mortality. Patients of lower socioeconomic status are often treated differently, and there is a need for improving quality and reducing inequities in their care [1, 2].
(b) Lack of knowledge regarding the role and variations of family structure and cohesiveness: recognizing the significance of the family dynamic and availability of social support is important in order to understand how patients interface with the healthcare delivery system.

2. How could this resident have handled the situation better?

Cross-Cultural Tools and Skills

(a) Avoid stereotyping and making quick judgments about new people and situations.
(b) Remain objective and manage his own emotions with respect to past personal/familial experiences.

3. Which components of the ACGME competencies are incorporated into this case [3]?

(a) *Professionalism*: Has professional and respectful interactions with patients, caregivers, and members of the interprofessional team.
(b) *Professionalism*: Responds to each patient's unique characteristics and needs [4, 5].
(c) *Interpersonal and communication skills*: Communicates effectively in interprofessional teams [6].

Case Outcome

The case manager, who is rounding with the patient's team, informs the resident that while the patient does receive Medicaid benefits, her children have expressed their commitment to handle fiscal responsibilities for her ongoing care needs. The case manager additionally informs the resident that the patient is a retired nurse, who is quite knowledgeable about her medication regimen and the importance of medication adherence and compliance. The patient is successfully transferred to an excellent assisted living facility. The attending physician schedules a meeting with the resident to provide feedback regarding his behavior. Using the Ask-Tell-Ask method [7], the attending first asked the resident for his self-reflection regarding the incident. The resident acknowledged his own bias and was embarrassed for making assumptions. The attending physician recounted his observation that the resident had not demonstrated professionalism but was encouraged that he was able to recognize his errors. Together, they developed a plan for improvement.

References

1. Fiscella K, Franks P, Gold MR, Clancy CM. Inequality in quality. JAMA. 2000;283(19):2579. https://doi.org/10.1001/jama.283.19.2579.
2. Balsa AI, McGuire TG. Prejudice, clinical uncertainty and stereotyping as sources of health disparities. J Health Econ. 2003;22(1):89–116. https://doi.org/10.1016/S0167-6296(02)00098-X.
3. Deslauriers J, Edgar L. Milestones guidebook for residents and fellows. Chicago: Accreditation Council for Graduate Medical Education; 2016. 41p.
4. Gillespie C, Paik S, Ark T, Zabar S, Kalet A. Residents' perceptions of their own professionalism and the professionalism of their learning environment. J Grad Med Educ. 2009;1(2):208–15. https://doi.org/10.4300/JGME-D-09-00018.1.
5. Ludwig S, Day S. Chapter 7, New standards for resident professionalism: discussion. In: The ACGME 2011 duty hour standards: enhancing quality of care, supervision, and resident professional development. Chicago: Accrediation Council for Graduate Medical Education; 2011. p. 47–51.
6. Accrediation Council for Graduate Medical Education. Advancing education in interpersonal and communication skills. Chicago: Accrediation Council for Graduate Medical Education; 2005. 19 p.
7. French JC, Colbert CY, Pien LC, Dannefer EF, Taylor CA. Targeted feedback in the milestones era: utilization of the ask-tell-ask feedback model to promote reflection and self-assessment. J Surg Educ. 2015;72(6):e274–9. https://doi.org/10.1016/j.jsurg.2015.05.016.

Chapter 23
Deaf Patient

Jason M. Rotoli and Trevor Halle

Case Scenario

A 42-year-old deaf female whose primary language is American Sign Language (ASL) presents to the emergency department for generalized abdominal pain, nausea, and vomiting. This is the third visit in 4 days for similar symptoms. She is 2 weeks status post-bilateral mastectomy for breast cancer.

Visit #1 The patient describes the pain as diffuse, sharp, and intermittent. She has vomited several times throughout the day. There are no exacerbating factors. She denies stool or urine changes. She denies chest pain or drainage from chest surgical wounds. She is communicating with the help of a distant family member who is struggling to interpret for her. No ASL interpreter is offered.

Labs appear normal. After IV fluids, IV analgesia, and IV antiemetics, the symptoms seem to transiently improve, and the patient is discharged with referral back to her primary care physician (PCP).

Visit #2 The patient returns with persistent, diffuse abdominal pain, and recurrent emesis. Again, she reports no exacerbating factors. She repeatedly denies stool or urine changes. She denies chest pain or drainage from chest surgical wounds. She is asked about working with an interpreter during the ED visit. A certified ASL interpreter is obtained for the interview. Although the provider empathizes with the patient by acknowledging her recent diagnosis of breast cancer, he does not inquire any further about the diagnosis for multiple reasons: the sensitive nature of the diagnosis, the impersonal environment of the emergency department, and the urge to move on to the next patient for fear of falling behind.

J. M. Rotoli (✉) · T. Halle
University of Rochester Medical Center, Rochester, NY, USA
e-mail: Jason_rotoli@urmc.rochester.edu; Trevor_halle@urmc.rochester.edu

© Springer International Publishing AG, part of Springer Nature 2019
M. L. Martin et al. (eds.), *Diversity and Inclusion in Quality Patient Care*,
https://doi.org/10.1007/978-3-319-92762-6_23

Labs appear normal. A CT scan of the abdomen and pelvis shows no acute pathology. Again, the patient is given IV fluids, IV analgesia, and IV antiemetics, and she feels well enough to reluctantly agree to discharge. She is discharged with antiemetics and oral analgesia and referred back to her PCP.

Visit #3 The patient returns to the ED for recurrent, persistent, and sharp abdominal pain despite taking the previously prescribed antiemetics and analgesia. The same family member who was present for the first visit accompanies her. The physician enters the room and begins using ASL to communicate directly with the patient. He asks the patient if she would like the family member stay or leave, and she prefers her to leave the room. The family member leaves the room and the interview continues. Again, she denies urinary or stool changes, reaction to food or medications, sick contacts, or fevers.

In ASL, the provider asks, "How are you coping with your surgery and recent diagnosis of breast cancer?" The patient begins to cry. "The diagnosis of cancer is really scary," she replies, "but I am even more scared to deal with this by myself." After asking about her support network, she cries even harder. The patient explains that she went in for surgery without telling her brother or mother about her diagnosis. The day after her surgery, she received a text from her mother informing her that her brother died unexpectedly the day before. "While I was having surgery, my brother died and I didn't get a chance to say goodbye. I can't tell my mother about my surgery because she is dealing with my brother's death. I have no one to talk to about this."

Review of Symptoms

The patient endorses abdominal pain, nausea, and vomiting. She also endorses feelings of helplessness and sadness but denies suicidal thoughts. All other systems are negative.

Past Medical History

She has a recent diagnosis of stage II breast cancer. She is 2 weeks status post-bilateral mastectomy. She has not started chemotherapy.

Family History

Noncontributory.

Social History

She lives alone. Mother is alive and lives out of state. Brother was her main support and recently died. Non-smoker, no alcohol.

Physical Exam

Vital Signs 37 °C, 110/60, 86, 12, 99% on room air

General Tearful, uncomfortable appearing, but nontoxic

Cardiovascular Regular rate, S1/S2, no murmurs

Respiratory Clear breath sounds bilaterally

Abdomen Soft, non-distended, non-tender; normal bowel sounds; no masses or rigidity

Extremities No cyanosis, no edema

Skin No rashes or lesions

Psych Tearful and sad, no active suicidal or homicidal thoughts, no audiovisual hallucinations

Questions for Discussion

1. Why did it take three visits to ascertain the true nature of the patient's visit?

Attitudes/Assumptions: The Physician

(a) It is acceptable to use a family member/friend to interpret for a non-English-speaking patient.
(b) The use of an interpreter will always result in the most accurate and useful information during a patient interview.
(c) Breast cancer seems unrelated to the patient's complaint of abdominal pain. The patient should be able to advocate for himself/herself if there is a mental health or social issue.
(d) There is nothing wrong if the labs and CT scan are negative.

Attitudes/Assumptions: The Patient

(a) I do not have a right to advocate for myself by asking for an interpreter if one is not offered.
(b) I do not want to ask questions about sadness and loneliness because they might be unrelated to my current visit, and I do not want to appear ignorant.
(c) My medical history and recent diagnosis are things that I have to deal with alone.

Gaps in Provider Knowledge

(a) Interpreters for non-English-speaking patients are required by law to allow for accessible health care and health information. Several policies and statutes have been written to provide equitable access to care and information including the Americans with Disabilities Act (1990), the civil rights statutes (1974), and the Joint Commission and Office of Minority Health national standards [1–4].

(b) Many Deaf patients have limited access to healthcare information, resulting in low health literacy levels and poor comprehension of their own medical problems. This contributes to increased risks of morbidities in comparison to the general hearing population, including depression and increased emergency department use [4, 5].

(c) Direct or concordant communication is communication in a patient's primary language. It allows for improved access to care and can foster the development of a strong physician-patient relationship through clear communication and understanding of a different culture. It results in increased use of primary care services and may reduce ED visits [5–7].

(d) Approximately 40% of deaf patients have mental illness (including depression) in comparison to 25% of the general hearing population. This can be difficult to recognize and is exacerbated by poor communication, inability to ask questions, the fear of appearing ignorant, and family dynamics [8].

2. What is the medical concern in this case?

(a) Failure to recognize the cultural differences and needs of the patient results in poor communication and potentially substandard care during the initial visit.

(b) Anchoring bias is the natural human tendency to focus too heavily or "anchor" on the first available piece(s) of information. During the first and second visits, this type of bias causes the providers to focus solely on the most likely physiologic causes of the patient's abdominal symptoms without considering other etiologies or work-ups.

(c) When discussing her health concerns, the patient was not asked about emotional or psychological issues and did not have the opportunity to discuss her brother's death privately until the third visit.

3. What actions could have been taken to improve the patient experience and outcome?

Cross-Cultural Tools and Skills

(a) Establish communication preferences in all patients. In the culturally deaf patient, it will likely be ASL. Utilize concordant communication with the patient whenever possible. If not possible, request an ASL interpreter for all deaf ASL users to help ensure adequate communication.

(b) Obtain a social history and perform a psychiatric evaluation as part of your physical exam, especially during a repeat visit for the same or a similar complaint. This is an opportunity to think outside the box and not simply repeat the same evaluation that was performed in the initial visits.

(c) Recognize that a culturally deaf patient is part of an underrepresented group and, like other vulnerable populations, has poor access to health care and poor health literacy. They often lack a primary care provider and emergency department visits may serve as their only source of medical care [4, 7].

Case Outcome

Diagnosis Abdominal pain secondary to psychosomatization due to home and life stressors

Disposition The patient is given time to discuss her cancer diagnosis, the impact of the diagnosis on her life, and the pain she is feeling from being unable to discuss this with her mother and recently deceased brother. The provider reviews her previous labs and imaging and finds no abnormalities. The patient and provider have a discussion about the somatic effects of emotional trauma, and how these symptoms might present in a person who is grieving about multiple different things. The patient and provider agree that her symptoms have a psychological component and that she is safe from a medical perspective. She agrees to contact her mother and discuss her diagnosis and emotional state. The patient is discharged from the emergency department with emergency crisis line information and primary care follow-up.

References

1. U.S. Department of Justice. Information and technical assistance on the Americans with disabilities act [Internet]. Washington, DC: U.S. Department of Justice; [cited 2017 Sep 1]. Available from www.ada.gov.
2. The Joint Commission. Joint commission: accreditation, health care, certification [Internet]. Oakbrook Terrace: The Joint Commission; 2017 [cited 2017 Sep 1]. Available from www.jointcommission.org.
3. National Association of the Deaf. National Association of the Deaf [Internet]. Silver Spring: National Association of the Deaf; 2017 [cited 2017 Sep 1]. Available from www.nad.org.
4. Richardson K. Deaf culture: competencies and best practices. Nurse Pract. 2014;39(5):20–8.
5. McKee M, et al. Emergency department use and risk factors among deaf American Sign Language users. Disabil Health J. 2015;8(4):573–8.
6. McKee M, et al. Perceptions of cardiovascular health in an underserved community of deaf adults using American Sign Language. Disabil Health J. 2011;4(3):192–7.
7. McKee M, et al. Impact of communication on preventive services among deaf American Sign Language users. Am J Prev Med. 2011;41(1):75–9.
8. Li C, et al. Hearing impairment associated with depression in US adults, national health and nutrition examination survey 2005–2010. Otolaryngol Head Neck Surg. 2014;140(4):293–302.

Chapter 24
African-American Pediatric Pain Patient

Matthew S. Lucas

Case Scenario

History of Presenting Illness and Review of Symptoms

A 6-year-old boy presents to the pediatric emergency department at a large, urban children's hospital at 11 am on a weekend morning. The child is accompanied by his mother, older brother, and younger sister. The waiting area is not busy, and the family is taken to a triage room immediately.

Triage Assessment

The patient's mother reports that approximately 30 min before arriving, she was preparing food in the kitchen, and, just as she turned away from the stove, the patient inadvertently pulled a medium-sized pot of boiling water onto himself while playing with his brother. The patient was the only one injured by the boiling water. The mother also reports changing him out of the wet clothes and then coming to the emergency department. The mother denies any other interventions at home or en route to the hospital.

The mother reports that her son screamed immediately and cried after being doused with the boiling water. The patient appears calm and attentive. When asked to indicate his level of pain using the Wong-Baker FACES® Pain Rating Scale [1], the child shyly looks at his mother. She states, "The nurse asked you a question. That's why we're here. It's okay to answer." He then points to the face on the right

M. S. Lucas
Department of Women, Children, and Family Health Science, College of Nursing, University of Illinois at Chicago, Chicago, IL, USA
e-mail: lucasm@uic.edu

© Springer International Publishing AG, part of Springer Nature 2019
M. L. Martin et al. (eds.), *Diversity and Inclusion in Quality Patient Care*,
https://doi.org/10.1007/978-3-319-92762-6_24

of the scale, which is crying and indicates 10/10 "hurts worst." When asked where the pain is, the child, while looking down, lifts his shirt to show the triage nurse his abdomen.

The triage nurse weighs the patient (21.2 kg) and administers 315 mg of acetaminophen oral suspension as guided by the triage protocol for pain management. She also documents the pain rating, her general impression of the patient, and the medication administration, as well as the brief history: "Report per mother: child pulled pot of boiling water on top of himself approximately 30 min prior to arrival. No redness. No signs of distress. Skin is clean, dry, and intact." This children's hospital categorizes triaged patients using the Emergency Severity Index (ESI), maintained by the Agency for Healthcare Research and Quality, which has five ratings: one requires immediate life-saving interventions; two is a high-risk situation, including patients with confusion or disorientation and patients with severe pain or distress; three requires many different resources for care, including medication administration and laboratory or radiology services; four anticipates only one resource needed; and five is a nonurgent situation anticipating no resource utilization [2]. The nurse categorizes the patient's triage level as a four, reflecting the acetaminophen administration. The family is instructed to return to the waiting area until called to be placed in a room.

Transfer to Room in ED

After 15 min, a nursing assistant brings the family to a room in the unit of the emergency department that is designated to attend to ESI level 4 and 5 patients. The nursing assistant orients the family to the room and helps the child change out of his shirt and into a gown. She then lets the treating nurse assigned to this room know that a patient has been placed in the room. Additionally, she states a brief history along with, "I changed him into his gown, and he doesn't look very good. I think you should see him soon."

The treating nurse enters the room to a quiet scene. After introducing himself, the nurse asks the patient to identify his pain using the FACES® rating scale, and the child again indicates the 10/10 crying face. The nurse performs a focused assessment of the areas of trauma and documents the following information.

Past Medical History

The patient is followed at the hospital's outpatient pediatric office, and the electronic medical record shows that he is up-to-date with well-child visits and vaccinations. He has one previous hospitalization, 2 years ago, for influenza-like illness. No past surgical history reported.

Family History

The patient lives with his family in an attached row home. Family consists of mother and father, older brother, younger sister, and maternal grandmother.

Social History

The patient is in first grade.

Physical Exam

Vital Signs Temperature, 99.2 °F (temporal); pulse, 136; BP, 124/78; respirations, 28; O_2 Saturation, 100% on room air; weight, 21.2 kg; pain, 10/10 FACES®

General Child intently focused on healthcare staff, sitting calmly on examination bed. When asked about how calmly he is presenting himself, the patient stated, "My mother told me to be good so that you can help me feel better, and it hurts to move."

Cardiovascular Tachycardia

Respiratory Clear and equal bilaterally, tachypnea

Skin The patient's skin is very dark and does not show a blanching response (tested on healthy skin of left arm). His skin is reddened on approximately 25% of his body, including most of abdomen, right side of chest, lateral and anterior sections of his right arm, entire right hand, right anterior and lateral thigh, and his groin. Most of the redness is flat and dry, with some areas of the right arm and abdomen that are raised. The patient's mother stated that she thinks most of the water hit these areas (with raised skin). The patient expresses increased pain upon palpation of burned areas.

After the physical exam, the treating nurse leaves the room and finds the unit's attending physician, stating, "Lisa, sorry to interrupt. We've just received a patient from waiting who you should probably see pretty soon. He's a six-year-old boy who was scalded by boiling water about 45 min ago and has burns covering about 25% of surface area—none to the face. He has very dark skin, and I think the extent of burns was missed in triage. He's also in quite a bit of pain. He had acetaminophen in triage, but we may need to add an opioid. And I think we need to transfer him to the main emergency department." Both nurse and physician enter the patient's room, and after a quick assessment, the physician enters an order for IV insertion, fluid administration, and IV morphine and requests that the nurse begin the transfer process after administering the pain medication.

Questions for Discussion

1. Why is it possible that the triage nurse missed the redness caused by the boiling water?
2. Why were the treating nurse and the physician able to identify the redness caused by the burn?
3. How can you reconcile the patient's self-reported pain rating with his demeanor?

Attitudes/Assumptions: The Mother

(a) Her child suffered an injury severe enough to require immediate medical attention.
(b) She wants the best outcome for her child and thus instructed him to "be good" for the clinicians so that they can help him feel better. Within the case, we learn that she told him to answer clinicians' questions and that to "be good" probably means to stay calm in spite of his distress, pain, and fear, in addition to referencing previous conversations about black bodies in the public realm.

Attitudes/Assumptions: The Patient

(a) The child trusts his mother.

4. What medical issues concern you about this case?
5. What concerns about implicit bias do you have in this case?
6. What assumptions were made by the triage nurse? How were these different from assumptions by the treating nurse and physician?

Attitudes/Assumptions: The Triage Nurse

(a) The patient is not in apparent distress and thus does not have as high a pain level as he indicated.
(b) The patient is black, and black people have high pain thresholds.
(c) Redness from burns is as readily visible on all skin as it is on white skin.
(d) Lack of discrepancy between skin color and redness from a potential burn indicates that there is either no burn or no pain.

Attitudes/Assumptions: The Treating Nurse and Attending Physician

(a) Pain ratings and apparent demeanor are individual to the patient.
(b) Trauma presentations may be different depending on skin color [3, 4].

7. Are the assumptions of the triage nurse the fault of the triage nurse? Think about what led her to have these assumptions. Why might the other clinicians not have the same assumptions?

Gaps in Provider Knowledge

(a) Inaccurate false beliefs about pain based upon a patient's race, including black patients having a higher pain threshold because their nerve endings are less sensitive, and their skin is thicker than whites' [5].

(b) False beliefs about pain contribute to race-based pain disparities in both pediatric [6–8] and adult populations [9].

(c) Trauma presentations may be different depending on skin color, and assessment techniques must be able to address these differences [3, 4]. For example, very darkly pigmented skin will not blanch before capillary refill as it does on skin without dark pigmentation. Lack of skill assessing bodies with darker skin color contributes to disparities in identification of trauma to the skin. These disparities include identification of developing pressure ulcers and can have forensic implications when attempting to identify abrasions after sexual assault.

(d) Inexperience with assessment of nonwhite bodies does not lay wholly with clinicians but also with health professions' educational programs and training texts that fail to deliver this information.

Cross-Cultural Tools and Skills

(a) While this case focused on the enactment of implicit racial bias by a nurse, the problem of implicit racial bias is intrinsic to the United States and thus pervasive throughout the health professions, including medicine. The majority of the research about implicit bias in health care has been conducted with physicians.

(b) The enactment of implicit racial bias is a part of communication, and management of implicit bias is the responsibility of the clinician. There are, unfortunately, very few options available to clinicians and clinician-trainees to individually and collectively address this problem; however, several suggestions from the existing literature are made below.

Implicit Racial Bias

(a) Implicit biases are automatic mental associations about attitudes or stereotypes that are unconscious and influence perceptions, decisions, behaviors, and other actions. These biases are learned through family and other social interactions, as well as through the media (e.g., television, advertising, movies, music, and books).

(b) Implicit racial bias is a form of unconscious racism.

(c) Implicit racial bias in healthcare settings interferes with clinicians' good intentions, including shared decision-making, and negatively affects health outcomes for patients of color, including less appropriate care [6, 10, 11], satisfaction [12, 13], and trust [13, 14], and ultimately premature morbidity and mortality [15, 16]. These outcomes are evident in treatment plan adherence and professional frustration, which often leads to clinician burnout.

(d) Patients recognize and internalize the biases even when clinicians are unaware that they exist.

(e) The compounded financial cost of unconscious racism to patients and the healthcare system is estimated to be in the hundreds of billions of dollars per year [17].

(f) Clinicians do not want to enact implicit racial bias or for patients to experience disparities in health. However, during the clinical encounter, clinicians are frequently influenced by implicit bias and may cause harm.

(g) Medical students learn, in part, through socialization [18], and students' implicit racial biases increase when hearing or seeing negative comments or behaviors about black patients from medical residents and attending physicians [19].

(h) Because implicit racial bias is learned, it can be unlearned.

(i) Implicit racial bias is unwanted by both patients and clinicians, and this is a good position to be in because everyone agrees that implicit bias should be eliminated or at least managed.

(j) Educational reform in response to implicit bias is underway, though approaches are time- and person-intensive and include interventions primarily through directive education [20–22] or discussion and reflection [23–25]. The interventions generally do not include medical education faculty [26], but faculty and staff should be included, as implicit biases are transferred through generations, which include those power hierarchies found in medicine.

Clinical Tools

(a) Clinicians and clinician-trainees should read, listen, and discuss with others—colleagues and patients alike—about implicit racial bias. Doing so will provide an entry into the experiences of patients receiving the bias and the clinicians who enact the bias.

(b) Ideas for discussion include: personal reflections compared to normative standards [23, 24], learning the skill of dialoging [27], constructive approaches to introspection and self-awareness [25, 26, 28], creating a more welcoming environment by reducing potential patients' "stereotype threat" [29], gaining understanding of antiracist pedagogies and structural competencies [30], and exploring other changes to medical education curricula [31].

(c) Discussions should not be a one-time event, but rather an evolving process. Implicit racial bias is learned over several years; anticipate that learning to manage implicit racial bias will take time.

(d) It is important to keep in mind that when a clinician questions why a patient is or is not responding or behaving as expected, a very important follow-up question should be: What is the clinician doing or not doing? Answers to this question can include the following possible responses: The clinician did not ask about structural impediments to implement the plan of care, or the clinician made an assumption about what the patient might or might not (be able to) do.

Case Outcome

Diagnosis First- and second-degree burns

Disposition Admission to trauma unit for pain control and hydration

The patient received morphine for pain control and had an IV line inserted to provide hydration. He was transferred to the main emergency department, which is better equipped to handle high-risk situations and patients with very high pain. The patient was reclassified as ESI level 2. The patient stayed in the inpatient trauma unit for 2 days before he was discharged to outpatient care.

The treating nurse followed up with the triage nurse in order to provide constructive feedback about how skin, trauma, and pain assessments may require assessment different from how it is learned on white patients. He also completed a report through the hospital's nonpunitive "patient event" reporting system.

References

1. Wong DL, Baker CM. Pain in children: comparison of assessment scales. Pediatr Nurs. 1988;14(1):9–17.
2. Gilboy N, Tanabe T, Travers D, Rosenau AM. Emergency Severity Index (ESI): a triage tool for emergency department care, Version 4. Implementation handbook 2012 edition. Rockville: Agency for Healthcare Research and Quality; 2011.
3. Sommers MS. Color awareness: a must for patient assessment. Am Nurse Today. 2011;6(1):6.
4. Everett JS, Budescu M, Sommers MS. Making sense of skin color in clinical care. Clin Nurs Res. 2012;21(4):495–516. https://doi.org/10.1177/1054773812446510.
5. Hoffman KM, Trawalter S, Axt JR, Oliver MN. Racial bias in pain assessment and treatment recommendations, and false beliefs about biological differences between blacks and whites. Proc Natl Acad Sci U S A. 2016;113(16):4296–301. https://doi.org/10.1073/pnas.1516047113.
6. Sabin JA, Greenwald AG. The influence of implicit bias on treatment recommendations for 4 common pediatric conditions: pain, urinary tract infection, attention deficit hyperactivity disorder, and asthma. Am J Public Health. 2012;102(5):988–95. https://doi.org/10.2105/AJPH.2011.300621.
7. Goyal MK, Kuppermann N, Cleary SD, Teach SJ, Chamberlain JM. Racial disparities in pain management of children with appendicitis in emergency departments. JAMA Pediatr. 2015;169(11):996–1002. https://doi.org/10.1001/jamapediatrics.2015.1915.
8. Lee HH, Lewis CW, McKinney CM. Disparities in emergency department pain treatment for toothache. JDR Clin Trans Res. 2016;1(3):226–33. https://doi.org/10.1177/2380084416655745.

9. Lazio MP, Costello HH, Courtney DM, Martinovich Z, Myers R, Zosel A, et al. A comparison of analgesic management for emergency department patients with sickle cell disease and renal colic. Clin J Pain. 2010;26(3):199–205. https://doi.org/10.1097/AJP.0b013e3181bed10c.

10. Green AR, Carney DR, Pallin DJ, Ngo LH, Raymond KL, Iezzoni LI, et al. Implicit bias among physicians and its prediction of thrombolysis decisions for black and white patients. J Gen Intern Med. 2007;22(9):1231–8. https://doi.org/10.1007/s11606-007-0258-5.

11. Haider AH, Schneider EB, Sriram N, Dossick DS, Scott VK, Swoboda SM, et al. Unconscious race and class bias: its association with decision making by trauma and acute care surgeons. J Trauma Acute Care Surg. 2014;77(3):409–16. https://doi.org/10.1097/TA.0000000000000392.

12. Blair IV, Steiner JF, Fairclough DL, Hanratty R, Price DW, Hirsh HK, et al. Clinicians' implicit ethnic/racial bias and perceptions of care among Black and Latino patients. Ann Fam Med. 2013;11(1):43–52. https://doi.org/10.1370/afm.1442.

13. Penner LA, Dovidio JF, Gonzalez R, Albrecht TL, Chapman R, Foster T, et al. The effects of oncologist implicit racial bias in racially discordant oncology interactions. J Clin Oncol. 2016;34(24):2874–80. https://doi.org/10.1200/JCO.2015.66.3658.

14. Penner LA, Dovidio JF, West TV, Gaertner SL, Albrecht TL, Dailey RK, et al. Aversive racism and medical interactions with black patients: a field study. J Exp Soc Psychol. 2010;46(2):436–40. https://doi.org/10.1016/j.jesp.2009.11.004.

15. Kochanek KD, Murphy SL, Xu JQ, Tejada-Vera B. Deaths: final data for 2014. Hyattsville: National Center for Health Statistics; 2016. Contract no.: 4. [cited 14 June 2018]. Available from: https://www.cdc.gov/nchs/data/nvsr/nvsr65/nvsr65_04.pdf.

16. Satcher D, Fryer GE Jr, McCann J, Troutman A, Woolf SH, Rust G. What if we were equal? A comparison of the black-white mortality gap in 1960 and 2000. Health Aff. 2005;24(2):459–64. https://doi.org/10.1377/hlthaff.24.2.459.

17. LaVeist TA, Gaskin D, Richard P. Estimating the economic burden of racial health inequalities in the United States. Int J Health Serv. 2011;41(2):231–8. https://doi.org/10.2190/HS.41.2.c.

18. Good BJ. How medicine constructs its objects. In: Medicine, rationality, and experience: an anthropological perspective. Cambridge: Cambridge University Press; 1994. p. 65–87.

19. van Ryn M, Hardeman R, Phelan SM, Burgess DJ, Dovidio JF, Herrin J, et al. Medical school experiences associated with change in implicit racial bias among 3547 students: a medical student CHANGES study report. J Gen Intern Med. 2015;30(12):1748–56. https://doi.org/10.1007/s11606-015-3447-7.

20. Gonzalez CM, Kim MY, Marantz PR. Implicit bias and its relation to health disparities: a teaching program and survey of medical students. Teach Learn Med. 2014;26(1):64–71. https://doi.org/10.1080/10401334.2013.857341.

21. Nelson SC, Prasad S, Hackman HW. Training providers on issues of race and racism improve health care equity. Pediatr Blood Cancer. 2015;62(5):915–7. https://doi.org/10.1002/pbc.25448.

22. Weech-Maldonado R, Dreachslin JL, Epane JP, Gail J, Gupta S, Wainio JA. Hospital cultural competency as a systematic organizational intervention: key findings from the national center for healthcare leadership diversity demonstration project. Health Care Manage Rev. 2018;43(1):30–41. https://doi.org/10.1097/HMR.0000000000000128.

23. Hernandez RA, Haidet P, Gill AC, Teal CR. Fostering students' reflection about bias in healthcare: cognitive dissonance and the role of personal and normative standards. Med Teach. 2013;35(4):e1082–9. https://doi.org/10.3109/0142159X.2012.733453.

24. Teal CR, Shada RE, Gill AC, Thompson BM, Fruge E, Villarreal GB, et al. When best intentions aren't enough: helping medical students develop strategies for managing bias about patients. J Gen Intern Med. 2010;25(Suppl 2):S115–8. https://doi.org/10.1007/s11606-009-1243-y.

25. White AA 3rd, Logghe HJ, Goodenough DA, Barnes LL, Hallward A, Allen IM, et al. Self-awareness and cultural identity as an effort to reduce bias in medicine. J Racial Ethn Health Disparities. 2017;5(1):34–9. https://doi.org/10.1007/s40615-017-0340-6.

26. Hannah SD, Carpenter-Song E. Patrolling your blind spots: introspection and public catharsis in a medical school faculty development course to reduce unconscious bias in medicine. Cult Med Psychiatry. 2013;37(2):314–39. https://doi.org/10.1007/s11013-013-9320-4.

27. Murray-Garcia JL, Harrell S, Garcia JA, Gizzi E, Simms-Mackey P. Dialogue as skill: training a health professions workforce that can talk about race and racism. Am J Orthopsychiatry. 2014;84(5):590–6. https://doi.org/10.1037/ort0000026.

28. Burgess DJ, Beach MC, Saha S. Mindfulness practice: a promising approach to reducing the effects of clinician implicit bias on patients. Patient Educ Couns. 2017;100(2):372–6. https://doi.org/10.1016/j.pec.2016.09.005.

29. Burgess DJ, Warren J, Phelan S, Dovidio J, van Ryn M. Stereotype threat and health disparities: what medical educators and future physicians need to know. J Gen Intern Med. 2010;25(Suppl 2):S169–77. https://doi.org/10.1007/s11606-009-1221-4.

30. Wear D, Zarconi J, Aultman JM, Chyatte MR, Kumagai AK. Remembering Freddie Gray: medical education for social justice. Acad Med. 2017;92(3):312–7. https://doi.org/10.1097/ACM.0000000000001355.

31. Sukhera J, Watling C. A framework for integrating implicit bias recognition into health professions education. Acad Med. 2017;93(1):35–40. https://doi.org/10.1097/ACM.0000000000001819.

Chapter 25
Sickle Cell Disease Patient

Gwendolyn Poles

Case Scenario

A 56-year-old African-American female with history of sickle cell disease (SCD) (Hgb SS) presents to the emergesncy department (ED) complaining of increasingly severe pain in her lower back and extremities over 2 days, unrelieved by oral hydromorphone and supplemental oxygen. She usually takes 2–6 mg hydromorphone as needed for pain unrelieved by acetaminophen or nabumetone. She informs the ED physician that she took a total of 40 mg hydromorphone over the preceding 24 h with no significant pain relief. She does not frequent the ED – her last ED visit was approximately 6 years prior. She rates her pain as 8/10.

Review of Symptoms

Patient denies fever, chills, and malaise. Remainder of review of symptoms is unremarkable except as noted above.

Past Medical History

Hgb SS, hypertension, sickle cell chronic lung disease, nocturnal hypoxemia, gout, chronic kidney disease stage III, osteoporosis, osteoarthritis, status post-total hip replacement due to avascular necrosis, GERD

G. Poles
PinnacleHealth System, Faculty, Internal Medicine Residency Program,
Medical Director Kline Health Center, Harrisburg, PA, USA

© Springer International Publishing AG, part of Springer Nature 2019
M. L. Martin et al. (eds.), *Diversity and Inclusion in Quality Patient Care*,
https://doi.org/10.1007/978-3-319-92762-6_25

Medications Hydroxyurea, folate, nadolol, chlorthalidone, telmisartan, allopurinol, alendronate/D, omeprazole, vitamins C and D, calcium carbonate, MVI, fluticasone nasal spray, loratadine, acetaminophen, vaginal estrogen ring, prn metoclopramide, zalephon, nabumetone, and hydromorphone

Family History

Positive for hypertension, type II diabetes mellitus, and sickle cell trait

Social History

Married; denies tobacco, alcohol, or illicit drug abuse; Employed as medical director of the Internal Medicine clinic and faculty member of this community hospital's Internal Medicine residency program, working 50–60 hours per week and as much as 18–20 consecutive days when working on the in-patient service.

Physical Exam

Vital Signs Temperature 99.7, pulse 72, respirations 20, BP 181/95

General Patient was in acute distress due to pain; grade II systolic murmur, occasional arrhythmias; exam otherwise unremarkable

Labs Hgb 7.3 g/dL, Hct 21.2%, WBC 13.17 K/uL, Plt 390 K/uL, MCV 119.1 fl, retic% 10.49, retic absolute 186,700/mm^3; sodium 140 mmol/L, potassium 4.5 mmol/L, chloride 108 mmol/L, carbon dioxide 26.0 mmol/L, BUN 23 mg/dL, creatinine 0.9 mg/dL, GFR 69.1 ml/min (uncorrected for race), glucose 109 mg/dL, calcium 9.6 mg/dL, LFT's normal

The patient is initially given 1 mg IV hydromorphone and IV fluids. The patient immediately shares with the ED physician, her colleague, that she usually receives a minimum of 2 mg of hydromorphone IV, reminding him that she has not received any significant pain relief with the unusually high amount of oral hydromorphone she took prior to coming to the ED. He then gives her an additional 1 mg IV hydromorphone.

The patient eventually receives another 1 mg of IV hydromorphone but does not receive relief with the total of 3 mg. She decides to endure the pain until her hematologist comes to see her. She has a long-standing relationship with her hematologist and knows he will ensure adequate pain relief. She is admitted, seen by her hematologist, and receives as needed dosing. She refuses several doses of hydromorphone during hospitalization to avoid the unwanted side effects despite her continued pain. During her hospitalization, cardiology is consulted due to shortness of breath and an episode of non-sustained ventricular tachycardia. She is diagnosed with congestive heart failure and mild ventricular hypertrophy, attributed to aggressive IV hydration and anemia, respectively. She responds well to gentle diuresis and red blood cell transfusion.

The length of this hospitalization is 7 days versus the customary 3–4 days in past decades.

One day after discharge to home, the patient is found by her husband unconscious on her bathroom floor. She is intubated in the field and transported to a different institution (level 1 Trauma Center) due to head trauma from the fall.

Labs Hgb 9.5 g/dL, Hct 27.7%, WBC 9.6 K/uL, sodium 141 mmol/L, potassium 2.8 mmol/L, chloride 102 mmol/L, bicarb 31 mmol/L, BUN 17 mg/dL, creatinine 0.88 mg/dL, glucose 155 mg/dL, calcium 7.8 mg/dL, magnesium 0.8 mg/dL, phosphorus 3.4 mg/dL

Imaging CT head, facial bones; cervical, thoracic, lumbar spine, right periorbital soft tissue swelling; otherwise no traumatic injury; no evidence of hemorrhage; CT chest, abdomen, pelvis, no acute injury; CXR, no obvious infiltrates; cardiopericardial silhouette mildly enlarged; endotracheal tube adjusted per CXR results

In the ED she is evaluated, intubated, and treated for status epilepticus, head trauma, severe hypomagnesemia, and other electrolyte abnormalities, and placed on empiric antibiotic treatment. She is admitted to the ICU. She is extubated on day 4 and transferred to the step-down unit. On day 13, she is cleared for transfer to in-patient rehabilitation. Clonidine and phenytoin are added to her preadmission medications.

During discharge planning from the trauma center, the case manager attempts to have the patient's husband transport her in his car to the outside rehabilitation center of her choice rather than arrange ambulance transport. She also assumes and overtly implies that the patient cannot afford the cash payment for ambulance transport. The patient and her husband insist upon ambulance transport given her severely deconditioned state (she could not stand without full assistance).

The patient pays by check and is transported via ambulance to the in-patient rehabilitation where she spends 2 weeks. She follows up with outpatient physical, occupational, speech, and neurocognitive therapy for 2 months and continues independent rehabilitation with the goal of returning to practice.

During home recovery, she requests copies of her medical records from both institutions to help facilitate posthospitalization follow-up care. Of note in her discharge summary from the trauma center was the phrase "Jane Doe is a 56y/o AA F, apparently a physician…"

Questions for Discussion

1. Implicit racial and gender biases by healthcare professionals impact minority and female patients regardless of socioeconomic status [1, 2]. What additional impact does this have on those who cannot advocate for themselves, due to socioeconomic status and/or mental state?
2. During the initial hospital presentation, what assumptions may the ED physician have made that led to inadequate pain control?

Attitudes/Assumptions: The Physician

(a) At the trauma center, inaccurate assumptions may have been made based on race combined with diagnosis (SCD), assumed class, and laboratory studies. There is a wide range of severity in SCD. Most physicians do not encounter patients with SCD, and those who do encounter those with more severe disease, thus creating unconscious biases [3–5]. If the physician suspected that the patient was an alcoholic due to extremely low magnesium, such conclusions may support the belief that this patient may not be a practicing physician. However, this patient rarely uses alcohol and has three plausible medical causes for hypomagnesemia: she is on omeprazole, has SCD, and was recently hospitalized [6–8].

(b) Regardless of the laboratory studies, the language in the discharge summary implies that the treating physicians were reluctant to believe this patient was a practicing physician. It was also unprofessional. This appears to be evidence of explicit bias based on race, diagnosis, presentation, and possibly gender.

(c) Additionally, some of the medications prescribed upon discharge were not appropriate for a physician planning to return to work after recovery. Two of the medications (clonidine for hypertension and phenytoin for new onset seizure disorder due to head trauma) required administration three times a day and caused somnolence. There were many once a day alternatives to the ones prescribed that do not cause somnolence. Physicians usually avoid prescribing medications that have to be taken several times a day and cause somnolence in patients that are employed.

(d) Patients are sometimes unaware of services not covered by their insurance. When a requested service is uncovered, healthcare professionals should share that information in a sensitive way. Physicians must not be presumptuous about a patient's ability or inability to pay. Physicians must be professional in dictating discharge summaries. Given the history of healthcare disparities in patients with SCD, minorities, and women, this only served to reinforce the patient's belief that the status quo in healthcare disparities remains. This patient can report her concerns to the hospital administration and/or patient advocate if she wishes.

3. What role could the diagnosis, race, or gender have played in the clinical decision-making?
4. How can physicians, other healthcare professionals, and institutions ensure equitable care for all patients?
5. How can a patient with this type of presentation be better cared for?
6. During the trauma center hospitalization, what considerations may explain the perceived difficulty in securing ambulance transfer to the in-patient rehabilitation facility?
7. During the trauma center hospitalization, what factors could have led to the statement in the discharge summary ("apparently a physician"), and is the statement appropriate?
8. What assumptions could explain the case manager's interaction with the patient?

Attitudes/Assumptions: The Case Manager

Inappropriate discharge arrangements suggested by the case manager could have placed this patient at risk for falling and the institution at risk for liability. It is unclear why the case manager did not approach the discharge planning for this patient in a more suitable manner. Other than attempting to steer the patient to this facility's in-patient rehabilitation facility, it is difficult to put forth an alternative explanation for her implying that the patient could not afford transport to the rehabilitation facility of her choice. It is also difficult to explain why the case manager did not take the initiative to ensure the safest transport method. The case manager appears to have demonstrated explicit bias and made some assumptions related to race and presumed class.

9. Why did the patient only come to the ED after taking such a high dose of oral hydromorphone? Why not come sooner?
10. Why did the patient choose to wait for her hematologist for adequate pain control instead of requesting more from the ED physician?
11. Why does the patient need such high doses of opioids?
12. Should this patient address the phrase "apparently a physician" in her discharge summary, and if so, how?
13. What assumptions or conclusions may the patient have made based on the above issues?

Attitudes/Assumptions: The Patient

It is documented that patients with SCD avoid going to the ED for a variety of reasons, but primarily due to how they are treated. They endure much stereotyping, such as being called a "drug seeker" and "the angry black man (or woman)." Some patients do become aggressive out of frustration, others may be viewed as "overreacting" during their painful episodes, and still some underreport their pain to avoid being labeled [9–12]. This patient avoided conflict with the ED physician by enduring the pain until her hematologist came to admit her.

Gaps in Provider Knowledge

At the first institution, there was probably a lack of knowledge on the proper dosing of the chosen opioid for a severe sickle cell crisis. In addition to the fact that the parenteral dose should have been much higher given the minimal response to the 40 mg of oral hydromorphone, studies have shown that patients with SCD, who are not opioid naïve, often require higher doses for adequate pain control than the general population [4, 5].

It is unclear whether any implicit or explicit bias based on gender, disease (SCD), or race played a role in this case. However, it has been well documented that patients with SCD suffer significantly more difficulty obtaining adequate pain control in all healthcare settings [5, 9–11]. There is also evidence that race, ethnicity, and gender do impact quality of health care including analgesia dosing [1, 2].

Cross-Cultural Tools and Skills

It is critical that healthcare professionals access readily available guidelines on the treatment of SCD as well as explore their implicit and/or explicit biases to avoid unnecessary patient suffering. Most patients with SCD (and/or their caretakers) can inform physicians which opioid and what dose usually works for them. Physicians should not assume a patient with SCD presenting with an acute painful event asking for a specific drug and dose is "drug seeking"; rather, they are trying to advocate for themselves. We do not conclude a diabetic patient is "insulin seeking" if they request what normally works for them. We do not assume that a patient with cystic fibrosis who knows the antibiotic their pathogens respond to is "antibiotic seeking."

Institutions need to have protocols in place to ensure discharge plans are appropriate for their patients. Continuing education and training on cultural competency, diversity, and inclusion should be an integral part of all healthcare practice settings. Methods of accountability must be implemented to ensure improvement in healthcare equality [1, 2].

Case Outcome

Diagnosis Initial hospitalization: Sickle cell anemia with sickle cell crisis, CHF, SVT, cardiac ischemia secondary to sickle cell crisis, gout

Subsequent hospitalization: Head trauma secondary to fall, post-concussion syndrome, sickle cell disease, hypertension, severe hypomagnesemia, hypokalemia, gout

Disposition After several months of recovery from physical deconditioning, cognitive impairment, and caring for her terminally ill husband, the physician-patient returned to her full-time position at her institution. She lost her husband 3 months after returning to work.

Fortunately, this patient had well-educated, outspoken advocates at her bedside during her second hospitalization (spouse, family, friends, and colleagues) when she could not initially advocate for herself. Due to her knowledge of the healthcare system and her financial resources, she was able to obtain ambulance transfer to the rehabilitation facility of her choosing.

This physician-patient had prior knowledge of cultural competency issues with the trauma institution where she was admitted. Most of the patient population she treated was economically and/or racially disenfranchised. As a result, this institution was her only option for most specialty care referrals.

She has worked over many years with her colleagues and local institutions to educate and sensitize clinicians on the care of patients with SCD and on issues of cultural competency, diversity, and inclusion. Sharing her own journey as a physician-patient who cares for many patients with SCD, she is hopeful some of the stereotypes and assumptions will decrease, and levels of demonstrable compassion and sensitivity will increase.

References

1. Smedley BD, Stith AY, Nelson AR, editors. Unequal treatment: confronting racial and ethnic disparities in health care. Washington, DC: National Academy Press; 2003. 432p.
2. Williams DR, Mohammed SA. Discrimination and racial disparities in health: evidence and needed research. J Behav Med. 2009;32:1–38. https://doi.org/10.1007/s10865-008-9185-0.
3. Marcus EN. More sickle cell patients survive, but care is hard to find for adults [Internet]. Menlo Park: Kaiser Family Foundation; 2016 [cited 2017 Nov 13]. Available from: https://khn.org/news/more-sickle-cell-patients-survive-but-care-is-hard-to-find-for-adults/.
4. National Heart, Lung, and Blood Institute (US). Evidence-based management of sickle cell disease: expert panel report, 2014. Washington, DC: U.S. Department of Health and Human Services National Institute of Health; 2014. 161p.
5. Solomon LR. Pain management in adults with sickle cell disease in a medical center emergency department. J Natl Med Assoc. 2010;102:1025–32.
6. Furlanetto TW, Faulhaber GAM. Hypomagnesemia and proton pump inhibitors: below the tip of the iceberg. Arch Intern Med. 2011;171(15):1391–2. https://doi.org/10.1001/archinternmed.2011.199.
7. Zehtabchi S, Sinert R, Rinnert S, Chang B, Heinis C, Altura RA, Altura BT, Altura BM. Serum ionized magnesium levels and ionized calcium-to-magnesium ratios in adult patients with sickle cell anemia. Am J Hematol. 2004;77:215–22.
8. Wong ET, Rude RK, Singer FR, Shaw ST Jr. A high prevalence of hypomagnesemia and hypermagnesemia in hospitalized patients. Am J Clin Pathol. 1983;79(3):348.
9. Shapiro BS, Benjamin LJ, Payne R, Heidrich G. Sickle cell-related pain: perceptions of medical practitioners. J Pain Symptom Manag. 1997;14(30):168–74. https://doi.org/10.1016/S0885-3924(97)00019-5.
10. Haywood C Jr, Tanabe P, Naik R, Beach MC, Lanzkron S. The impact of race and disease on sickle cell patient wait times in the emergency department. Am J Emerg Med. 2013;4:651–6.
11. Begley S. 'Every time it's a battle': in excruciating pain, sickle cell patients are shunted aside [Internet]. Boston: STAT News; 2017 [cited 2017 Nov 13]. Available from: https://www.statnews.com/2017/09/18/sickle-cell-pain-treatment/.
12. Drayer RA, Henderson J, Reidenberg M. Barriers to better pain control in hospitalized patients. J Pain Symptom Manag. 1999;6:434–40. https://doi.org/10.1016/S0885-3924(99)00022-6.

Chapter 26
Rage Attack and Racial Slurs

Marcus L. Martin, DeVanté J. Cunningham, Leigh-Ann J. Webb, and Emmanuel Agyemang-Dua

Case Scenario

Ms. Meghan Eller is a 25-year-old white female who presents to the emergency department (ED) early Saturday morning. Ms. Tracy Smith, a close family friend accompanying Ms. Eller, has noted increasingly strange behavior over the past few days and has encouraged Ms. Eller to seek medical attention. The triage nurse documents her chief complaint: "I have run out of medicine and must see a doctor immediately." When asked what medicine she is prescribed, she raises her voice and repeats, "I need to see a doctor, *now*!" Ms. Eller begins to pace and mumble. The nurse and Ms. Smith are unable to calm her. Ms. Eller is placed on security precautions and quickly transferred from triage to a room in the ED.

Dr. Alvin Hairston, an African-American, is the attending emergency physician on duty supervising three emergency medicine residents and two medical students. He is made aware of Ms. Eller immediately after she is placed on security precautions. Dr. Hairston and a medical student approach Ms. Eller in the exam room and immediately notice her odd behavior. She continues to pace back and forth in her room. Upon approach, she repetitiously screams "doctor nigger" with intermittent expletives ("f-you," "f-me"). Although offended, Dr. Hairston maintains a professional demeanor and addresses the expletives directly by emphasizing to the patient that he is there to help her but will not tolerate derogatory language against any of

M. L. Martin (✉) · L.-A. J. Webb · E. Agyemang-Dua
University of Virginia, Charlottesville, VA, USA
e-mail: mlm8n@virginia.edu; lcj2p@virginia.edu; ea9cf@virginia.edu

D. J. Cunningham
Clinical Psychology, Montclair State University, Montclair, NJ, USA
e-mail: cunninghamd3@montclair.edu

© Springer International Publishing AG, part of Springer Nature 2019
M. L. Martin et al. (eds.), *Diversity and Inclusion in Quality Patient Care*,
https://doi.org/10.1007/978-3-319-92762-6_26

the staff in the ED. Ms. Eller refuses to cooperate with Dr. Hairston. She twists away in defiance as he attempts a physical exam. Dr. Hairston leaves the room for a quick chart review, and an African-American female resident, Dr. Ellen Benson, steps in to evaluate the "new patient," unaware of the patient's encounter with Dr. Hairston. The patient's agitation intensifies, and she spits and yells out, "F-all nigger doctors." Several security officers are now at the bedside.

Dr. Benson makes futile attempts to verbally de-escalate the situation before discussing treatment options with Dr. Hairston, who has returned to the bedside. Dr. Hairston's review of the electronic medical record indicates a previous diagnosis of Tourette syndrome (TS) with similar presentations to the ED. Drs. Benson and Hairston presume the patient is having another "rage attack" and agree to administer intramuscular Haldol and Ativan. Ms. Eller is chemically sedated and sleeps in the department with continuous cardiac monitoring and one-to-one security observation. Collateral information obtained from friends and family indicates that the patient's previous rage attacks were precipitated after periods of medication nonadherence.

Three hours later, Ms. Eller is slightly groggy but remains calm and cooperative. She informs her nurse that she has not taken her current medication, Paxil, for about 2 weeks and has not seen a psychiatrist in at least 6 months. Two weeks ago, following an argument with her mother about her lifestyle, she discarded her medications. At this time, the ED team is able to reassess her. The patient is able to affirm that she has no suicidal or homicidal ideation. She denies alcohol and illicit drug use prior to arrival and is cooperative with both a complete history and physical examination.

Review of Symptoms

Negative for head trauma, no recent illness

Past Medical History

Major depressive disorder, anxiety, Tourette syndrome (TS) diagnosed at age 16, history of rage attacks
   Past Medications: Paxil
   Past Surgical History: Appendectomy

Family History

Type II diabetes

Social History

Drinks two beers daily, smokes a half pack of cigarettes per day, denies illicit drugs; ran out of her medication 2 weeks ago; no doctor's visit in at least 6 months; frequently argues with her family

Physical Exam

Vital Signs Temp 98.9, BP 130/80, HR 107, RR 16, oxygen saturation 95% RA

General Slightly unkempt appearance

HEENT Pupils equal, round, reactive to light, normal oropharynx

Neck Supple, no lymphadenopathy

Cardiovascular Regular rate and rhythm, no murmurs/rubs/gallops

Respiratory Lungs clear to auscultation bilaterally

Abdomen Soft, non-tender, non-distended

Neuro Alert, oriented, cranial nerves II-XII intact

Skin Normal

Extremities Normal, no edema

Psychiatric Agitated, nonlinear thought process on arrival, now calm and cooperative

Questions for Discussion

1. What is the Tourette's disorder, or Tourette syndrome (TS)?
      The DSM-5 diagnostic criteria for Tourette syndrome is (A-D) [1].
   (a) Two or more occurrences of motor tics and one or more vocal tics, although not necessarily concurrently.
   (b) The tics may be daily or intermittent for at least 1 year.
   (c) The onset is prior to 18 years old.
   (d) The disturbance is not attributable to the physiological effects of a substance, medication, or another medical condition.

2. What precipitates this "rage attack"?

Attitudes/Assumptions: The Physician

(a) Ms. Eller has a history of rage attacks. Medication nonadherence, anxiety, arguments with her mother, and possibly a change in environment are potential catalysts or triggers for this attack [2].
(b) It is important that the physicians manage the care of Ms. Eller in a professional manner and provide the highest quality care.
(c) Ms. Eller's negative comments about African-American physicians may have been without ill intention, but it is unclear if she has unconscious racial bias.

Attitudes/Assumptions: The Patient

(a) Sometimes I just get so tense and anxious that I explode. My medicine doesn't work most of the time. So I drink a few beers and smoke to take off the edge, but I still take my pills almost every day. I just can't help it. I don't want my doctors to judge me.
(b) I moved back home 2 weeks ago, and my mom and I got into an argument about my lifestyle and about taking my medications. So I flushed my medications down the toilet because I'm an adult, and she can't tell me what to do anymore.
(c) I have no clue why those words were coming out my mouth. I wasn't trying to be racist or direct hurtful slurs at anyone. I couldn't help it. I'm so embarrassed when this happens.

Case Outcome

Diagnosis Tourette syndrome with acute rage attack

Disposition The patient is discharged from ED in stable condition with her friend. After a lengthy discussion with her psychiatrist, the decision is made to renew her prescription for paroxetine, and she is advised to follow up with both her primary care physician and psychiatrist. Additionally, the patient allows Dr. Benson to discuss her presentation to the ED, interventions, and future plans with her mother over the telephone. Her mother agrees to assist with follow-up appointments.

References

1. American Psychiatric Association. Section II, Tic disorders. In: Diagnostic and statistical manual of mental disorders. 5th ed. Washington, DC: APA; 2013. p. 81–5.
2. Cath DC, Ludolph AG. Chapter 4, Other psychiatric comorbidities in Tourette syndrome. In: Tourette syndrome. New York: Oxford University Press; 2013. p. 74–106.

Chapter 27
Use of Interpreter Phone

Denee Moore

Case Scenario

A 38-year-old Latino female, whose preferred language is Spanish, comes to the primary care office for a well-woman exam with Papanicolaou (Pap) test. The Spanish telephone interpreter is used during the entire visit. When obtaining the OB-GYN history, the patient informs the physician that she has a Mirena intrauterine device (IUD) that was inserted by a physician at another office 11 months ago. She tells the physician that she returned to the office 1 month after insertion for routine IUD monitoring and was told that "everything is okay." When the physician performs a pelvic exam to obtain a cervical sample for the Pap test and to confirm the placement of the IUD, the physician is unable to visualize the IUD strings. When the physician informs the patient that the IUD strings are not visualized, the patient expresses great surprise regarding the physician's findings. Also, the patient voices her concerns about the device's effectiveness and the potential medical complications that could arise from a malpositioned IUD. The physician requests records from the physician who inserted the IUD, and the records are obtained and reviewed with the patient during the office visit. The records indicate that during the IUD monitoring appointment, the physician who inserted the IUD was not able to visualize the IUD strings. A pelvic ultrasound was performed the same day by the physician who inserted the IUD which confirmed that the IUD was in the correct position inside the uterus. The physician who inserted the IUD recommended routine office follow-up. There is no documentation that interpreter services were used during that visit.

D. Moore
Central Virginia Health Services, Charlottesville, VA, USA

© Springer International Publishing AG, part of Springer Nature 2019
M. L. Martin et al. (eds.), *Diversity and Inclusion in Quality Patient Care*,
https://doi.org/10.1007/978-3-319-92762-6_27

Review of Symptoms

The patient denies abdominal pain, pelvic pain, heavy menstrual periods, or irregular menstrual periods. All other systems are reported negative.

Past Medical History

Seasonal allergies, non-morbid obesity, cervical intraepithelial neoplasia (CIN) I

Family History

Family members are healthy.

Social History

She does not smoke, drink, or use alcohol. She lives with her significant other and their children.

Physical Exam

Vital Signs Temp, 97.9 F; pulse, 61; BP, 110/80; respirations, 18; O_2 Sat 99% on room air

General In no acute distress

Cardiovascular Regular rate and rhythm; no murmurs, rubs, or gallops

Respiratory Clear breath sounds throughout

Abdomen Bowel sounds present, soft, non-tender, non-distended

Genitourinary Chaperone present in room, external genitalia normal without rashes or lesions, vaginal mucosa without lesions, no vaginal discharge present, cervix normal in appearance and without lesions, IUD strings are not visualized in the cervical os.

Questions for Discussion

1. Why was the patient unaware of the details surrounding her IUD?

Attitudes/Assumptions: The Physician Who Inserted the IUD

(a) The pelvic ultrasound shows that the IUD is in the correct position within the uterus, which means that it is effective.
(b) Patients do not need to know all the details about a medical device or treatment; the basics are usually sufficient.
(c) Using interpreter services during routine, basic office visits such as this one can slow workflow; most patients know basic words/phrases such as "okay" or basic gestures that signal positivity such as a "thumbs up" regardless of their primary language.

Attitudes/Assumptions: The Patient

(a) The physician who inserted the IUD and initially discovered the missing IUD strings should have notified me about this finding during my visit with them.
(b) Although I have not experienced any problems so far, I am very concerned that I may experience problems in the future due to the missing IUD strings.
(c) I am no longer sure if I can trust physicians to give me all the information I need regarding my health care.

Gaps in Provider Knowledge

(a) Lack of knowledge regarding a patient's need for information: Some patients prefer basic information about their health conditions, while other patients prefer extensive details about the same.
(b) Lack of knowledge of communication barriers: Effective communication is key to improving healthcare outcomes and improving patient satisfaction with healthcare delivery.
(c) Lack of knowledge of disparities: Some groups of patients, particularly those of ethnic minorities, limited English proficiency, and low socioeconomic backgrounds, are more likely to endorse experiencing negative interactions with the healthcare system than other groups. These perceived negative interactions can affect understanding of and compliance with the treatment plan which can then lead to negative health outcomes [1].

2. What actions could have been taken by the physician who inserted the IUD to avoid/prevent this outcome?

Cross-Cultural Tools and Skills

(a) Assume that the patient wants to be an active participant in her health care.

(b) Assume that if you communicate with the patient effectively, she will understand any potential implications of your findings and will be able to notify you promptly if a problem were to arise.

(c) Assess the patient's need for healthcare information and deliver the information in an appropriate fashion.

3. What medical issues concern you about this case?

(a) The physician did not communicate with the patient in her preferred language which can lead to misunderstandings about findings and the treatment plan. Title VI of the Civil Rights Act mandates that professional interpreter services be available for all patients who have limited English proficiency [1–3].

(b) The physician who inserted the IUD should discuss with the patient the potential implications of missing IUD strings, perform the tests necessary to confirm correct positioning of the IUD, inform the patient as to whether the IUD is positioned correctly, and if the IUD is positioned correctly, reassure the patient that the device is still effective and give the patient information on the symptoms of a malpositioned IUD that would warrant further evaluation.

4. Which components of the Milestones of the ACGME competencies are incorporated in the case?

(a) Demonstrates humanism and cultural proficiency [4].
(b) Develops meaningful, therapeutic relationships with patients and families [4].
(c) Communicates effectively with patients, families, and the public [4].

Case Outcome

Diagnosis IUD in place

Disposition Home

After reviewing the pelvic ultrasound results which confirmed the correct positioning of the IUD in the uterus, the physician informs the patient that the IUD is still effective, and a minor surgical procedure will need to be performed to remove the IUD in the future. The patient was given information regarding symptoms that could occur if the IUD is malpositioned, and the patient was instructed to return to the physician's office immediately if these symptoms occur. The patient verbalized understanding.

References

1. Juckett G, Unger K. Appropriate use of medical interpreters. Am Fam Physician [serial on the Internet]. 2014 [cited 2017 Sept 24];90(7):476–80. Available from: http://www.aafp.org/afp/2014/1001/p476.html.
2. The United States Department of Justice. Executive order 13166 [document on Internet]. Washington, DC: The Department of Justice; 2015 [cited 2017 Sept 24]. Available from: https://www.justice.gov/crt/executive-order-13166.
3. The United States Department of Justice. Limited English proficiency (LEP): a federal inter-agency website [document on Internet]. Washington, DC: The Department of Justice; 2017 [cited 2017 Sept 24]. Available from: https://www.lep.gov/.
4. The Family Medicine Milestone Project [Internet]. Chicago: The Accreditation Council for Graduate Medical Education and the American Board of Family Medicine; 2013 [cited 20 Jul 2017]. Available from: https://www.acgme.org/Portals/0/PDFs/Milestones/FamilyMedicineMilestones.pdf.

Chapter 28
Labeling Patients

Gwyneth Milbrath

Case Scenario

A 53-year-old white American female arrives with her two grandchildren 10 min late for her first appointment with her primary care provider at a federally qualified health center. Today is her third scheduled appointment, having missed the first appointment, canceled the second appointment, and rescheduled for today. The healthcare provider reviewed the patient's records from her last primary care provider and pain management clinic, both of which had "fired" her for being "drug-seeking," "non-compliant," and a "no show." The patient has several documented chronic medical conditions. Since being "fired" from her former healthcare providers last month, she has been to the emergency department four times: twice for panic attacks and twice for severe, non-traumatic back pain, where she was prescribed a short 2–3-day course of lorazepam and hydrocodone-acetaminophen, respectively. Today, the patient is asking for an assessment of her chronic back pain and fatigue, and a refill of her pain and anxiety medications. The provider investigates her record of controlled drug use and notes that she has asked for and been granted refills for oxycodone more frequently than would be expected based on her prescription.

G. Milbrath
College of Nursing, University of Illinois at Chicago, Chicago, IL, USA
e-mail: gwyneth@uic.edu

© Springer International Publishing AG, part of Springer Nature 2019
M. L. Martin et al. (eds.), *Diversity and Inclusion in Quality Patient Care*,
https://doi.org/10.1007/978-3-319-92762-6_28

Review of Symptoms

Subjectively, the patient reports ongoing fatigue and insomnia that have not worsened but have not improved over the past several weeks since she saw her former healthcare provider. She reports mid-lower back pain radiating down both legs with weakness and tingling in both her legs. She rates her pain at a 9/10 and states that the only thing that helps is her pain medication. She says she has had two panic attacks this month from an unknown trigger and often wakes up in the morning with a headache.

Past Medical History

Depression, anxiety, fibromyalgia, hypertension, obesity, hyperlipidemia, degenerative disk disease, type II diabetes, stage one renal failure, history of non-healing surgical wounds.

Medication List (unverified) Acetaminophen 650 mg every 6 h as needed for pain, alprazolam 0.5 mg every 8 h as needed for panic attacks, aspirin 81 mg daily, duloxetine hydrochloride 20 mg twice daily, estradiol 0.5 mg daily, gabapentin 600 mg three times daily, insulin glargine 28 units at bedtime, metformin 1000 mg twice per day, metoprolol tartrate 50 mg daily, oxycodone 10 mg every 6 h as needed for severe pain, quetiapine 50 mg daily at bedtime, simvastatin 40 mg daily, zolpidem 5 mg at bedtime

Past Surgical History Hysterectomy, cholecystectomy, right inguinal hernia repair, left total knee replacement

Family History

The patient states she was adopted at age 4 and has no known medical history from her biological family.

Social History

The patient states she lives in a two-bedroom apartment with her daughter, her daughter's boyfriend, and their two children, aged 6 months and 3 years. She has been disabled for the last 5 years and is dependent on Social Security and her daughter's boyfriend for income. She has a high school education and most recently worked at a call center until she became disabled due to her back pain and fibromyalgia. Her daughter's boyfriend has a vehicle, which he primarily uses to get to and from work and transport his children and girlfriend when needed.

Physical Exam

Vital Signs Temp, 98.4 °F; pulse, 72; BP, 182/104; respirations, 16, O_2 Sat 97% on room air; height, 5 ft. 5in; weight, 230lbs; BMI, 38.3; blood glucose, 274

General Obese female, ambulates with a walker

Cardiovascular S1 and S2, rate of 72 with no murmurs, gallops, or rubs

Respiratory Clear and equal bilaterally, no apparent distress, no increased work of breathing

HEENT Tympanic membranes not visualized due to excessive wax, nose clear, throat clear, no erythema, uvula midline; Neck is non-tender, no adenopathy

Abdomen Rounded, non-tender with hypoactive bowel sounds, no palpable masses, or organomegaly

Extremities No cyanosis, mild 1+ non-pitting edema noted to bilateral lower extremities

Skin No rashes or lesions

Neuro CN I–XII intact; PERRLA; 5/5 strength noted to bilateral upper extremities, 5/5 strength bilateral lower extremities; Tingling reported in bilateral lower extremities L > R. Sensation intact; Patient is tender to palpation along her spine from L1– L5. No deformities noted.

Psych Patient appears disheveled, body odor noted during exam, patient has poor eye contact and states she is feeling anxious. She denies any suicidal or homicidal ideation.

After the physical exam, the physician reviews the patient's medication and finds out she has not been taking her insulin glargine, metformin, estradiol, simvastatin, or metoprolol because she cannot afford her prescriptions. She states her other medications are up to date, except she is also out of her alprazolam and oxycodone. The provider confronts her about her frequent refills on her oxycodone and alprazolam and expresses concerns that she is abusing the medication. The patient vehemently denies abusing or misusing her prescriptions but cannot give the provider a reason to explain her "drug-seeking behavior." The physician then educates the patient about the importance of taking her other medications to manage her diabetes and high blood pressure and that some of her symptoms may be due to her not taking her medications as directed. The patient appears withdrawn with poor eye contact, holds her belongings in her lap, and keeps looking toward the door like she is ready to leave.

Questions for Discussion

1. What patterns of behavior are concerning?
2. What medical issues concern you about this case?
3. What social issues concern you about this case?
4. What assumptions were made by the patient? By the provider?

Attitudes/Assumptions: The Provider

(a) This patient is on public insurance and abuses the healthcare system by doctor shopping and looking for drugs. There is probably nothing medically causing her pain, and it would be a waste of resources to order tests that I know will just be normal.
(b) Maybe if she took her other medications and tried to take care of her health I would be more inclined to give her pain medication.
(c) This patient is going to take up so much of my time and I won't get paid what I deserve for trying to help her.

Attitudes/Assumptions: The Patient

(d) None of the other doctors will listen to me or take me seriously, so this person is probably no different. Even if I tell the doctor the truth, she won't believe me.
(e) I know the doctor says I should take my other medications, but they don't always make me feel better when I take them, and they are too expensive.
(f) I came here for help with my pain and anxiety, and the doctor won't help me; she only wants to talk about what is important to her. No one will help me.
(g) I know I should only go to the ER for emergencies, but they treat my pain and are better doctors because they order more tests.

5. What actions could have been taken by the doctor to avoid/prevent this unfortunate outcome?

Gaps in Provider Knowledge

(a) "Drug-seeking" is often used when discussing patients, but the term is rarely used in documentation, and it is not well defined. Often, the term is applied to people who have a perceived major social flaw, such as chemical dependency, or the provider feels the patient is challenging him or her for control of the interaction [1].

(b) Most of the patient's perceived stigma associated with poverty or being drug-seeking is based on their experience with their provider; however, occasionally it can come from an internal sense of shame related to being uninsured or on public insurance [2].

(c) Patients with inconsistent stories are not always being deceptive. Their lack of knowledge of their medical history could be due to cognitive impairment, medication side effects, psychiatric illness, or difficulty communicating due to language or cultural differences. Their level of pain intensity can also affect their ability to recall their past pain or medication usage over the past days or weeks [1].

(d) Some people may not be aware of the "street value" of their medications and may not protect their medication from theft or abuse by family members [1].

Cross-Cultural Tools and Skills

Negative Consequences of Stigma

(a) According to sociologists Link and Phelan, stigma occurs when a label associated with a negative stereotype is attached to a characteristic, causing people with this characteristic to be seen as separate from and lower in status than others [3].

(b) The process of stigmatization discounts the multidimensionality of a person and reduces them to be defined by a single, negative characteristic, causing the individual to be discredited, devalued, rejected, and socially excluded [4].

(c) If people are deemed responsible for their condition, they are judged with anger and blame and stigmatized. Those deemed not responsible for their condition are judged with more sympathy and acceptance. This can be applied to patients who are seen as impoverished or in pain. If they are deemed not responsible for their situation in life, they are more likely to be treated with sympathy and acceptance [5].

(d) When patients are labeled as drug-seeking, healthcare professionals are less likely to believe a patient is in acute pain or that their pain is undertreated [1].

(e) When patients' pain is undertreated, patients are less honest with their provider and are more likely to change their behavior to a behavior they believe is more likely to get them out of pain, causing them to become manipulative [1].

Health Disparities in Poverty

(a) With the expansion of Medicaid in several states, an estimated 12 million low-income adults became newly eligible for health insurance. However, access became a major issue as many primary care providers could not accept many new patients with Medicaid [2].

(b) Low socioeconomic status (SES) is associated with large health disparities across the lifespan including health status, morbidity, and mortality [6].

(c) Pregnant women with a low SES have a higher rate of adverse birth outcomes, including unplanned pregnancy, single parenthood, smoking, urinary tract infections, inadequate prenatal care, low birth rate, and infant mortality [6].

(d) Children living in poverty are more likely to die from infectious disease or suffer from sudden infant death syndrome, accidents, child abuse, lead poisoning, household smoke, asthma, developmental delay, learning disabilities, conduct disturbances, preventable hospitalizations, and exposure to violence at a young age [6].

(e) Adolescents with low SES homes have higher rates of pregnancy, sexually transmitted infections, depression, obesity, suicide, sexual abuse, and accidental or violent death [6].

(f) Adults with a low SES are more likely to experience chronic morbidity, disability, and earlier onset of hypertension, diabetes, cardiovascular disease, obesity, arthritis, depression, poor dental health, and several types of cancer [6].

(g) A lack of resources, including educational, financial, and access to health care, is more prevalent for those with a low SES and associated with chronic stress. Exposure to chronic stress increases allostatic load, causing adverse metabolic, autonomic, and neurologic effects [6].

(h) Low income is also associated with reduced access to health care, fewer cardiac procedures, less preventative care for children and adults, and worse outcomes following medical procedures [6].

(i) Medicaid reimburses at a significantly lower rate than other insurances, despite the higher risk and more work and time often required to medically manage these patients [6].

Clinical Tools

(a) Before passing judgment on someone that may be drug seeking, the provider should stop and think, "What would the patient have to say or do to make me relieve the pain?" [1].

(b) Instead of labeling patients as "drug-seeking," the behaviors can be described as "concern-raising" which can alert the provider to unusual behavior while still conveying a caring and positive attitude toward the patient [1].

(c) Instead of dictating the nature of the interaction, use the experience of both the clinician and the patient in a shared space, where neither is considered an expert, and discussions can take place with an open mind. In this shared space, both the clinician and the patient can resist socially or culturally determined stereotypes [4].

(d) Rather than avoiding the issue, discuss the concerning behavior with the patient in a respectful manner to determine the meaning and cause of the behavior and to work together to develop a solution [1].

(e) To help those feeling stigmatized, providers can refer them for educational and counseling interventions, which provide information and support to help people make good decisions. Journaling or other forms of expression can help a person cope with their feelings of stigma [7].

(f) Other interventions to help decrease the feeling of stigma include addressing the stigmatized person's sense of belonging, connecting with the person who feels stigmatized on a personal level, and affirming that the person is valued in society [7].

Case Outcome

Diagnosis Anxiety disorder, unspecified; chronic back pain greater than 3 months; insomnia, unspecified; failed compliance with medical treatment or regimen; diabetes, poorly controlled; unspecified essential hypertension

Disposition The provider writes new prescriptions for insulin glargine, metformin, estradiol, simvastatin, and metoprolol but does not refill her alprazolam or oxycodone and refers the patient to a pain management specialist.

Although the patient showed concerning behavior that indicated she may be abusing narcotics, the urine drug screen on the patient was negative for narcotics. The office care manager completed a home visit and assessment on the patient and discovered that her daughter's boyfriend was stealing her pain and anxiety medications. The patient did not feel safe enough to trust her provider with the information and is afraid that she will no longer be able to live with her daughter if she reports her daughter's boyfriend to the police. According to the care manager, the patient was able to get her other medications refilled and is taking them as directed, and her future narcotic and anxiety medications will be kept in a locked medication box. The care manager also scheduled a follow-up appointment to reassess her progress in 3 weeks.

References

1. McCaffery M, Grimm MA, Pasero C, Ferrell B, Uman GC. On the meaning of "drug seeking". Pain Manag Nurs. 2005;6(4):122–36.
2. Allen H, Wright BJ, Harding K, Broffman L. The role of stigma in access to health care for the poor. Milbank Q. 2014;92(2):289–318.
3. Link BG, Phelan JC. Conceptualizing stigma. Annu Rev Sociol. 2001;27(1):363–85.
4. Cohen M, Quintner J, Buchanan D, Nielsen M, Guy L. Stigmatization of patients with chronic pain: the extinction of empathy. Pain Med. 2011;12(11):1637–43.
5. Decety J, Echols S, Correll J. The blame game: the effect of responsibility and social stigma on empathy for pain. J Cogn Neurosci. 2010;22(5):985–97.
6. Fiscella K, Williams DR. Health disparities based on socioeconomic inequities: implications for urban health care. Acad Med. 2004;79(12):1139–47.
7. Cook JE, Purdie-Vaughns V, Meyer IH, Busch JT. Intervening within and across levels: a multilevel approach to stigma and public health. Soc Sci Med. 2014;103:101–9.

Chapter 29
Waiting for a Miracle

Kevin Adams, Rebecca Adrian, Mildred Best, Jamie L. W. Kennedy, Swami Sarvaananda, and Yoshiya Takahashi

Case Scenario

Mr. M, also referred to as M, is a 73-year-old African-American male who presents to the emergency department (ED) of a level 1 trauma center complaining of severe shortness of breath. Mr. M was brought into the ED via emergency medical service (EMS) subsequent to a 911 call made by the patient's younger sister with whom the patient currently resides. Upon arrival, the patient is receiving supplemental oxygen by face mask. On examination by the ED staff, the patient is becoming increasingly lethargic and minimally responsive.

Mr. M has congestive heart failure (CHF) and is known to this medical center and to the ED from previous admissions over the past 12 years, most recently with three admissions in the past 6 months. With each admission, the patient's health has declined, with worsening cardiac function and progressive end-organ dysfunction despite all appropriate medical therapies. At his best, he is able to walk from room to room in his home with a walker. During his last admission, the cardiology fellow's record of a conversation with Mr. M indicated his desire that

K. Adams (✉) · R. Adrian · M. Best · Y. Takahashi
Chaplaincy Services and Pastoral Education, University of Virginia Health System, Charlottesville, VA, USA
e-mail: kea3a@virginia.edu; raa8n@virginia.edu; mb3aq@virginia.edu; yt8gG@virginia.edu

J. L. W. Kennedy
Cardiovascular Medicine, University of Virginia Health System, Charlottesville, VA, USA
e-mail: JLK4B@hscmail.mcc.virginia.edu

S. Sarvaananda
Clinical Pastoral Education Programs, University of Virginia Health System, Charlottesville, VA, USA

© Springer International Publishing AG, part of Springer Nature 2019
M. L. Martin et al. (eds.), *Diversity and Inclusion in Quality Patient Care*,
https://doi.org/10.1007/978-3-319-92762-6_29

no extraordinary measures be taken to resuscitate him should he suffer an arrest. Per Mr. M's request, a do-not-resuscitate (DNR) order was placed in his chart. Mr. M's desire for no extraordinary measures was reinforced in a note by his attending cardiologist at a follow-up clinic appointment 1 week post-discharge. Mr. M does not have a healthcare power of attorney, living will, or durable DNR. Of note, an implantable cardioverter defibrillator for primary prevention of sudden cardiac death has been discussed with Mr. M several times over the last few years which he has consistently declined because he does not want artificial things in his body.

Mr. M is not married and has no children. His parents died over 20 years prior, father from lung cancer and mother of complications from a cerebral vascular accident (CVA). The patient has three siblings, two younger sisters and an older brother. He lives with one sister, and both sisters are in good health. His brother died 6 months prior of complications due to a ST-elevation myocardial infarction (STEMI).

Both sisters arrived together to the ED approximately 15 min after the patient. As ED staff were assessing the patient, Mr. M demonstrated increasing difficulty breathing and weak heart function. The ED attending physician assessed that there was a slim likelihood the patient could return to baseline from his previous discharge. The treatment options were to intubate Mr. M for pulmonary support and start inotropes and vasopressors to temporarily augment cardiac heart function or to keep the patient comfortable and not interfere with the dying process.

Review of Symptoms

Significant for unintentional weight loss of 30 lbs. over the last 6 months, poor appetite, frequent nausea and occasional vomiting, dyspnea with minimal exertion, orthopnea, paroxysmal nocturnal dyspnea, edema, fatigue, and depression.

Past Medical History

Significant for hypertension diagnosed in his 30s, heart failure due to nonischemic cardiomyopathy diagnosed at age 61, and progressive renal insufficiency over the last 2 years.

Family History

His brother died 6 months prior of complications due to a ST-elevation myocardial infarction (STEMI).

Social History

Nonsmoker, does not drink alcohol or use illicit drugs.

Physical Exam

Vital signs Pulse 115, respiratory rate 28, BP 98/70, SpO$_2$ 90% on 15 LPM

General Cachectic African-American gentleman, tachypneic, and somnolent

Head No scleral icterus, clear oropharynx, temporal wasting

Neck Marked jugular venous distention, no carotid bruits, supple, no lymphadenopathy

ENT Unremarkable

Cardiovascular Tachycardic but regular, S3 gallop present, II/VI holosystolic murmur at the apex

Respiratory Coarse crackles halfway up

Abdomen Bowel sounds present, soft, tender liver edge palpable 2 inches below the costal margin, mildly distended with ascites

Extremities Cool, 2+ bilateral lower extremity edema, radial pulses 2+ bilaterally, pedal pulses 1+ bilaterally

Skin Stasis dermatitis changes of the bilateral lower extremities

What Was Said?

The ED attending approached Mr. M's sisters, who were waiting in a consult room. The attending summarized the patient's medical history, including his current condition and his documented conversations during his previous admission and clinic visit. The attending then recommended that the previous DNR order be reinstated and Mr. M be transitioned to comfort care.

The patient's sisters refused the recommended plan of care despite knowledge of the patient's stated wishes to the healthcare team. Mr. M has had heart failure for over 12 years, has had episodes just like this before, and has always come back. The sisters said that God has had many opportunities to "take him home to heaven" and has not chosen to do so. They went further to say that if God had wanted to take M, there is nothing anyone would be able to do about it, so God must want M to stay around a while longer. Mr. M is a deacon in their church and is well-loved and respected by everyone in the community, both inside and outside the church. He has done a lot of work on God's behalf, and there are people all over the world in constant prayer for his healing. They have been assured by godly people they know and respect that God is going to heal Mr. M. Further, they dispute that Mr. M said these things to anyone. Not only is Mr. M a fighter and has never given up on life, Mr. M would never give up on God and God's promise to heal him so that he can continue on in service to God and the church. The sisters both reinforced that it was up to all of God's people to remain steadfast and have faith in God's promise by continuing to do everything for Mr. M.

Mr. M was not showing any indication of improving, so the ED team intubated him and started inotropes and vasopressors. He was admitted to the cardiac care unit (CCU) pending bed availability. Because of the resistance to comfort care based on religious reasons, a chaplain consult was requested and the ED chaplain was immediately paged.

After a consult with the ED team regarding Mr. M's history, current condition, and the attending's conversation with the family, the chaplain went to an ED consult room to meet with the sisters, both of whom who were open to her presence. Mr. M and his sisters are active members of a Pentecostal Christian church in the local area. He and his siblings grew up attending this church, and their parents were charter members when the church started over 75 years prior. A central tenet of their church's faith is in God's power to affect direct change in creation, one manifestation of this activity being miraculous physical healing. God's power and love are absolute, and it is the duty of God's people to believe in God's power to heal and to never allow doubt to diminish this faith.

During their conversation, the chaplain asked the sisters if Mr. M had ever spoken with them about his worsening condition and what he wanted to do should he ever be so sick that he could not speak for himself. They said he did not talk much about his condition to them, but they knew him to be someone who loved life. He would never give up on trying to live and be with his family as long as he could. They felt there was no way that he ever told the doctors he wanted to stop. They thought it was something the doctors decided, or maybe they pressured or manipulated Mr. M into agreeing to the DNR. After all, it would not be the first time. When the chaplain asked them what they meant, they replied that their brother who died 6 months prior was just someone's research project, and those people did not really care what happened to him. They said they were determined to not let that happen to M. They were going to keep pushing the doctors to do everything until God intervened in God's own time.

What Was Done?

The chaplain consulted with the ED team and with members of the CCU team who were in the ED assessing the patient for transfer. An ED physician and the chaplain returned to speak with the sisters. The physician provided an update of M's condition and queried his sisters for more information about the other brother and his death. They explained that about 3 months after his death, they received a letter from the emergency medical service that transported him to the hospital informing them that their brother was part of a research study on emergency transportation. It seemed to them that people were still being treated as research subjects without their knowledge and that some things never change.

M was transferred to the CCU. Over the next 72 h, the CCU team explored all possible treatment options. During that time, M's condition deteriorated, and he became increasingly dependent on vasopressors. Unfortunately, his renal function declined precipitously, and renal replacement therapy was considered. As his sisters were M's next of kin, the team provided them with regular updates of all test results and consulted with them on the plan of care. During that same time, the CCU physicians were available for as-needed consults with family. There were also two interprofessional goals of care conversations that included cardiology, nephrology, nursing, chaplaincy, social work, the two sisters, and various extended family members. The second of these meetings also included palliative care and M's/the family's pastor. The team worked to hear family concerns and maintained transparency about all their assessments and actions throughout the process.

After M was transferred to the CCU, the chaplain followed up with the family daily and participated in the goals of care meetings. Per family consent, she consulted with M's pastor when the pastor was in the hospital visiting M and his family. During the chaplain contacts, she explored M's and his family's religious faith, including their God image and how they understood God's presence in creation. The family expressed the firm belief that God's presence and authority in creation are absolute, and God will have the final say in M's healing. Part of the chaplain's intervention was exploring other ways God may affect M's healing, including this healing taking place in the next life, in God's presence, especially if medicine should reach the limit of what it can do to help and support M. The family seemed open to this consideration but were resistant to that being the case with M.

The family was consistently at M's bedside. M's condition continued to worsen despite the medications and other medical interventions. On day three of admission, the team held a third goals of care meeting with the family. During this meeting, the family acknowledged M's deteriorating condition. The cardiology attending physician provided an overview of everything that had happened since admission and a summary of M's current status. She then admitted that the team had reached the end of any therapeutic options they could offer, and she feared that anything else they did would have no positive effect for M and would instead be subjecting him to unnecessary discomfort. Palliative care added that perhaps they should consider other options for his care to make him as comfortable as possible for whatever time M was still with us.

The sisters indicated that, since the previous meeting, they had been talking about this with each other, other family members, and their pastor. They saw that the CCU team had done everything they could, and more than they imagined could be done, but M just kept getting sicker. They began to be tearful and said they were beginning to think that God may, indeed, be calling M to heaven. They said that perhaps they needed to let go of M and let him and God decide what was best.

The team recognized and empathized with the sisters and the painful process they worked through to come to this decision. The team validated the family's desire to provide M every chance to improve and supported their decision as a humane and compassionate one. The team committed to doing everything possible to keep the patient comfortable and support the family throughout this next step in the process.

Following the meeting, the CCU team collaborated with the sisters to continue pulmonary and pressor support to M until more of his family and their pastor could be present. Once family and the pastor arrived and had an opportunity to say their goodbyes, M was administered comfort care medications, extubated, and had his vasopressors turned off. The pastor prayed with M and his family at the bedside and continued to hold a vigil while M's heart rate slowed. M died approximately 1 h later surrounded by his family, his pastor, and his healthcare team.

Question for Discussion

1. What underlying attitudes and assumptions are present in this case?

Attitudes/Assumptions: The Provider

During Mr. M's stay in the medical center, there were family interactions with numerous members of the interprofessional team. The focus of this part of the discussion will be the admitting CCU attending physician, the CCU nurses, and the chaplain who followed the patient/family throughout the admission.

In the context of the Hippocratic oath pledge to "do no harm," the CCU attending physician had difficulty providing this type of care. In this case the chances of recovery were remote, the interventions aggressive, and the risks of aggressive treatment in an inpatient setting no longer outweighed any potential benefit. The physician felt like they were doing harm. As a result, the CCU attending physician found it difficult going against the patient's stated wishes even though his sisters disagreed with these wishes. In retrospect, the physician could have requested an ethics consultation.

CCU nurses are well acquainted with patients affected by heart failure, and it is likely they cared for Mr. M during several of his multiple admissions especially in the latter stages of his disease. The relationships the CCU nurses built with Mr. M presented both emotional and ethical challenges for them during his care. There was a mixture of empathy, sadness, and foreboding of when death may occur. As the people providing most of the direct care to the patient, the nurses experienced the tension between what the healthcare delivery team felt and what the family felt was in the patient's best interest. In that tension, they also carried a "burden of foreknowledge," having experienced similar patient scenarios and outcomes. In this circumstance while maintaining a professional, caring relationship with the patient and family, they have a deep desire to spare the patient and family the rigors of escalating therapies that are not only not helpful but are often futile and even painful.

Early in the interactions with the family, the chaplain recognized the gap between Mr. M's family's and the medical team's respective understandings about his condition and prognosis. She recognized the family as interpreting his prognosis through the lenses of grief and their understanding of their religious faith. The chaplain's intent was to serve in the role of a nonmedical healthcare professional who can bridge some of the distance between faith and science. She saw her role in the situation as facilitating communication between the family, the family's pastor, and the medical team. This bridge building was accomplished through listening to the family's hopes and fears and collaborating with them and the medical team to identify and access appropriate spiritual and emotional coping and meaning-making resources.

Attitudes/Assumptions: The Patient

In the current situation, the patient was unable to speak for himself. According to medical staff and chart documentation, Mr. M did not want extraordinary measures taken to extend his life. It can be inferred that his attitude was that these wishes would be carried out by his medical team. In the state of Virginia, in the absence of a formal advance directive, such as a living will or healthcare power of attorney, healthcare decisions that need to be made when a patient is incapacitated rest with the legal next of kin. In the case of Mr. M, the next of kin are his adult siblings, and decisions are made by majority consensus [1]. In this situation, therefore, the attitudes and assumptions of the family most directly affect the treatment plan. And, according to the sisters, Mr. M has never discussed with them his wishes regarding treatment options.

Lunney et al. proposed four trajectories for dying: sudden death, terminal illness, organ failure, and frailty (Fig. 29.1) [2]. Mr. M, diagnosed with CHF, had shown evidence of the organ failure trajectory through repeated hospital admissions and declining health. There is a point in disease progression at which life-extending therapies are no longer beneficial. In the case of organ failure, heart failure in particular, "...prognosis for survival remains ambiguous. For example, half of heart failure patients who die from their disease do so within 1 week of the point at which a multivariable prognostic model would assign them at least a 50% probability of living 6 months longer" [2].

Mr. M and his cardiologist seemed to have concluded that his prognosis was poor and there was need for a change in the treatment plan. On the other hand, Mr. M had never discussed his condition with his family. As a result, they were unaware of his health decline. This altered their perception of his illness. Since they saw that he always recovered, their perception would be more of a modified sudden death tra-

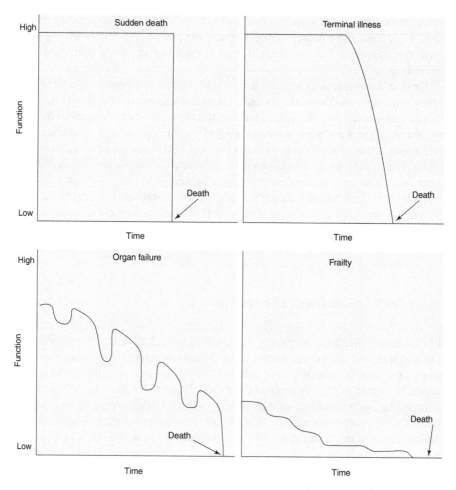

Fig. 29.1 Proposed trajectories of dying. Lunney et al. proposed four trajectories for dying: sudden death, terminal illness, organ failure, and frailty [2]

jectory that would have been interspersed with episodes of illness followed by full recovery (Fig. 29.2). This modified trajectory would end only with God's direct intervention at which time no medical therapy would be able to alter it.

Family attitudes seemed to have been influenced by three additional factors: family interpretation of their religious faith, the history of tension between medicine and the African-American community, and the recent death of Mr. M's and the sisters' brother. One of the central features of the Pentecostal church is divine healing from illness [3]. For example, the belief statement of the Church of God in Christ, regarding divine healing, says, "Therefore, we believe that healing by faith in God has scriptural support and ordained authority. St. James' writings in his epistle encourage Elders to pray for the sick, lay hands upon them and to anoint them with oil, and that prayers with faith shall heal the sick and the Lord shall raise them up" [4].

Fig. 29.2 Family perception of patient's decline and end of life. Family perceived that patient would return to previous baseline of functioning until God decided the time of patient's death

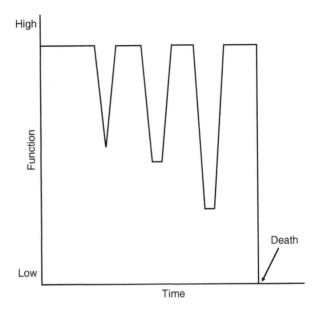

There is a historical tension between the African-American community and health care. This dynamic is evident in the sisters' concerns about the other brother being treated as a research subject without their knowledge, most likely a direct reference to the Tuskegee Syphilis Study, which ran from 1932 to 1972. "In content and form, the historical Tuskegee episode has been central to boundaries of modern African American trust in the medical system…" [5]. The relevance of Tuskegee speaks to African-Americans as a collective in that it places emphasis on the worth of black bodies, with particular emphasis on that experience with medicine, both clinical and experimental [5]. It should not be surprising, then, that Mr. M's sisters, informed by this collective experience, see parallels between Mr. M's condition and that of his brother (Fig. 29.3).

Cross-Cultural Tools and Skills

George Fitchett's 7 × 7 model for spiritual assessment identifies seven dimensions of care: holistic, medical, psychological, family systems, psychosocial, ethnic/racial/cultural, social, and spiritual. There are seven aspects within the spiritual dimension: belief and meaning, vocation and consequences, experience and emotions, doubt (courage) and growth, ritual and practice, community, and authority and guidance [6]. The chaplain was aware of and sensitive to the family systems dimension in the lack of communication between Mr. M and family regarding his health. She was also sensitive to the ethnic, racial, and cultural dimension regarding the sisters' concerns related to the other brother being part of a research study

Fig. 29.3 Family perception of parallels between Mr. M and his brother. Culturally influenced family perception of parallels between Mr. M's and his brother's outcomes

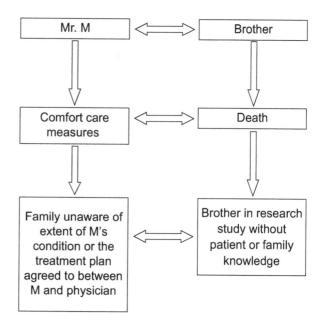

Table 29.1 Key spiritual aspects identified in the care of Mr. M's family

Key Aspects in Spiritual Dimension
Belief and Meaning – healing power of God
Vocation and Consequences – Mr. M's lifelong contributions to his community and church
Experience and Emotions – family's recent loss of Another Brother
Authority and Guidance – providence of God in all matters of life

without their prior knowledge. The chaplain shared these with the ED and CCU teams. There were several key aspects identified in the spiritual dimension (Table 29.1). In response, the chaplain and other members of the interprofessional team worked to honor and validate the family's belief system. The chaplain helped the family explore their belief in God and God's role in Mr. M's health, involving their home spiritual care leadership in the exploration.

There are eight domains in the clinical practice guidelines for quality palliative care (Table 29.2) [7]. The key domains pertinent to this case are: physical aspects of care (Domain 2); spiritual, religious, and existential aspects of care (Domain 5); cultural aspects of care (Domain 6); and care of the imminently dying patient (Domain 7). The interprofessional team addressed these domains by providing interprofessional collaboration with the family both individually in in goals of care meetings. They also validated and supported the family's beliefs and concerns through listening, education, and transparency.

Table 29.2 Eight domains of care for quality palliative care [7]

Clinical practice guidelines for quality palliative care	
Domain 1	Structure and processes of care
Domain 2	Physical aspects of care
Domain 3	Psychological and psychiatric aspects of care
Domain 4	Social aspects of care
Domain 5	Spiritual, religious, and existential aspects of care
Domain 6	Cultural aspects of care
Domain 7	Care of the imminently dying patient
Domain 8	Ethical and legal aspects of care

Pearls and Pitfalls

Pearl The interprofessional team demonstrated integration in their collaboration across disciplines especially between the medical and psychosocial-spiritual provision of care.

Pearl The team demonstrated care and concern for the family, supporting them as they came to understand the extent of Mr. M's condition and prognosis.

Pitfall There was a lack of communication between Mr. M and his family regarding his prognosis and wishes related to medical care in light of this prognosis. Was there ever conversation between Mr. M and his cardiologist regarding including his family in conversations about his health?

Pearl/Pitfall Considering the amount of time the patient was in the hospital, there was no indication that the family interacted with more than one chaplain. This may be because the family was receiving appropriate spiritual care through the staff chaplain and family pastor, but the assessment of the plan for spiritual care did not directly address this aspect.

Pearl/Pitfall While it may have been addressed indirectly through the transparency in the plan of care, there is no indication that the question of the brother being a research subject without his knowledge and the implications for the family's concerns for Mr. M were addressed directly. This dynamic was a mixture of good outcome that could have been done with more intentionality to more effectively address the underlying causes of the family's concern.

Case Outcome

The family was supported through sensitivity to their concerns, a transparent medical process, and support and validation of their feelings and spiritual beliefs. Mr. M died while being supported through palliative comfort care measures with the support of his family and pastor.

References

1. Summary of Virginia health care decisions act-effective 2009 [Internet]. Richmond: Health Law Section of the Virginia State Bar; 2009 [cited 2017 Nov 28]. Available from http://m.vsb.org/docs/sections/health/Summary-HCDA-2009.pdf.
2. Lunney JR, Lynn J, Hogan C. Profiles of older medicare decedents. J Am Geriatr Soc. 2002;50(6):1108–12. doi:jgs50268 [pii].
3. Pentecostalism [Internet]. London: BBC; 2009 Jul 2 [cited 2017 Nov 28]. Available from http://www.bbc.co.uk/religion/religions/christianity/subdivisions/pentecostal_1.shtml.
4. What we believe. Memphis: Church Of God In Christ, Inc.; 2017 [cited 2017 Nov 28]. Available from http://www.cogic.org/about-company/what-we-believe/.
5. Laws T. Tuskegee as sacred rhetoric: focal point for the emergent field of African American religion and health. J Relig Health. 2017. https://doi.org/10.1007/s10943-017-0505-y.
6. Fitchett G. Assessing spiritual needs: a guide for caregivers, revised edition. 2nd ed. Lima: First Academic Renewal Press; 2002. 134 p.
7. National Consensus Project for Quality Palliative Care. Clinical practice guidelines for quality palliative care. 2nd ed. Pittsburgh: National Consensus Project for Quality Palliative Care; 2009. 74 p.

Chapter 30
Patients with Mental Health History

Audrey Snyder and Julie Deters

Case Scenario

A 43-year-old Caucasian female presents to the urgent care after hours clinic with a complaint of neck and midscapular back pain worsening over the last 2 days, which she rates as an 8/10. She states she has had a lot of stress lately. She has had similar pain in the past with stress but not this bad. The pain is worse when she does anything over her head with her arms raised. The pain is not improved with heat, massage, or acetaminophen. She complains of generalized "muscle aches that have been going on for a while, but no one wants to address it." The patient is tearful as she describes what she calls her "struggles." She is dressed in a spaghetti-strap top and shorts. She is slightly diaphoretic. The outside temperature is in the high 80s. A neighbor brought her to the urgent care clinic. A nurse practitioner student assesses the patient first and reports her findings to the provider. The exam is remarkable for an obese Caucasian female with prominent buffalo hump, or dorsocervical fat pad, over lower cervical and upper thoracic posterior processes; diffuse striae over upper arms, legs, and abdomen; and galactorrhea. The remainder of the physical exam is unremarkable. The patient has a history of type II diabetes mellitus, which is uncontrolled. She was in the office last month for her annual exam with her primary care provider. When asked about the reported fasting blood glucose that was in the 300s at her last visit, she states she has had trouble keeping a job because of depression and anxiety. She states the week this lab was drawn, she only had $5 in her checking account and could not buy food, so she drank soda with sugar in it. She feels her anxiety is worse because of the unrelieved pain and financial concerns.

A. Snyder (✉) · J. Deters
University of Northern Colorado, Greeley, CO, USA
e-mail: audrey.snyder@unco.edu; julie.deters@unco.edu

© Springer International Publishing AG, part of Springer Nature 2019
M. L. Martin et al. (eds.), *Diversity and Inclusion in Quality Patient Care*,
https://doi.org/10.1007/978-3-319-92762-6_30

Review of Symptoms

The patient reports she has trouble losing weight but does not think she has gained any recently. She reports difficulty walking due to generalized muscle pain. Depression is reported as baseline on current medications. Anxiety is worse as noted above. She denies difficulty swallowing, respiratory distress, and chest or abdominal pain. She reports galactorrhea, which has been persistent for several months. All other systems are reported negative.

Past Medical History

Depression, anxiety, schizoaffective disorder, type II diabetes uncontrolled, hyperlipidemia, metabolic syndrome, morbid obesity, post-traumatic stress disorder, sleep apnea, and vitamin D deficiency

Gynecologic history: P2, 1 live, 1 tubal, last pap 3 years ago, last mammogram 4 years ago

Surgical history: Left ulnar nerve transposition

Immunizations are up-to-date except for tetanus and diphtheria, which are 3 years overdue.

Medications Zocor 20 mg daily at bedtime, aripiprazole 15 mg daily at bedtime, metformin Hcl 1000 mg extended release daily, fexofenadine 180 mg daily, alprazolam 0.5 mg daily as needed, chlorpheniramine maleate 4 mg every 4–6 hours, Depakote ER 500 mg, 2 tablets at bedtime

Allergies Amoxicillin and penicillin

Health screenings Immunizations, tetanus 3 years overdue; last diabetic monofilament exam 11 months ago, due in 1 month; dilated eye exam 10 months past due; microalbumin due in 1 month; hemoglobin A1C (14%) last month; lipid panel last month

Family History

Type II diabetes in paternal grandfather; no mental health concerns, hypertension, cancer, or other illnesses

Social History

Occupation: Not working currently, on unemployment

Marital status: Single

Children: One son

No history of tobacco, alcohol, marijuana, or illicit substance use reported. Caffeine: coffee 3 servings per month, tea 1 serving per week, and soda 1–2 liters per day

Health insurance: Currently has a policy with a high deductible

Physical Exam

Vital signs Temp, 98.7 °F; pulse, 69; BP, 100/66; respirations, 18; O_2 sat 97% on room air; Ht 5 ft. 4 inches, weight 226 lb., BMI 38.8

General Obese Caucasian female appears stated age, appropriately dressed for weather, tearful and anxious but cooperative, good eye contact

HEENT Normocephalic, moon facies, CN II-X12 intact, trachea midline, no thyromegaly, nares clear, TMs with good light reflex bilaterally

Neck Supple, tender over lower cervical posterior processes, paraspinous muscle tenderness cervical and upper thoracic region, buffalo hump present, no adenopathy

Neuro Grossly intact, alert, and oriented x 3, intact memory for recent and remote events, upper extremities strength 4/5, no obvious sign of deficit

Mental health/psych Depressed affect, expressed anxiety about current symptoms, denies suicidal thoughts, no agitation, normal thought processes

Cardiovascular S1S2 regular rate and rhythm, no murmurs, gallops, or rubs

Respiratory Bilateral breath sounds equal and clear

Abdomen Obese, round, soft, non-tender with normoactive bowel sounds all four quadrants, no hepatosplenomegaly

Extremities No cyanosis, no edema

Skin No rashes or lesions, reddish-purple striae over inferior aspect of upper arms, abdomen, and medial aspect of thighs

Breast No erythema, no palpable lumps, milky discharge from nipples bilaterally

The patient's medical record is reviewed for the past year. There is no record of the physical exam findings of dorsocervical fat pad, recent thyroid-stimulating hormone (TSH) lab, or endocrine workup. The patient denies being told about the fat pad on her back. She is prescribed cyclobenzaprine 10 mg every 8 h as needed to help her muscles relax and placed on ibuprofen 600 mg every 6–8 hours for 2 days and then as needed for pain. TSH and adrenocorticotropic hormone (ACTH) levels and a 24-h urine free cortisol level are ordered. The patient is scheduled for a follow-up visit in 2 weeks with her primary care provider. The patient's primary provider is sent an electronic message through the medical record indicating the abnormal findings and expressing concern for Cushing's syndrome, as well as mentioning scheduling an appointment and the possible need for MRI and endocrine referral. The primary provider responds, "You know she drinks sodas every day. She has lots of complaints that have no basis. She frequently cancels her appointments and will probably be a no show" [1].

Questions for Discussion

1. What was said by whom, to whom?
   The patient said, "Muscle aches that have been going on for a while but no one wants to address it."

Attitudes/Assumptions: The Patient

(a) My high deductible insurance plan prevents me seeing a doctor when I am sick until it is really bad.
(b) Doctors just think my physical complaints are all in my head.

The doctor wrote, "You know she drinks sodas every day. She is a very noncompliant patient. She has lots of complaints that have no basis. She frequently cancels her appointments and will probably be a no show."

Attitudes/Assumptions: The Primary Care Provider

(a) This patient is not adherent to an ADA diet or recommendations.
(b) This patient has a psychiatric history and creates complaints.
(c) This patient is not working and is probably drug seeking with the complaint of "back pain."

Gaps in Provider Knowledge

(a) Lack of awareness of Cushing's syndrome constellation of symptoms.
(b) Lack of knowledge of patient's financial situation impacting food choices and ability to keep appointments in clinic. Assess patient reasons for nonadherence versus labeling patient as noncompliant.
(c) Lack of knowledge of disparities/discrimination: Persons with a medical history of mental health diagnoses are often subject to bias [2].

2. What was done?

Urgent care provider identified that patient has a conglomeration of symptoms that may reflect Cushing's syndrome. She ordered the appropriate lab test. She followed up with the patient on lab results, encouraged her to keep the primary care provider follow-up appointment, and asked about the patient's ability to obtain a ride to the clinic.

3. What actions could have been taken by the primary care provider for earlier identification of a potential problem?

(a) Perform a comprehensive physical exam every year.
(b) Assume a patient with a mental illness who presents with medical complaints is ill.
(c) Do not assume that all patients who present with back pain are drug seeking [3].
(d) Check the Controlled Substance Prescription Monitoring Program online to see if the patient is receiving narcotics from other sources.

4. What medical issues concern you about this case?

(a) The patient has significant persistent physical findings for Cushing's syndrome that have not been previously documented or evaluated. Signs and symptoms of Cushing's syndrome include truncal obesity, moon face, hypertension, skin atrophy and bruising, diabetes or glucose intolerance, gonadal dysfunction, muscle weakness, hirsutism/acne, mood disorders, osteoporosis, edema, polydipsia/polyuria, and fungal infections. Truncal obesity is the most common manifestation [4]. Clinical suspicion of Cushing's syndrome "arises in the presence of central obesity with face and supraclavicular fat accumulation, a cervical fat pad, thinned skin, purple striae, proximal muscle weakness, fatigue, hypertension, impaired glucose metabolism and diabetes, acne, hirsutism, and menstrual irregularities" [4].
(b) In a fast-paced primary care environment, patients may not be fully undressed for physical exams.
(c) Social circumstances should be evaluated with patient encounters. Ancillary staff may be helpful in updating this information.

Pearls and Pitfalls

Pearl The urgent care provider completed a comprehensive history and physical exam, not just a problem-focused exam, when the patient presented in the urgent care environment. A detailed social history was also obtained.

Pearl The urgent care provider listened to the patient's concerns even though the patient felt previous providers were not listening. Mental health history was not the focus of the chief complaint.

Pitfall This patient could be lost to follow-up since she presented in an urgent care environment.

Case Outcome

Diagnosis Muscle spasms in neck and back, concern for Cushing's syndrome, depression, anxiety, type II diabetes mellitus

Disposition The patient returned to the primary care clinic for her follow-up appointment. Her pain was tolerable at a rating 3–4/10 while on muscle relaxants and NSAIDS. TSH was elevated at 6.5, and she was started on levothyroxine. ACTH level was assessed as intermediate at 13. A MRI of the pituitary was ordered, and the patient was referred to endocrinology. She expressed gratitude for her symptoms being assessed and addressed.

References

1. Keeling A, Utz SW, Shuster GF 3rd, Boyle A. Noncompliance revisited: a disciplinary perspective of a nursing diagnosis. Nurs Diagn. 1993;4(3):91–8.
2. Kaplan A. Bias against schizophrenic patients seeking medical care [Internet]. [place unknown]: Psychiatric Times; 2013 [cited 2017 Nov 6]. Available from: http://www.psychiatrictimes.com/apa2013/bias-against-schizophrenic-patients-seeking-medical-care.
3. Grover CA, Eder JW, Close RJH, Curry SM. How frequently are "classic" drug-seeking behaviors used by drug-seeking patients in the emergency department? West J Emerg Med. 2012;13(5):416–21.
4. Boscaro M, Arnaldi G. Approach to the patient with possible Cushing's syndrome. J Clin Endocrinol Metab. 2009;94(9):3121–31.

Chapter 31
International Victim of War

Lisa Moreno-Walton

Case Scenario

Ms. Hiba Tahir, a woman appearing to be about 20 years old but whose exact date of birth is unknown, presents to the emergency department (ED) with a man appearing to be in his late forties, who identifies himself as her husband and explains to the triage nurse that Ms. Tahir complains of constipation, which is causing her some lower abdominal bloating and cramping. Both the patient and husband are dressed in traditional sub-Saharan African attire, including a head covering for Ms. Tahir. The man identifies himself as Abdul and states that he will act as her translator, since she speaks no English. The triage nurse attempts to use the translator phone service, but Abdul tells her that Ms. Tahir speaks "a rare language" and that it will be unlikely that a phone translator can be found. Abdul answers all questions on behalf of Ms. Tahir, stating that she had no fevers, vomiting, or diarrhea; only that she had not had a bowel movement in 3 days, and for a couple of weeks prior to that, her stools were hard and difficult to pass. Ms. Tahir appears in no apparent distress, so the nurse places her in an exam room. Abdul goes out of the room and paces, complaining that they are being made to wait for the doctor.

Dr. Sally Morales, a Latina attending emergency physician, is supervising Dr. Quintorris Brookes, the African-American male resident who picked up the case with the Caucasian male medical student who was assigned to work with him that day. She overhears a loud exchange between Dr. Brookes and Abdul taking place outside of Ms. Tahir's room. Abdul says that no men, and especially men "who are not even real doctors," are going to take care of his wife. Dr. Brookes replies calmly, addressing the patient's husband as "sir" and inquires as to his last name, to which the husband replies, "That's not your business." Dr. Brookes explains that he only

L. Moreno-Walton
Department of Medicine, Section of Emergency Medicine, Louisiana State University
Health Sciences Center-New Orleans, New Orleans, LA, USA

© Springer International Publishing AG, part of Springer Nature 2019   225
M. L. Martin et al. (eds.), *Diversity and Inclusion in Quality Patient Care*,
https://doi.org/10.1007/978-3-319-92762-6_31

wants to know Abdul's name in order to address him more respectfully, but Abdul replies, "Just call me 'Abdul,' and get a real doctor in here." Dr. Morales approaches and introduces herself as the supervising physician who will be responsible for the patient's care and asks if there is a problem. Abdul replies that he and his wife are devout Muslims and that she cannot be examined by a man. Dr. Morales informs the male trainees that she will assess Ms. Tahir while they see other patients, and the three will talk later. Abdul follows her into the room, and after introducing herself to Ms. Tahir, smiling and shaking her hand, Dr. Morales obtains the history from him. During the history taking, Ms. Tahir's eyes remain downcast, although she frequently steals a look at Abdul. She sits on the bed on her left hip, with her buttocks off the mattress.

Review of Symptoms

No fevers, chills, nausea, vomiting, diarrhea, weight loss, or decreased appetite

Past Medical History

Mother of two children whom she had delivered by normal spontaneous vaginal route at home, under the care of the village midwife

Past medications None, including no oral contraception

Past surgical history Negative

Family History

Abdul states that he does not have this information, since Hiba was from a distant village, and he only met her during the diaspora that resulted from the civil war in the Sudan.

Social History

He denies that the patient has ever smoked or used alcohol or drugs. He volunteers that she is one of his four wives, that he is in the import-export business, and that he comes to New York City about once every 2 months for business and brings one of the wives with him each time. This is Hiba's first time accompanying him.

Physical Exam

Vital signs Temp 98.9, BP 118/76, HR 72, RR 16, oxygen saturation 100% RA

General Thin, well-appearing African female who appears nervous and uncomfortable

HEENT EOMI, anicteric, no oral exudates

Neck Supple, no lymphadenopathy

Cardiovascular Regular rate and rhythm, no murmurs/rubs/gallops

Respiratory Lungs clear to auscultation bilaterally

Abdomen NABS, soft, with diffuse mild tenderness to palpation but no rebound or guarding

Neuro Alert, oriented

Skin Warm, dry, supple, without rashes

Extremities No edema

Genitalia A large cluster of warty, papillated skin-colored lesions is noted to surround and almost obscures the anus, growing anteriorly across the perineum into the posterior portion of the vaginal introitus.

Dr. Morales lowers the patient's skirt and informs Abdul that she needs to do a pelvic examination, to which he replies, "Go ahead." She tells him that these exams are done privately, without family observation, and when he insists that he must remain, she tells him that the patient will have to consent to that. Abdul shouts, "She speaks Fur. You can't communicate with her. Only I can!"

Dr. Morales excuses herself, telling Abdul that she will return shortly. She reconvenes with Dr. Brookes and the medical student and instructs them to order basic labs and a rapid HIV test, to locate Sgt. Paxton, the hospital police officer who is an African-American, Muslim male, and to get a Fur translator on the language line. Sgt. Paxton is able to move Abdul to the waiting room without incident. A full history is taken using the translator phone, and the pelvic examination is completed.

The physician team assures Ms. Tahir that her story will be kept confidential from Abdul and that if she is in any danger from him, she will not be released from the hospital, and police will be notified. She is then able to communicate to the physician team that just about 2 months prior to arrival in New York City, she had been in a displaced persons camp near Darfur with her two children. Abdul's brother was a guard at the camp, and he gave her extra food for her children in exchange for sexual intercourse, threatening that they would receive no food at all if she failed to cooperate. A few days later, Abdul came to the camp and removed her and the children, claiming that she was his wife and had become displaced. He took her to his village, where she lived with several other women, all of whom were expected to service various men brought to their tents by Abdul and who were beaten or denied food if they refused. One of the women was suffering from "the falling down sickness that many African people have" where she became cachectic, developed oral lesions and diarrhea, and was too ill to walk. Hiba's children are currently in the care of one of her "sister wives" in the Sudan. She does not know how long Abdul will keep her in New York, although all the other women he brought here had returned with him. She is relieved not be required to have sex with men unknown to her while in New York and to be receiving medical care.

Questions for Discussion

1. How common is human trafficking in the United States?

(a) The US State Department identified 77,823 victims of sexual and labor trafficking in the USA in 2015 [1].
(b) Sex trafficking occurs in every US state. It is most common in California, Texas, and Florida and least common in Vermont, Rhode Island, and Idaho [2].
(c) The Polaris Project Hotline received phone calls which led to the identification of 8,042 cases of sexual trafficking in 2016, an increase of 35% from 2015 [1].
(d) Trafficked patients come to the ED every day, but are usually not identified.

2. What are the signs of a trafficked patient?

Trafficked patients often present with abdominal complaints, a chief complaint often seen in all depressed patients, females more often than males. They frequently exhibit poor eye contact and/or scripted responses and have untreated injuries or sexually transmitted diseases. A thorough examination should be performed since many of these patients have been branded by their traffickers, sometimes even with bar codes that are scanned to keep track of how much money they are earning for their captors. Traffickers tend to either fail to leave the room or hover in the vicinity, making frequent checks on the patient [1, 3].

Attitudes/Assumptions: The Physician

(a) Dr. Brookes approached the patient's husband respectfully and attempted to engage him. When this did not work, he appropriately deferred to Dr. Morales.
(b) Dr. Morales was familiar with the Muslim culture and worked with her team to accommodate the patient/family's culture until it became apparent that the patient's best interest was not being served by the husband's requests.

(c) Sgt. Paxton shared a common gender, religion, and race with the family member. He used these common factors and his communication skills to diffuse the situation.

Attitudes/Assumptions: The Patient

(a) The patient understood her role and cooperated with her trafficker in order to protect herself and her children.
(b) A safe environment was created in which the patient was given the opportunity to share her story in a bid for freedom.

Case Outcome

Diagnosis Condylomata accuminata, human immunodeficiency virus, human trafficking victim

Disposition The patient is admitted to the colorectal service for fulguration of the lesions. She is started on stool softeners and a laxative. The crime of trafficking is reported to the police and Abdul is taken into custody from the waiting room. The police department engages the Department of Immigration, which sends a social worker to interview Hiba Tahir and assist her with post-discharge planning, including exploring how to reunite her with her children. The infectious disease team was consulted while Hiba was an inpatient. They started her on anti-retroviral therapy and explained how to take the medication and how to prevent HIV transmission. They advised her to have her children tested.

References

1. Polaris [Internet]. Washington, DC: Polaris; 2017 [cited 2017 Dec 21]. Available from: https://polarisproject.org/.
2. Addressing human trafficking and exploitation in times of crisis – evidence and recommendations for further action to protect vulnerable and mobile populations I December 2015 [Internet]. Geneva: International Organization for Migration; 2015 [cited 2017 Dec 21]. Available from: https://publications.iom.int/system/files/addressing_human_trafficking_dec2015.pdf.
3. CaeBaca L, Sigmon JN. Combating trafficking in persons: a call to action for global health professionals. Glob Health Sci Pract. 2014;2(3):261–7.

Chapter 32
Pregnant Incarcerated Heroin User

P. Preston Reynolds, Patricia Workman, and Christian A. Chisholm

Case Scenario

SA is a 23-year-old woman who was arrested for possession of drug paraphernalia and brought to the local jail. She noticed 1 month ago that she felt a kicking sensation in her abdomen and wondered if she was pregnant. A urine pregnancy test during routine jail intake screening is positive. She has had no recent medical care but is expressing a concern to the intake nurse that she will withdraw from heroin.

The intake nurse calls to inform the medical director of the local jail of her concerns. The medical director decides to go in that evening to evaluate SA. The medical director has the basic equipment necessary to take vital signs, test her blood sugar, and do a urinalysis. There is a fetoscope in one of the drawers. It has not been used by the medical staff in several years. There is no other equipment.

The medical director begins the examination by asking her about her living situation and her drug use. She was living with her boyfriend when she was arrested. She believes he is the father of her unborn baby. Their housing situation is tenuous, and they have experienced homelessness. They do not have transportation and also face challenges with their food supply. She reports she is currently injecting four grams of heroin daily. She last used that morning, just prior to her arrest. They support their drug habit by taking donations at street corners, and her partner deals in drugs when they are short of money. She denies partner abuse or exchanging sex for drugs.

She has not previously been pregnant. She did not notice any nausea with the pregnancy but is beginning to feel nauseous this evening.

P. Preston Reynolds (✉) · C. A. Chisholm
University of Virginia, Charlottesville, VA, USA
e-mail: pprestonreynolds@virginia.edu; cac2u@virginia.edu

P. Workman
Fluvanna Correctional Center for Women, Troy, VA, USA

© Springer International Publishing AG, part of Springer Nature 2019   231
M. L. Martin et al. (eds.), *Diversity and Inclusion in Quality Patient Care*,
https://doi.org/10.1007/978-3-319-92762-6_32

She is not taking any prescribed or over-the-counter medications and does not have any known drug allergies.

Review of Symptoms

General She received all of her childhood vaccinations as scheduled and was seen by a pediatrician until high school. She has no known history of any medical illnesses.

HEENT No visual changes, no hearing loss or tinnitus, no history of strep throat or seasonal allergies. She has had several months of dental pain. She has never seen a dentist. She is beginning to have some rhinorrhea.

Cardiovascular No chest pain, palpitations, or lower extremity edema   ·

Respiratory No asthma, wheezing, shortness of breath, hemoptysis, cough, pneumonia

Abdomen No constipation, diarrhea, bloody stool; she is beginning to feel some nausea and abdominal cramping and notes the baby is moving a lot.

Extremities No history of fractures, focal weakness, loss of strength, joint swelling or warmth, or neck pain; she does have some lower back discomfort.

Neurological No history of seizures, problems with balance, numbness or tingling, or headaches; she has had symptoms of previous withdrawal from opiates but no hospitalizations for withdrawal.

GU No history of sexually transmitted diseases, no knowledge of HIV or Hep C status, recurrent UTIs; she is having a smelly, mostly white vaginal discharge. She has never had a Pap smear. She denies performing sex acts in exchange for drugs.

Skin History of acne during adolescence, no history of skin abscesses

Past Medical History

Acne as a teenager, treated for 6 months with topical solutions and antibiotics obtained from a dermatologist

Family History

No illicit drug use; no miscarriages or birth defects; no cancer, diabetes, coronary artery disease, strokes, or neurologic disease; no mental health disease

Social History

Marital status: Single; living with boyfriend, history of other sexual partners, random use of condoms

Drug use: She started using heroin 6 months ago and has escalated from snorting to shooting up daily. She has been using about four grams of heroin a day for about 2 months. She often reuses needles and shares with her boyfriend. She denies alcohol, tobacco, marijuana, or other drugs.

Education: Graduated from high school

Children: None.

She is not currently working.

Physical Exam

Vital signs BP = 150/95, P = 110, R = 14, T = 98.6

HEENT PERRL, EOMI, hearing intact, dental caries involving two maxillary molars on right and three teeth on lower left, no posterior pharyngeal erythema or exudate, no cervical or supraclavicular adenopathy, no skin lesions on face or scalp; mild rhinorrhea present

Cardiovascular S1S2, no murmurs, rubs, or gallops

Respiratory Clear to auscultation and percussion

Abdomen Distended uterus on palpation, diminished bowel sounds, no focal tenderness; Fetoscope registered heart rate of 166 bpm

Extremities Track marks on left forearm, antecubital fossa, and hand; no signs of infection with red streaking, no skin abscesses; lower extremities without signs of injection on feet or legs; 5/5 strength throughout upper and lower extremities and hands

Neurological Cranial nerves II–XII intact, normal reflexes throughout, normal cerebellar coordination, normal sensation to light touch, and pinprick in lower extremities; she is beginning to show piloerection.

What Was Said?

The medical director informs the inmate that she is trained in internal medicine, not obstetrics, and so it would be necessary to involve a specialist from the nearby university's medical center to provide her and her unborn child the best care possible. The patient is also made aware of the jail policy to assist patients through withdrawal using medical protocols to help control withdrawal symptoms. However, this would potentially present a problem for the fetus. Opioids easily cross the placenta and enter the fetal circulation, leading to the development of physiologic dependence of the unborn baby [1, 2].

With her daily heroin use, the fetus is also addicted, and withdrawal could present a problem for the unborn baby. The medical director must ensure the safety of all inmates. Since it is the responsibility of the jail to provide all medically necessary care to all of the inmates, the medical director recommends that the expertise of someone trained in high-risk obstetrics be consulted to determine the safest way to care for her and her unborn child through the remainder of the pregnancy.

The inmate thanks the medical director for her compassion and concern and, again, informs the medical director that she is beginning to feel nauseous and have a sensation of all-over muscle pain.

What Was Done?

Since the medical director came in that evening to evaluate SA, she first calls the chief resident in obstetrics, who refers the medical director to the chief of maternal/fetal medicine. The chief of maternal/fetal medicine quickly calls the medical director back, and together they develop a plan for care of SA and her unborn child.

Questions for Discussion

1. Should the medical director obtain additional training? If so, in what areas?
2. Is the medical director aware of standards of care for withdrawing addicted pregnant patients?

3. Is the medical director aware of legal limitations that exist that can hamper the treatment of these patients?

4. Do physicians in the community have a responsibility to assist the medical director of the jail in delivering care to inmates if their area of expertise is vital to the safety of an inmate?

5. Has the medical director established liaisons within the community for transfer of care in the event of the patient's release? (The average incarceration at a local jail will be about 2 days.)

   1. The maternal-fetal medicine physician recognized a barrier (incarceration) to providing the patient with the standard of care (medication-assisted therapy). The multidisciplinary team had to devise a plan to safely withdraw the patient from opioids in a medically supervised manner [1, 2].

6. How does a provider reconcile the inability to provide standard of care management to a patient due to external factors (incarceration, lack of insurance coverage, patient refusal)?

7. Does the inmate want to be free completely of opiates, or does she want to try an opiate substitute, such as buprenorphine or methadone?

8. Are there legal limitations to administration of buprenorphine or methadone in a correctional facility? What are the policies of this jail with regard to administration of buprenorphine or methadone? Is the medical director licensed to administer buprenorphine?

9. Can the inmate obtain addiction-counseling services while in jail?

10. Are there facilities where she can be transferred that provide the addiction services she may need while incarcerated if they are not available at the correctional facility where she is housed?

11. What if she is not ready to quit?

12. What if she later admits she is experiencing partner violence and has been forced into prostitution?

13. What if the patient is released from the jail soon after she arrives? What will be the medical recommendations to her for care of her addiction and safe delivery of the unborn child?

14. Are there local agencies to which our patient can be referred?

15. How can the medical director ensure inmates receive the services they need if he/she is unable to deliver them because of lack of training in these specialized areas of medical care, addiction medicine, and obstetrics?

16. Is it the right of inmates to have access to medical care, dental care, and mental health services that are available to other people in the same community?

17. Should this inmate be treated differently because she is using heroin?

18. Should this inmate be treated differently because she is pregnant and using heroin?

Attitude/Assumptions: The Provider

The internist recognized her limitation in knowledge and skill related to high-risk pregnancies. She sought input from experts because SA's daily heroin use required a need to ensure safe withdrawal of the patient and fetus from an opiate.

Attitude/Assumptions: The Patient

The patient is addicted to heroin and is uncertain she can quit. She wants the baby to be born healthy and eventually wants to raise the baby. While she is feeling very sick, she wants to get clean and stay off heroin in the future.

Gaps in Provider Knowledge

Clinicians must know the limits of their knowledge and seek assistance from experts when faced with clinical situations beyond their scope of competence. This is a fundamental principle of professionalism. While the internist recently recertified in internal medicine, there are several areas that are beyond the training of this specialty: medical care of a viable fetus in an addicted mother with a substance abuse disorder, withdrawal of a pregnant woman from narcotics, and addiction counseling for pregnant women.

Case Outcome

Disposition All correctional facilities withdraw inmates from illicit drugs under close supervision. If there is concern about multiple drug ingestions, inmates will often be transferred to a nearby hospital for closer observation because the need for intensive services may arise suddenly.

SA is now an inmate in a correctional facility where it is standard procedure to withdraw her from heroin, using a clonidine taper protocol [3]. The issue in this case is that heroin withdrawal in an unborn child may cause harm to the fetus; and thus, the decision is made to call the experts in maternal/fetal medicine at the nearby university for assistance.

Under close monitoring, with special technologies, of both the fetus and the mother in the delivery suite, SA and her unborn child underwent an uneventful heroin withdrawal, receiving IV fluids, clonidine, and other symptomatic care. SA remained in the hospital until the clonidine protocol was completed. She was seen by psychiatry and evaluated for substance use disorder. She was discharged back to the local jail. She was kept in the medical unit for a week and then placed in general population with the other female inmates. While in jail, SA participated actively in drug addiction classes and expressed a strong desire to remain drug-free upon release. She delivered a healthy baby at the university; the baby at birth had no signs of addiction or further drug withdrawal. SA's parents were given custody of the baby after she was discharged from the hospital. SA returned to the jail until she was released to a long-term drug addiction facility where she was reunited with her baby. At the inpatient facility, she was scheduled to receive both parenting classes and further drug addiction treatment.

Ethics, do no harm to an unborn fetus; beneficence, ensuring the health and safety of both mother and fetus; justice, wanting to ensure long-term health of mother and baby with access to drug treatment facilities; inmates have a legal guarantee of receiving medically necessary care [4]. Most inmates at local jails have not yet been to court and have not yet been found guilty. Many will be found not guilty. Provision of medical care to inmates is further guided by the American Correctional Association and the National Commission on Correctional Health Care [5, 6].

References

1. Jones HE, Martin PR, Heil SH, Kaltenbach K, Selby P, Coyle MG, Stine SM, O'Grady KE, Arria AM, Fischer G. Treatment of opioid-dependent pregnant women: clinical and research issues. J Subst Abus Treat. 2008;35(3):245–59. https://doi.org/10.1016/j.jsat.2007.10.007. Epub 2008 Jan 14.
2. American College of Obstetricians and Gynecologists. Opioid use and opioid use disorder in pregnancy. Committee opinion 711. Obstet Gynecol. 2017;130:e81–94.
3. Detoxification of chemically dependent inmates: Federal Bureau of Prisons clinical practice guidelines [Internet]. Washington: Federal Bureau of Prisons; 2014 [cited 2017 Nov 29]. Available from: https://www.bop.gov/resources/pdfs/detoxification.pdf.
4. Estelle v Gamble, 429 U.S. 97; 1976.
5. Standards for health services in jails. Chicago: National Commission on Correctional Health Care; 2014. 200p.
6. Publications and resources related to specific populations [Internet]. Rockville: SAMHSA; [cited 2017 Nov 29]. Available from: https://www.samhsa.gov/specific-populations/publications-resources.

Chapter 33
Offensive Tattoo

Sybil Zachariah

Case Scenario

A 46-year-old male presents to the emergency department with epigastric abdominal pain, vomiting, and weight loss for 6 weeks. He saw his primary care doctor 4 weeks earlier, who started a proton pump inhibitor, and he is scheduled for follow-up there in 2 weeks. He has ongoing epigastric abdominal pain, a progressive inability to tolerate food, and is currently on a liquid diet. He vomits or regurgitates any solid food. He has unintentionally lost 20 pounds in the past month. The patient is accompanied by his wife, and both are visibly upset and angry regarding the lack of improvement and progression of his symptoms. He states, "I've tried calling my doctor but she's not doing anything! I'm just getting worse, I can't eat anything!" His wife continues, "Doc, you have to help him. This isn't like him, he usually eats a ton, and he's losing so much weight!" The patient says, "You have to do something today, doctor. Please help me. I'm not leaving till we figure this out."

Review of Symptoms

Notable for weight loss, fatigue, night sweats, vomiting, and constipation/decreased bowel movements; all other symptoms reviewed are negative.

S. Zachariah, MD
Stanford University, Stanford, CA, USA

© Springer International Publishing AG, part of Springer Nature 2019
M. L. Martin et al. (eds.), *Diversity and Inclusion in Quality Patient Care*,
https://doi.org/10.1007/978-3-319-92762-6_33

Past Medical History

Hypertension

Family History

Noncontributory

Social History

Social alcohol, one pack per day of smoking for 10 years

Physical Exam

Vital signs Temperature normal, blood pressure 140/80, pulse 89

General No acute distress

HEENT Normal

Cardiovascular Normal

Respiratory Normal

Abdomen Soft, non-tender, non-distended, no masses, no flank tenderness

GU Deferred

Extremities Normal range of motion, no deformities or pitting edema

Skin No jaundice, rashes, or wounds; large "White Power" tattoo covering most of back, featuring an eagle and an American flag

Neuro Normal

What Was Said?

The physician in this case is of Indian heritage. She elected not to comment on the tattoo. The patient did not address the tattoo either.

What Was Done?

The physician completed the examination and ordered labs and an abdominal CT scan. The CT demonstrated a large mass at the distal esophagus with multiple masses in the liver and enlarged retroperitoneal lymph nodes, concerning for metastatic malignancy.

Question for Discussion

1. What are some issues that could impede the doctor-patient relationship?

Attitudes/Assumptions: The Provider

As a woman of color, the physician was offended by the tattoo. She felt it was directly antagonistic toward people of her heritage and that the patient is likely a white supremacist. She was tempted to state something to this effect and express her discomfort with this body art.

The physician was also concerned that the patient may discriminate against her due to his presumed white supremacist beliefs. He was already visibly angry, and after seeing the tattoo she was concerned the situation had the potential to become increasingly hostile. She considered reaching out to another physician to assume the case.

However, the physician also realized that the patient, although demanding, had not directed any anger or offensive language toward her. His anger stemmed from being distraught and fearful with regards to his medical condition, not toward her ethnicity. She continued with the patient interaction.

Attitudes/Assumptions: The Patient

This doctor of color may not provide me the best care after seeing the "White Power" tattoo on my back.

Research demonstrates that tattoos in general can negatively affect the perception of an individual and that tattoos with certain designs or placement can invoke this negative perception more strongly [1–3]. A racist or offensive tattoo can be expected to elicit negative feelings from a practitioner, particularly if it is offensive toward a group of people with whom the practitioner identifies. Being aware of this bias can help a provider avoid succumbing to it and allow them to treat their patients objectively and appropriately.

In this case, the attending physician does not take the implications of a displayed racist tattoo personally and instead inwardly acknowledges that the patient has been polite and deferential toward her during their interaction. Addressing the tattoo out of turn could make the patient defensive, prompt him to leave the ED, or cause him to grow aggressive toward the physician, all of which are not beneficial toward caring for the patient and could harm the doctor-patient relationship. In a related scenario where a physician finds him or herself unable to ignore the tattoo, or if the patient is additionally being offensive toward the physician, it would be acceptable to assign the patient to another provider if possible to deescalate the situation and still provide quality care for the patient.

Case Outcome

The physician discussed the concern for metastatic cancer with the patient and his spouse, both of whom were angry and upset with the findings but grateful for the care provided. The patient was admitted to the hospital for further care.

References

1. Resenhoeft A, Villa J, Wiseman D. Tattoos can harm perceptions: a study and suggestions. J Am Coll Heal. 2008;56(5):593–6.
2. Degelman D, Price ND. Tattoos and ratings of personal characteristics. Psychol Rep. 2002;90:507–14.
3. Hawkes D, Senn C, Thorn C. Factors that influence attitudes toward women with tattoos. Sex Roles J Res. 2004;50:125–46.

Part III
Medical Student and Nursing Student Cases

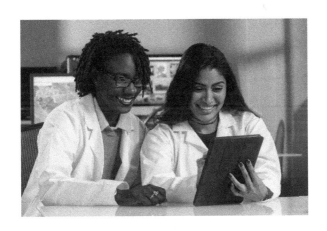

Chapter 34
Medical Student Experiences

Marianne Haughey, Erick A. Eiting, Sarah Jamison, and Tiffany Murano

The years of being a medical student are a significant time of transition in the formation of professional identity. Cruess et al. proposed a definition specific to physician development as: "A physician's identity is a representation of self, achieved in stages over time during which the characteristics, values and norms of the medical profession are internalized, resulting in an individual thinking, feeling and acting like a physician" [1].

Students might have idealized and altruistic thoughts of what it means to be a physician. After all, they have written essays for their applications filled with the goals of "helping people" and "giving back." However, students typically begin medical school identifying as lay people with patients' perceptions of the healthcare interaction [2]. They also have all the complexities of their personal identity, with some components fairly formed but with others still in flux. This can include gender

M. Haughey (✉)
CUNY School of Medicine, Department of Emergency Medicine, SBH Health System, New York, NY, USA

Albert Einstein College of Medicine, Bronx, NY, USA
e-mail: mhaughey@sbhny.org

E. A. Eiting
Icahn School of Medicine at Mount Sinai, New York, NY, USA

David B. Kriser Department of Emergency Medicine, Mount Sinai Beth Israel, New York, NY, USA
e-mail: erick.eiting@mountsinai.org

S. Jamison
CUNY School of Medicine, Department of Emergency Medicine, SBH Health System, New York, NY, USA
e-mail: sjamison@sbhny.org; mhaughey@sbhny.org

T. Murano
Department of Emergency Medicine, Rutgers New Jersey Medical School, Newark, NJ, USA
e-mail: Tiffany.Murano@rutgers.edu

© Springer International Publishing AG, part of Springer Nature 2019
M. L. Martin et al. (eds.), *Diversity and Inclusion in Quality Patient Care*,
https://doi.org/10.1007/978-3-319-92762-6_34

identity, sexual identity, racial or ethnic group identity, or geographical or place of origin identity [1]. The process of acculturation occurs through a level of intense involvement in studies and expectations that are both expressed and unexpressed through clinical exposures as being essential in the process of forming a professional identity. This is a merging of the new professional identity and the previous personal identity based on one's prior life experiences. Ideally, values from all identities can be integrated fully and consistently applied.

Mentors, instructors, residents, more senior students, and attendings, as well as the expectations of patients and nurses, are essential to the formation of one's perception of their identity as a physician. In Keegan's levels of development in professional identification, Stage 3 is "understanding and expectations of the professional role is externalized, shaped by interpersonal relationships, observing others and following the norms and status quo within the organization without question" [2, 3]. Of course, the hope would be that there would be many wonderful mentors who would help shape the individual young physician's development of their professional identity in this new culture. But medicine is still very much an apprenticeship, and those who train others do not do so in a vacuum. They are also individuals with their biases, beliefs, and stereotypes, both recognized and unrecognized. Individual trainers' biases can become apparent through personal interactions, such as clinical, small group, or individual interactions [4]. These interactions are not monitored like those in front of a large auditorium might be. Thus, inappropriate actions, including microaggressions, can be more easily expressed without the microaggressor being called out on their inappropriate behavior, due to the power dynamic between students and teachers and the usual privacy of the interaction.

Students caught in the moment of the microaggression are particularly vulnerable, due to both the power dynamic and their lack of experience of the world of medicine. The pressure to succeed is extremely strong, and opposing a teacher's expressed bias can be terribly challenging as it can risk the student's success in that course. In addition, given the unfamiliarity with much of the culture of medicine, it can seem that in order to become "part of the club," there is a need to "go along with the group," even when "going along" conflicts with the student's personal identity, belief system, and past experiences [1]. Individual small personal interactions can also create a challenge because one biased individual can make a significant impact on their students, as their exposure to others with different viewpoints might be limited.

These are stories of students who came across situations or microaggressions demonstrating the biases of those they were meant to honor as teachers. This develops a particular challenge as it discredits the role of that teacher for that student. The mature student can realize they need to develop their own identity separate from the one being modeled poorly, but it can be difficult to draw that line in the midst of the competition of medical school. There are tools being developed to help in this process for healthy development of the medical student's professional identity [5].

Female Medical Student Is Given Roles Different from Male Students

Case Scenario

A 25-year-old male presents to the emergency department of a level 1 trauma center with right hip pain immediately following a motor vehicle crash in which he was the restrained driver of a vehicle that lost control on icy pavement and struck a tree. The airbags in the vehicle were deployed, and there was significant damage to the vehicle. There was no loss of consciousness. The right hip pain is described as constant, sharp, 8/10 in intensity, and is worsened when he attempts to move the extremity.

Review of Symptoms

He denies neck, chest, and abdominal pain.

Past Medical History

Negative

Social History

Denies tobacco, alcohol, and recreational drug use.

Physical Exam

Vital signs Temperature normal; blood pressure, 140/86; heart rate, 105; respiratory rate, 16; oxygen saturation, 99% on room air

General Well-developed and well-nourished male in moderate discomfort

Head Normal

Neck There is no posterior midline tenderness or bony step-offs to palpation of the cervical spine.

Cardiovascular Tachycardic and regular; no murmurs, rubs, or gallops appreciated

Lungs Breaths are normal and symmetric.

Abdomen Bowel sounds are normal. There is ecchymosis to the lower abdomen with tenderness in the right lower quadrant. There is no rebound or guarding.

Extremities The right lower extremity is held at 90° flexion at the hip. Distal pulses are palpable and are +2.

Neuro GCS is 15. Neurologic examination was grossly non-focal.

Skin There were various abrasions to the scalp, trunk, and extremities. Again, noted is the area of linear ecchymosis to the lower abdomen.

What Was Said?

The emergency department and trauma service consult the on-call orthopedics service for evaluation of a suspected posterior dislocation of the right hip. The on-call orthopedics consulting team is comprised of a male resident, a female medical student (Ashley), and a male medical student (John). A posterior hip dislocation is confirmed by radiographic imaging. The orthopedics resident says to the students, "This looks like it is going to be a tough one. John, I'm going to need your muscles, you can help me with this reduction." John knows that his fellow student is a triathlete and is interested in practicing orthopedics as a career. John is interested in going into pediatrics and feels that Ashley would gain valuable experience from participating in this procedure. John says, "You know, Ashley is stronger than she looks. Plus, she wants orthopedics." The resident responds by saying, "That's great. I want you for this, John. This is going to take a while and the cafeteria is about to close. Ashley, would you mind picking up dinner for us while we reduce this hip?" Angry and frustrated, Ashley agrees but is clearly unhappy about this.

What Was Done?

The resident and John perform the procedure while Ashley retrieved food for them. When she returns with the food, her fellow student is apologetic and uncomfortable. Ashley goes to the call room to study and reflect on the interaction. She feels that maybe she should reconsider her choice of orthopedics, as it appears to be a specialty for men. John tells the resident, "I think Ashley is unhappy about not doing the procedure. She went to the call room to read and she didn't even eat dinner." The resident replies, "She's being too sensitive. This was a really tough procedure and I was only trying to protect her from getting hurt! Maybe it's that time of the month for her. You know how irrational girls can be during that time."

Ashley later sought guidance from advisors in the medical school, as well as the clerkship director. These advisors encouraged Ashley to report her experience in an evaluation and assured her that the resident would be spoken to about his behavior and further educated. Ashley was also connected with female mentors who were orthopedic specialists.

Question for Discussion

1. What are some attitudes and assumptions of the resident and medical students?

Attitudes/Assumptions: The Resident

There were clear gender stereotypes and gender role restrictions that the resident exhibited. He reasoned that the male student was better suited for the procedure because it required strength that he assumed the male student possessed and the female student did not. There is a societal assumption/belief that all men are physically stronger and better suited for physical tasks, while women are better suited for nurturing roles [6]. In addition, there is a stereotype that women are emotional and illogical. The resident thought the student was overreacting. There is also the benevolent sexism that was demonstrated here: the feeling that Ashley was being protected by not being allowed to engage in the procedure.

Attitudes/Assumptions: The Male Medical Student

The male medical student recognized the behavior by the resident. However, even in his defense of his fellow student, he unwittingly engages in microaggression by stating that the female resident is "stronger than she looks."

Attitudes/Assumptions: The Female Medical Student

The female medical student, Ashley, recognizes that the behavior is unfair and inappropriate. However, she complies with the unreasonable request of her resident and gets food for the male members of her team. She may have done this because she felt that she was in a subordinate situation and did not realize that this may be reinforcing the gender stereotype that women are better suited for a more nurturing and supportive role.

Gaps in Provider Knowledge

The resident demonstrated a lack of sensitivity and knowledge of the roles that women play in the medical field as well as in society. This, combined with his unfounded beliefs in societal assumptions about gender stereotypes, led to his microaggressions. The resident would benefit from cultural sensitivity training and promotion of diversity and inclusion.

Although the medical students knew that the resident's behavior was inappropriate and spoke up, they would both benefit from communication and advocacy in difficult situations.

Cross-Cultural Tools and Skills

Aliya Khan, writer for *Everyday Feminism*, suggests six ways to respond to people who engage in microaggression [7]:

1. Present another way of viewing the situation.
2. Challenge the microaggression.
3. Express your disagreement.
4. Explain to them why you disagree.
5. Change or redirect the conversation.
6. Do nothing.

Pearls and Pitfalls

Pearl Informing supervising physicians of incidents allows the medical student to not only voice her concern but also raise awareness that this behavior exists.

Pearl Microaggressions are commonly unintentional, and the microaggressors are unaware that they are being offensive. By informing the clerkship director, the resident will have the opportunity to be educated on gender discrimination and microaggression.

Pitfall Repetitive microaggression can have long-term effects both mentally and physically. While opting to do nothing or "go with the flow" may be appropriate for a certain set of circumstances, it should probably not be a standing practice for all situations.

Case Outcome

The patient was admitted to the hospital for observation and was discharged home within 48 h.

Resident Physician Uses a Derogatory Term During a Shift

Case Scenario
An 8-year-old presents to an inner city emergency department with a chief complaint of left ankle pain. The patient was running when she tripped and landed on the everted joint.

Review of Symptoms

Denies headache, knee pain, or abdominal pain

Past Medical History

Asthma

Medications Ventolin inhaler as needed

Family History

Noncontributory

Social History

The patient lives at home with her grandmother, mother, and three siblings. She is in the third grade.

Physical Exam

Vital signs Temperature normal, blood pressure 93/60, pulse 120

General Well-groomed, healthy-appearing African-American girl, tearful, lying on stretcher

Head Normocephalic, atraumatic

Neck Supple, no midline tenderness; no bony step-offs

ENT Oropharynx within normal limits

Cardiovascular Heart regular rhythm with tachycardia

Respiratory Lungs clear

Abdomen Abdomen soft, non-tender, non-distended; bowel sounds normal

Extremities Left mildly swollen and tender to palpation at the posterior lateral malleolus; range of motion slightly decreased; +2 dorsalis pedal pulse; capillary refill less than 2 s

Skin No abrasions, contusions, or lacerations

Neuro Normal

What Was Said?

After interviewing and examining his patient, the emergency medicine resident Eric, who is being shadowed by rotating medical school student Nicole, steps out of the patient's room to place orders in the computer. He sits down at the doctor's station where he takes out a chlorohexidine wipe and begins to clean the keyboard at his selected work station. "What are you doing?" asks one of his co-residents. "Oh nothing…just wiping off all of the reggin germs before I settle in." Noticing the perplexed look on his colleague's face, Eric leans in and whispers, "Reggin. R-E-G-G-I-N. Spell it backwards." With looks of both shock and amusement, the two residents glance at each other and begin to laugh hysterically. "That's awesome. I'm stealing that, man," says the other resident. Nicole, who is an African-American woman, overhears the entire conversation in disbelief.

What Was Done?

Eric ordered an ankle X-ray and pain medication for his patient. The study is read as negative, and Eric places the patient in a bulky Jones dressing before discharging her home. Nicole, who feels very upset and uncomfortable, leaves the shift to attend a previously scheduled lecture. While sitting in her classroom, Nicole decides that while the conversation Eric had with his co-resident was inappropriate, she does not want to risk receiving a poor evaluation from him. She has 2 more weeks in her emergency medicine rotation and does not want to earn negative attention during her remaining time. She resolves to keep the incident to herself and simply avoid working with Eric in the future.

Question for Discussion

1. Had Nicole been unaware of the conversation, would Eric's language be perceived as more, less, or equally as racist?

Attitudes/Assumptions: The Resident

Although hidden under the guise of another word, Eric used a derogatory term that has roots in overt, undeniable racism. Eric felt safe to use that microaggression in the presence of another young, white male, who, instead of denouncing Eric's behavior, applauded it. In fact, Eric's colleague was so accepting of Eric's behavior that he decides to adopt the racist term into his own vocabulary.

Attitudes/Assumptions: Medical School Student

Nicole finds herself at conflict with her feelings. She knows she heard a conversation not intended for her ears; however, what Eric said was wrong, and she feels compelled to confront him. Further complicating the matter, Eric is her superior and can impact how well or poorly Nicole is graded in her rotation. She is aware of the stereotype featuring the "angry black woman" and feels that she will be perceived as a troublemaker or a difficult person to work with if she chooses to speak up.

Cross-Cultural Tools and Skills

Mary C. Gentile, senior research scholar at Babson College, is the author of 2010's *Giving Voice to Values: How to Speak Your Mind When You Know What's Right* [8]. She gives the following tips on how to deal with offensive language in the workplace:

1. Ask yourself what you find offensive and why.
2. Think about what you may or may not accomplish by confronting the issue.
3. Change the subject if you think the offensive mentality behind the behavior cannot be changed.
4. If you decide to confront the offensive behavior, take time to collect your thoughts and defuse your emotion before speaking.

Pearls and Pitfalls

Pearl Nicole took time to sort through her feelings rather than confronting Eric with an emotional response. An off-the-cuff response may have interrupted patient care and possibly created an environment that made the patient feel unsafe.

Pitfall Eric's behavior is unprofessional, insensitive, and unfortunately, was not confronted. On a large scale, his use of derogatory language perpetuates negative thoughts and behaviors that serve to oppress others. On a smaller, yet equally important scale, Eric's actions may compromise the cohesion of his team and thereby compromise patient care. Furthermore, Eric inadvertently used his position of authority to marginalize, rather than mentor Nicole. Nicole feels uncomfortable in her work environment and no longer feels as though she is a part of the team. She also feels helpless and at conflict with her beliefs – speaking up against what she knows is wrong could potentially have negative effects on her personal advancement.

Case Outcome

The patient followed up with her primary care provider 1 week later where she reported improved symptoms and return to full functional status.

Attending Physician Makes Inappropriate Comments About a Gay Patient to a Medical Student Who Is Also Gay

Case Scenario
A 28-year-old male presents to a small, community emergency department (ED) complaining of low-grade fever, gradually worsening headache, and intolerance to bright lights over the past 6 h. He has vomited once and continues to have nausea. The pain is worse with movement of head and neck. He denies cough, nasal congestion, or sore throat. He has no recent sick contacts. He is accompanied to the ED by his male partner who is asymptomatic.

Review of Symptoms

He denies chest pain, shortness of breath, or abdominal pain.

Past Medical History

Negative

Medications Truvada for PrEP, intermittent compliance due to monogamous relationship

Social History

Reports social alcohol, occasional marijuana use, and admits to trying GHB 6 months prior. Denies tobacco use. Last HIV test 1 year ago was negative. Reports being sexually active with only his male partner for the past year.

Physical Exam

Vital signs Temperature 102.7; blood pressure, 130/82; heart rate, 109; respiratory rate, 18; oxygen saturation, 99% on room air

General Well-developed and well-nourished male in moderate discomfort

Head Eyes closed, +photophobia bilaterally

Neck There is nuchal rigidity.

Cardiovascular Tachycardic and regular; no murmurs, rubs, or gallops appreciated

Lungs Breaths are normal and symmetric.

Abdomen Bowel sounds are normal. Abdomen is soft, non-tender, and non-distended. There is no rebound or guarding.

Extremities There is full range of motion at all joints. Distal pulses are palpable and are +2.

Neuro GCS is 15. Neurologic examination was grossly non-focal.

Skin Unremarkable, no rashes

What Was Said?

The attending emergency physician, a 56-year-old male, discusses the case with Mark, a third-year medical student interested in emergency medicine. The attending tells Mark that the patient is probably sexually promiscuous, noting the previous use of GHB. The attending says, "We'll have to order an HIV test, I'm sure he has it given his lifestyle." Mark mentions the negative test HIV test from 1 year ago, and the attending says it cannot be trusted. He says, "He's probably lying about getting tested so his partner doesn't find out." Mark is uncomfortable with the interaction with the attending, who does not know that Mark is gay.

What Was Done?

A CT of the head is done, and a lumbar puncture is performed to evaluate for acute bacterial meningitis. An HIV test is done with a negative result. When the attending and Mark go to tell the patient about the negative test, they ask the partner to leave the room. The patient insists that the partner stay. When they give the patient the negative result, he is upset that HIV testing was done without his consent. Mark is visibly uncomfortable with the interaction. "Don't worry, we did the right thing," the attending tells Mark. "HIV could make his infection much more severe if he has meningitis, and we just can't trust some people."

Mark discusses the case with a faculty member at the medical school who is also gay. While Mark does not purposefully hide his sexuality, he also does not feel the need to disclose being gay to each attending he works with. He felt the interaction would have been different if the attending knew he was gay. He also expressed feeling helpless and regretted not responding more forcefully to the negative comments made by the attending.

Question for Discussion

1. What are some attitudes and assumptions in this case?

Attitudes/Assumptions: The Attending

The attending had a clear bias toward a gay patient who came to the ED with his partner. He assumed that the patient was promiscuous and even stated that the information he provided could not be trusted. While studies suggest that gay men are more likely to use tobacco, alcohol, and recreational drugs, use of these substances cannot be universally applied to all patients [9]. Additionally, the attending assumed that testing for HIV was in the patient's best interest and that consent was not necessary. While advanced HIV or AIDS make patients immunocompromised, it would not greatly impact the treatment for acute bacterial meningitis. Patients who have capacity should consent before HIV testing is done. Partners should be asked to leave the room when discussing the merits of HIV testing. As part of the discussion, providers should discuss with patients whether results can be shared with partners before the test is performed. If the patient in this case had tested positive for HIV, the already awkward interaction with the attending could have been much worse.

Attitudes/Assumptions: The Medical Student

Mark was clearly bothered by the comments of the attending and assumes he would not have said them if he knew Mark was gay.

Gaps in Provider Knowledge

The attending physician in this case expressed some clear knowledge gaps. He drew conclusions about patient behavior based on stereotypes and perpetuated them when discussing the case with Mark. Additionally, the attending assumed that testing for HIV was in the patient's best interest and that consent was not necessary. While advanced HIV or AIDS make patients immunocompromised, it would not greatly impact the treatment for acute bacterial meningitis. Patients who have capacity should consent before HIV testing is done. Partners should be asked to leave the room when discussing the merits of HIV testing. As part of the discussion, providers should discuss with patients whether results can be shared with partners before the test is performed. If the patient in this case had tested positive for HIV, the already awkward interaction with the attending could have been much worse.

Cross-Cultural Tools and Skills

According to Boroughs et al. [10]:

> Cultural competence with sexual and gender minority groups involves: (a) awareness of one's own beliefs, biases, and attitudes regarding LGBT populations; (b) knowledge and understanding of LGBT populations, including expectations for the counseling relationship and how one's own sexual orientation and gender identity come into play; and (c) skills and tools to provide culturally-sensitive interventions for LGBT populations. Training programs should increase LGBT-specific knowledge both of theories of identity formation, minority stress, and the current state of the literature (which changes at rapid pace) about LGBT-specific concerns and health disparities.

Pearls and Pitfalls

Pearl HIV testing in the ED should include a separate discussion with the patient before being performed, including a discussion of who can be present when giving results. Several states do not require a separate consent for HIV testing, but this does not remove the need to discuss this delicate subject before performing the test [11].

Pitfall Do not allow attending physicians who make inappropriate assumptions about patients based on gender, race, religion, ethnicity, sexual orientation, and/or gender identity to go unchallenged. Understanding epidemiology of specific populations can help identify risk factors for certain diseases, but be careful not to apply assumptions to all patients within these groups [12]. If the student does not feel comfortable discussing this with the attending, speak to the clerkship director, advisory, or other appropriate supervisor.

Case Outcome

Cerebrospinal fluid came back with no white blood cells and no organisms identified on Gram stain. The patient felt much better after hydration with IV fluids and was discharged.

References

1. Cruess RL, Cruess SR, Boudreau JD, et al. Reframing medical education to support professional identity formation. Acad Med. 2014;89:1446–14511.
2. Kalet A, Buckvar-Keltz L, Harnik V, et al. Measuring professional identity formation early in medical school. Med Teach. 2017;39:255–61.
3. Kegan R. The evolving self. Cambridge, MA: Harvard University Press; 1982. 335p.
4. Sue DW, Capodilupo CM, Torino GC, et al. Racial microaggressions in everyday life; implications for clinical practice. Am Psychol. 2007;62:27–286.
5. Wald HS, Anthony D, Hutchinson TA, et al. Professional identity formation in medical education for humanistic, resilient physicians: pedagogic strategies for bridging theory to practice. Acad Med. 2015;90:753–60.
6. Sue DW. Microaggressions in every day life: race, gender and sexual orientation. Hoboken: Wiley; 2010. 352 p.
7. Khan A. 6 ways to respond to sexist microaggressions in everyday conversations [Internet]. [place unknown]: Everyday Feminism; 2015 [cited 2017 Nov 13]. Available from: https://everydayfeminism.com/2015/01/responses-to-sexist-microaggressions/.
8. Gentile MC. Giving voice to values: how to speak your mind when you know what's right. New Haven: Yale University Press; 2010. 329p.
9. Cochran S, Keenan C, Schober C, Mays V. Estimates of alcohol use and clinical treatment needs among homosexually active men and women in the U.S. population. J Consult Clin Psychol. 2000;68:1062–71.

10. Boroughs MS, Bedoya CA, O'Cleirigh C, Safren SA. Toward defining, measuring, and evaluating LGBT cultural competence for psychologists. Clin Psychol. 2015;22(2):151–71.
11. Conron KJ, Mimiaga MJ, Landers SJ. A population-based study of sexual orientation identity and gender differences in adult health. Am J Public Health. 2010;100(10):1953–60.
12. Eckstrand KL, Ehrenfeld JM. Lesbian, gay, bisexual, and transgender healthcare: a clinical guide to preventive, primary and specialist care. 1st ed. New York: Springer; 2016. 483p.

Chapter 35
Colored Girl Student

Mekbib Gemeda and Anthonia Ojo

Case Scenario

A 62-year-old Caucasian male presents to the emergency room after a witnessed seizure. He is difficult to arouse and accompanied by his wife. As per his wife, the patient was eating breakfast when he had generalized rigidity followed by upper and lower extremity convulsions lasting 2 min. The incident was followed by bowel and bladder incontinence. His wife denies head trauma or signs of aspiration. The patient is in a drowsy postictal state.

After the emergency room team treats the patient, the neurology resident instructs the medical student to start an admitting history and physical. The medical student, an African-American female, enters the room and introduces herself and her role.

The patient's wife refuses to let the medical student see the patient, claiming, "This is not Obama's America anymore. I can decide who can or cannot touch my husband." "I do not want the colored girl to care for my husband," the patient's wife said to the nurse. The medical student returns to the resident and attending to explain the incident.

Review of Symptoms

Provided by the wife: New-onset headaches and lower back pain for 2 months, reports 10-pound unintentional weight loss in 2 months; no fever, chills, or changes in vision or hearing

M. Gemeda (✉) · A. Ojo
Eastern Virginia Medical School, Norfolk, VA, USA
e-mail: gemedam@evms.edu

© Springer International Publishing AG, part of Springer Nature 2019

M. L. Martin et al. (eds.), *Diversity and Inclusion in Quality Patient Care*,
https://doi.org/10.1007/978-3-319-92762-6_35

Past Medical History

Prostate cancer diagnosed 2 years ago and in remission.

Family History

Noncontributory

Social History

Denies alcohol, drug, or tobacco use. Lives at home with wife.

Physical Exam

Vital Signs Temperature 98.7F, pulse 60, respiration 12, BP 157/87, O_2 sat: 99% room air

General Frail male, drowsy postictal state

HEENT Head normocephalic, atraumatic; pupils equal and reactive to light and accommodation, no signs of papilledema; ear canals and tympanic membrane clear bilaterally, nose clear, throat clear; oropharynx reveals no inflammation, swelling, exudate, or lesions. Teeth and gingiva in general good condition; lacerations on lateral tongue

Cardiovascular Regular rate and rhythm, no murmur, rubs, or gallops

Respiratory Clear breath sounds

Skin No rashes or lesions

Neuro Not oriented to time, place, or situation; drowsy, confused; sensation to pain and touch normal; deep tendon reflexes 2+ in upper and lower extremities; no focal deficits

What Was Said?

The patient's wife says, "This is not Obama's America anymore. I can decide who can or cannot touch my husband. I do not want the colored girl to care for my husband." The student leaves the room, visibly upset by the comments. The student finds the resident and relates to her that she is unable to take the history and administer a physical examination. The student describes the reaction and comments of the patient's wife while she was attempting to conduct her assigned duty. The resident, who was looking at the chart of a patient for discharge, listens to the student inattentively and says to the student, "No problem, I will take care of it." The resident enters the room to take the history and administer the physical examination. The patient's wife is courteous and friendly in providing the information needed. The patient was not in a state to respond and did not directly refuse to see the medical student – the wife did, and situation is not emergent. The patient's wife does not mention what transpired with the student, and the resident does not ask.

What Was Done?

The student reports the incident to the resident. The resident takes the history and administers the physical in place of the student. The resident does not entertain the broader problem, which is the student's concern and altruism, the possible psychological stress, and denial of opportunity for learning because of her race [1, 2]. The resident does not report it to the attending, considering it a routine case of rogue racist patients that "we need to be equipped to handle" [3, 4].

The student did not report the case to the attending. She did not want to ruffle any feathers and affect the evaluation of her clerkship negatively. The student did not want to create the impression that she was going above the resident or questioning in any way how he dealt with the situation [2]. She was also not sure how the attending would react to the problem. Would he be sympathetic to her feelings of disempowerment and discrimination? Would he support the decision of the patient's wife from the perspective of valuing the patient and family's choice or from a hidden bias that he himself may possess?

The issue came up 2 weeks later, without much detail as to who and what was involved, when the nurse mentioned it in passing regarding outrageous demands by patients and families. The attending, resident, and student were all present. The student did not say anything. The attending agreed that patients at times make outrageous requests, and as providers "we try to accommodate in the best way possible" [3, 5–7].

Questions for Discussion

1. Was the comment by the wife actually "racist"?

Attitudes/Assumptions: The Patient

The actions of the patient's wife certainly suggest a racial bias toward the student who was preparing to take the history and conduct the physical examination of her husband. She responded aggressively to the student's presence in the care environment and demanded that she be removed. The reason for the student's removal was her race and not her competency or her ability to perform the task at hand.

2. What should the attending and resident tell the student?

The issue reported by the student, who was asked to leave her duty, should have been escalated by the resident to the attending for immediate intervention.

Attitudes/Assumptions: The Provider

Unfortunately in this case, the attending did not seem to respond to the lighthearted indication of a bias incident that the nurse shared. The resident did not see it as important enough to escalate to the attending. The student was afraid to report it to the attending after sharing with the resident without any action [8].

3. What should the attending and resident tell the wife?

The attending and resident should have addressed the issue with the patient's wife directly. They should have informed the patient's wife that the student is a trainee who is part of the team prepared to provide the best care to the patient and address the patient and family's needs. They should inform the patient's wife that the institution takes pride in selecting the best and brightest to the school to participate in the training program, and the student is one of these best and brightest students.

Gaps in Provider Knowledge

There are a number of issues at play here that relate to the student, the resident, and the attending. The student should realize that there should be levels of protection for her against discrimination in her learning environment. Realizing that unconscious biases and the subjective nature of clerkship evaluation could be difficult to navigate, she should have tools to enable her to address issues of bias with her resident and attending. The resident should have an understanding of racial, ethnic, and other forms of bias in health care that affect not only patients but providers as well. In that context, she should be able to intervene to provide the best care for patients and the best learning environment for trainees. The attending should have the necessary sensitivity to detect bias and discrimination, even when incidents are not officially reported. The attending also must explore and intervene immediately in order to ensure an environment of high-quality care, safety, and excellent training for students.

Cross-Cultural Tools and Skills

A knowledge level of racial and ethnic bias in the healthcare system that affects patients, trainees, and providers seems to be deficient in this scenario. Understanding of systemic biases and how they manifest in healthcare settings would be recommended as best practice interventions.

Pearls and Pitfalls

Pearl The reaction of the patient's wife should not be foreign to anyone if we were to translate it into various settings. We all might make biased assumptions or stereotype others from different groups based on their race, ethnicity, sexual orientation, gender identity, or even professional or functional groups. We also tend to mask these underlying biases or discomforts with broader ideological or political blankets as rationale. This is in large part how implicit bias works. Research and education on implicit bias in health care is not as robust as we would like it to be in relation to bias against providers or trainees based on their race, ethnicity, or association with any other identity groups.

Pitfall Providers may be unequipped to address the difficult issues that relate to racial bias in the healthcare environment. It is important to note that what is central in the scenario here is quality of care and education that has been compromised. As we are engaged in delivering both, we can, and in fact we must, address the issue that seems to compromise them directly.

Case Outcome

Diagnosis Prostate cancer metastasis to brain

Disposition The patient was admitted to the hospital in care of the oncology team.

References

1. Ansell DA, McDonald EK. Bias, black lives, and academic medicine. N Engl J Med. 2015;372:1087–9. https://doi.org/10.1056/NEJMp1500832.
2. Brooks KC. A silent curriculum. JAMA. 2015;313(19):1909–10.
3. Betancourt JR. Not me! Doctors, decisions, and disparities in health care. Cardiovasc Rev Rep. 2005;25(3):105–9.
4. Ewen SC, Barret JK, Paul D, Askew DA, Webb G, Wilkin A. When a patient's ethnicity is declared, medical students' decision-making processes are affected. Intern Med J. 2015;45(8):805–12.
5. Azevedo RT, Macaluso E, Avenanti A, Santangelo V, Cazzato V, Aglioti SM. Their pain is not our pain: brain and automatic correlates of empathic resonance with the pain of same and different race individuals. Hum Brain Mapp. 2012;34:3168–81. https://doi.org/10.1002/hbm.22133.
6. Hirsh AT, Hollingshead NA, Ashburn-Nardo L, Kroenke K. The interaction of patient race, provider bias, and clinical ambiguity on pain management decisions. J Pain. 2015;16(6):558–68.
7. Penner LA, Dovidio JF, West TV, Gaertner SL, Albrecht TL, Dailey RK, Markova T. Aversive racism and medical interactions with black patients: a field study. J Exp Soc Psychol. 2010;46(2):436–40.
8. Teal CR, Gill AC, Green AR, Crandall S. Helping medical learners recognise and manage unconscious bias toward certain patient groups. Med Educ. 2012;46(1):80–8.

Chapter 36
Gay Student

Timothy Layng and Joel Moll

Case Scenario

A 52-year-old Caucasian male presents to the preoperative area of the endoscopic suite for a routine colonoscopy. Trevor, a third-year medical student, enters the preoperative bay to meet Dr. Kline, an attending anesthesiologist. Dr. Kline hands over the patient's chart and says, "I'm going to go check on another patient, look over Mr. Price's chart, and I'll be right back." As the student is examining the chart outside the patient's bay, a nurse enters the bay and loudly exclaims, "Trevor! I saw that picture of you and your boyfriend from this weekend, it was very cute!"

Trevor replies, "Thank you! Cole and I had a great weekend," just as Dr. Kline returns and gestures Trevor into the room by pulling back the curtain to Bed 1. Dr. Kline introduces himself to the patient and informs him that Trevor will be part of the team today. The patient does not reply, and Trevor begins obtaining the patient's history.

Review of Symptoms

Asymptomatic, anxious about the examination.

T. Layng · J. Moll (✉)
Department of Emergency Medicine, Virginia Commonwealth
University, Richmond, VA, USA
e-mail: joel.moll@vcuhealth.org

Past Medical History

Type II diabetes mellitus, hyperlipidemia, obstructive sleep apnea, hypertension.

Family History

Type II diabetes mellitus, coronary artery disease.

Social History

Drinks socially, has used chewing tobacco for 30 years, works as a farmer on his large family owned farm in a local rural town.

Physical Exam

Vital Signs Temp 37.1, BP 143/93, HR 113, RR 20, SpO2 98% on room air.

Head Head is normocephalic and atraumatic; cranial nerves II–XII are grossly intact.

ENT The patient has poor dentition and a small area of leukoplakia.

Neck Non-tender.

Cardiovascular Tachycardia, but no murmurs are appreciated.

Respiratory Lungs are clear to auscultation bilaterally.

Abdomen Obese but non-tender.

Extremities Patient has good peripheral pulses and good muscle strength.

Neuro Non-focal neurologic examination.

What Was Said?

After eliciting the history and performing the physical exam, Trevor states, "This patient doesn't have a peripheral IV." Dr. Kline replies, "Ah yes, he'll need one for the procedure. Mr. Pierce, do you mind if my student attempts to place the IV?" The patient becomes uneasy and does not initially reply. After a few seconds, Dr. Kline asks, "I'm sorry sir, is there a problem?" Mr. Pierce replies, "Can't the nurse just put it in? I don't want the gay student poking me with a needle."

What Was Done?

The attending identifies that the patient is uncomfortable with the student and asks him to please leave the encounter. The attending reminds the patient of the hospital's role in educating future physicians; however, it is up to the patient to decide who participates in his care. The attending asks Trevor to leave the bedside and begin the interview on the next patient. A female nurse enters the bay and starts a peripheral line. The attending informs the student about the school's LGBT support group.

Questions for Discussion

1. What was implied or assumed, and by whom?

Attitudes/Assumptions: The Nurse

(a) The nurse assumes Trevor is comfortable talking about his personal life in a professional setting.
(b) She may also assume that no one else is listening or could hear the conversation.

Attitudes/Assumptions: The Patient

(a) The patient implies that he is uncomfortable with the gay student performing a procedure.

Attitudes/Assumptions: The Physician

(a) The physician implies that the patient has a right to decide who participates in his care by asking the student to proceed to the next patient.

2. Is this encounter likely to affect the well-being of the medical student?
   Trevor is stereotyped as being high risk to the patient due to his sexual orientation, making him feel discriminated against and isolated. A 2015 study compar-

ing the mental health and well-being of sexual minority and heterosexual medical students revealed that sexual minority students were at a significantly greater risk of social stressors such as harassment and isolation [1].

3. Is the student at a higher risk for depression than his heterosexual classmates?
A survey of osteopathic medical students performed in 2014 by Lapinski and Sexton demonstrated higher levels of depression in students who identified as lesbian, gay, or bisexual (no study participants self-identified as transgender) [2]. There were also statistically significant lower levels of perceived social support, and these students reported an increased level of discomfort with disclosure of sexual orientation, as well as a campus climate described as "noninclusive."

4. Does the student's sexual orientation place him at a disadvantage for his choice in residency education?
LGBT Health published a study that reiterated the unique stressors that sexual and gender minorities (SGM) face in their training. They extrapolate on this with data supporting the notion that specialty prestige inversely correlated with percentage of SGMs that ultimately matched to such specialties as orthopedics, neurosurgery, thoracic surgery, general surgery, and colorectal surgery. This finding paralleled previous data that identified surgery, OB/GYN, pediatrics, and anesthesiology as the most biased specialties for SGMs [3].

Gaps In Provider Knowledge

(a) The attending physician provides a very simple response to the event, with resources for local LGBT groups within the school. He misses an opportunity to provide information about national groups, such as the American Medical Student Association's Committee on Gender and Sexuality [4].

(b) The attending physician misses an opportunity for further education of the patient. Instead, he reinforces the patient's beliefs by quickly ordering the student to leave and telling the patient he can choose who participates in his care.

Cross-Cultural Tools and Skills

(a) The National LGBT Health Education Center, a program of the Fenway Institute, has a number of patient handouts (educational resources) on their website, specifically for LGBT patients [5].

(b) The Fenway Institute also publishes an evidenced-based review guide that highlights current issues LGBT patients experience, which can serve as an integral resource to any practicing physician [6].

Pearls and Pitfalls

Pearl The attending decision to have the student leave the room was within his purview. The attending counseled the patient on his right to choose whether students can participate in his care.

Pearl The attending supports the student's sexual orientation and offers information about social support groups.

Pitfall The nurse assumes the medical student is comfortable discussing his personal life in a professional setting and that others in the area are also comfortable with the subject.

Pitfall The attending physician could have asked the patient what his concern is for allowing the student to care for him, perhaps missing an opportunity to educate the patient.

Case Outcome

Procedure Dr. Reynolds, the attending gastroenterologist, performs the colonoscopy with anesthesia administered by Dr. Kline.

Diagnosis Normal routine screening colonoscopy.

Disposition Home with follow-up with primary care physician.

Dr. Kline approaches the student after the encounter and asks if the student is aware of the school's LGBT support group. Trevor is already an active member of the group and states he is aware that such bias is still present in certain areas of the country. He reports that similar situations have made him feel isolated in the past, but he has felt strong support from friends and family that have helped him through such experiences. Dr. Kline informs him that he is a strong student and looks forward to their last week on the rotation together.

References

1. Przedworski JM, Dovidio JF, Hardeman RR, et al. A comparison of the mental health and well-being of sexual minority and heterosexual first-year medical students: a report from medical student CHANGES. Acad Med. 2015;90(5):652–9. https://doi.org/10.1097/ACM.0000000000000658.
2. Lapinski J, Sexton P. Still in the closet: the invisible minority in medical education. BMC Med Educ. 2014;14(1). https://doi.org/10.1186/1472-6920-14-171.

3. Sitkin NA, Pachankis JE. Specialty choice among sexual and gender minorities in medicine: the role of specialty prestige, perceived inclusion, and medical school climate. LGBT Health. 2016;3(6):451–60. https://doi.org/10.1089/lgbt.2016.0058.
4. Gender & Sexuality Action Committee [Internet]. Sterling: American Medical Student Association; 2017 [cited 2017 Nov 7]. Available from: www.amsa.org/advocacy/action-committees/gender-sexuality/.
5. Patient Handouts [Internet]. Boston: National LGBT Health Education Center, Fenway Institute; [cited 2017 Nov 7]. Available from: www.lgbthealtheducation.org/lgbt-education/publications/patient-handouts-2/.
6. Makadon HJ, et al. The Fenway guide to lesbian, gay, bisexual, and transgender health. 2nd ed. Philadelphia: American College of Physicians; 2015. p. 603.

Chapter 37
Jewish Student

Shana Zucker

Case Scenario

A 70-year-old black male presents to a federally qualified health center with the complaint of episodes of dizziness and weakness. He has lived in New Orleans his entire life and was among the evacuees during Hurricane Katrina that were harbored in the Mercedes Super Dome. Prior to Hurricane Katrina, he lived in the Lower Ninth Ward, but he has since moved to Gentilly. When approached by a Jewish medical student, he says, "The Jews and 'em don't care about us." After taking the patient history, the first year medical student, who is Jewish, explains to the patient that she will proceed to the physical examination. The patient responds, "No offense, but can you let the doctor do it? I know you're learning and all, but I don't want no kike touching me." The examination is discontinued, and the Jewish medical student asks the attending physician if she would see the patient and complete the examination. The attending is an African-American female.

Review of Symptoms

Chief complaint of dizzy spells that are alleviated by rest and eating. They have been happening sporadically over the last 4 years but have been occurring several times a day over the last 2 weeks, prompting his wife to bring him in to the health center.

S. Zucker
Tulane University School of Medicine, New Orleans, LA, USA
e-mail: szucker@tulane.edu

© Springer International Publishing AG, part of Springer Nature 2019
M. L. Martin et al. (eds.), *Diversity and Inclusion in Quality Patient Care*,
https://doi.org/10.1007/978-3-319-92762-6_37

Past Medical History

The patient's past medical history is questionable for diabetes mellitus type II. On initial interview, the patient states that he has never taken medication for diabetes and that he was diagnosed with the condition 4 years ago. Outside the patient's room, his wife discloses that he was diagnosed 30 years ago.

Family History

Mother and father died at ages 80 and 76, respectively, of unspecified heart problems. The patient's 64-year-old sister has diabetes. The patient's two maternal aunts have diabetes, and the patient's maternal uncle has diabetes and has had a stroke.

Social History

Drinks alcohol, heavily for many years; smoked two packs a day for 4 years in his youth but quit cold turkey 40 years ago. Smokes about one joint of marijuana a week for the last year. The patient has been married for 47 years and has two adult children.

Physical Exam

Vital Signs Temperature normal, blood pressure 170/97, pulse 103.

General NAD, well appearing.

HEENT No changes in vision, no congestion, no changes in hearing.

Cardiovascular Aortic valve regurgitation is appreciated; axillary artery and external carotid artery are noted for pulsatile distention.

Respiratory Lungs are clear to auscultation bilaterally.

Abdomen Soft, non-tender; bowel sounds are normal.

Extremities Hammertoes on right foot, tinea pedis noted between toes of right foot; four slowly healing wounds described as "blisters" by the patient on the bilateral feet and right leg, ranging in age from 1 week to 6 months; sensation intact.

What Was Said?

The patient said, "I don't want no kike touching me." This prompted the medical student to respond, "Let me find my attending." The patient also said, "The Jews and 'em don't care about us."

What Was Done?

The medical student reported patient history and vitals and informed the attending that the patient requested another physician to complete the physical exam due to the student's ethnicity. The attending returned to perform the physical exam and asked the patient if the medical student may observe. The patient seemed hesitant. The physician encouraged the patient to allow the medical student to observe so that she can learn. The patient complied. The attending performed the physical exam and measured the patient's non-fasting blood glucose. The glucometer reading was 418 mg/dl. The physician concluded that, given the combination of the patient's uncontrolled diabetes, newly diagnosed hypertension, large pulse pressure, and aortic valve regurgitation, the patient needed to be referred for a full workup at the local hospital.

Question for Discussion

1. What may be contributing to some underlying attitudes and assumptions in this case?

Attitudes/Assumptions: The Patient

Black-Jewish relations post-Katrina resulted in widely disparate attitudes toward Jewish people. Fifty-one percent of Katrina-related deaths were of black individuals; zero Jews died of Katrina-related causes [1]. On the other hand, the shared diaspora of both groups in the hurricane's aftermath contributed to a sense of unity, with many describing rescuers making no distinction of ethnicity [2]; still, the recovery rate of white, upper-middle class neighborhoods was quadruple that of black, working-class neighborhoods, specifically the Lower Ninth Ward [3]. In the wake of Katrina, many groups encouraged "voluntourism," and the presence of Jewish groups was particularly publicized [4]. However, these altruistic notions "ignored the deeply entrenched political, economic, and social equalities," and perpetuated the "white savior complex" (note: while, historically, both blacks and Jews experienced discrimination in early New Orleans, the Jewish people benefited from upward mobility and slowly came to be considered "white" in American society) [5]. Black survivors' attitudes toward this "humanitarianism" ranged from gratitude for help with small tasks [4, 5] to general apathy or frustration as "such assistance was temporary and would not singlehandedly transform deeply entrenched issues that affected the Lower Ninth Ward every day" [4, 5]. Additionally, the partnership between the Jewish Federation and the St. Bernard Parish Project, which was found in contempt for intentional racial discrimination in post-Katrina rebuilding, foddered contempt toward Jews [6]. The black-Jewish relations in New Orleans are further complicated by political division within the Black Lives Matter (BLM) movement. While 57% of Jews support BLM, the incorporation of Israel-Palestine policy into the vision of BLM has caused subdivision and added nuanced complexity to race relations [7]. The attitudes of this patient cannot be assumed.

Attitudes/Assumptions: Providers

The medical student felt the need to excuse herself after the initial interaction with this patient. She was caught off-guard by the patient's use of an anti-Semitic slur and his correct assumption of her religion/ethnicity based off of her appearance alone that she is Jewish, and thought that disputing the patient's wishes would be unproductive.

Gaps in Provider Knowledge

The medical student did not know the best way to handle the situation. Further, the medical student was unfamiliar with the historical context of Black-Jewish relations, and their particular intricacy in New Orleans.

Cross-Cultural Tools and Skills

The medical student sought out the attending, who took the lead on the rest of the case. The medical student was not equipped with cross-cultural tools and skills.

Pearls and Pitfalls

Pearl Mature medical student decision to politely excuse herself without arguing with the patient's request or beliefs and to seek the attending's assistance to accommodate the patient's wishes [8].

Pearl The attending physician continued to provide excellent care regardless of the patient's differing views and did not allow her own implicit bias to impact treatment.

Pitfall In an emergency situation, finding another care provider may not be appropriate. However, in this case, this was the best outcome.

Pitfall The medical student should have taken the opportunity after the patient left to ask the attending to debrief the situation in order to depersonalize the experience and emotionally prepare for a future similar encounter. Likewise, the attending physician should have taken the opportunity to debrief about the interaction with the student and any other trainees on this case [9].

Case Outcome

The patient and his wife are educated about the seriousness of pursuing follow-up care. The physician schedules a follow-up appointment for the patient at the local hospital and also hands the patient and his wife her card in case they have any concerns between now and the follow-up appointment. The physician encourages the medical student to offer her contact information, so the medical student asks if the patient would like her contact information. The patient declines. The physician calls the local hospital the next week; the patient did indeed follow up and is now linked into necessary care.

References

1. Brunkard J, Namulanda G, Ratard R. Hurricane Katrina deaths, Louisiana, 2005. Disaster Med Public Health Prep. 2008;2(04):215–23.
2. Schuman J. Children of exile [Internet]. Washington: Religious Action Center; 2009 [cited 2017 Jul 28]. Available from: http://blogs.rj.org/rac/2009/07/27/children_of_exile/.
3. Adams V, Hattum TV, English D. Chronic disaster syndrome: displacement, disaster capitalism, and the eviction of the poor from New Orleans. Am Ethnol. 2009;36(4):615–36.
4. Kornfeld MHG. The chosen universalists: Jewish philanthropy and youth activism in post-Katrina New Orleans. Dissertation, University of Michigan, Ann Arbor; 2015. 308 p.
5. Smithson ME. Disaster, displacement, and voluntourism: helping narratives of college student volunteers in post-Katrina New Orleans. Undergraduate thesis, University of Mississippi, Oxford; 2014. 82 p.
6. Ochieng A. Black-Jewish relations intensified and tested by current political climate [Internet]. Washington: NPR; 2017 [cited 2017 Aug 1]. Available from: http://www.npr.org/sections/codeswitch/2017/04/23/494790016/black-jewish-relations-intensified-and-tested-by-current-political-climate.
7. Alexander-Bloch B. Federal judge again finds St. Bernard Parish in contempt for racial discrimination [Internet]. New Orleans: NOLA.com; 2011 [cited 2017 Jul 30]. Available from: http://www.nola.com/crime/index.ssf/2011/10/federal_judge_again_finds_st_b.html.
8. Whitgob EE, Blankenburg RL, Bogetz AL. The discriminatory patient and family. Acad Med. 2016;91:S64–9.
9. Paul-Emile K, Smith AK, Fernández A. Dealing with racist patients. N Engl J Med. 2016;374(8):708–11.

Chapter 38
Resident to Student Barriers and Bias

J. Bridgman Goines

Case Scenario

As the attending is seeing patients, the senior level emergency medicine resident is assigning cases to two medical students who are part of the emergency department (ED) treatment team for the evening shift. Both students are cisgender females, with one identifying as masculine-presenting (she/her pronouns). Given her interest in cardiac pathology, the masculine-presenting medical student requests to see a 30-year-old cisgender male with chest pain who is on the ED track board. However, the resident, a cisgender male, assigns the masculine-presenting medical student to a transgender female patient presenting with abdominal pain. He assigns the other student to the chest pain case. When the masculine-presenting medical student begins to explain her specific interest in cardiac pathology, the resident interrupts and states, "He...she...it...whatever...will probably do better with you. It's just easier this way and will help everybody be more comfortable." The masculine-presenting medical student's attitude visibly changes, but she completes the exam and reports findings to the resident. The interactions between the medical student and resident continue to be tense and uncomfortable throughout the shift. The student requests that the resident add a note to the patient medical record indicating the patient's preferred name and gender identifier. Additionally, the masculine-presenting medical student informs the resident that she is uncomfortable being assigned patients based on her gender presentation and do not want such instances to impede learning opportunities for all members of the team. Future interactions between the resident and masculine-presenting medical student appear tense, and in reviews, the resident refers to the masculine-presenting medical student as "aggressive in demeanor" and "uncooperative – not a team player."

J. Bridgman Goines
Department of Emergency Medicine, Emory University School of Medicine,
Atlanta, GA, USA
e-mail: jgoines@emory.edu

© Springer International Publishing AG, part of Springer Nature 2019
M. L. Martin et al. (eds.), *Diversity and Inclusion in Quality Patient Care*,
https://doi.org/10.1007/978-3-319-92762-6_38

Questions for Discussion

1. What caused the medical student's attitude change?

Attitudes/Assumptions: The Resident

(a) This masculine-presenting medical student looks as though they are gay or transgender.
(b) Given the medical student's assumed identity, they are probably interested in treating a transgender patient.
(c) Medically speaking, this patient is male.

Attitudes/Assumptions: The Medical Student

(a) The resident judged me by my appearance and decided that I am a member of the LGBT community without caring to talk to me about my identity.
(b) The resident ignored my petition to see the cardiac patient and sees me only by my minority status.
(c) The resident's misgendering of the patient shows that he is transphobic and unable to take corrective feedback.
(d) It is my obligation to advocate for this patient (e.g., note her gender identity accurately on her medical chart).
(e) I just need to get through this rotation. I will remember this encounter and be sure to not apply here when applying for residencies.

Gaps in Provider Knowledge

Pertaining to the patient:
(a) "It" is never an appropriate pronoun for a human and can specifically be dehumanizing for members of the transgender community (e.g., the patient) and those who closely identify with it (e.g., the medical student).
(b) Knowledge of gender and sex are both important aspects of an individual's case and may be pertinent to their care.
(c) As gender is self-determined, providers should be sure to use the gender assigned by the individual when discussing the case (e.g., in this case the individual identifies as female and should be referred to by the pronouns she and her).

Pertaining to the medical student:

(a) Never assume the LGBT status of an individual. Allow the individual to divulge this information if they deem it necessary.

(b) Members of the LGBT community are extremely diverse in identity, concerns, and stigma against them.

Pertaining to the transgender population generally:

(a) Transgender individuals are generally not as well understood or legally protected as even lesbian and gay individuals and are thus more vulnerable to legal, medical, and socioeconomic status discrimination.

(b) Understanding the various terminology surrounding transgendered individuals is important.

2. What misunderstandings and biases were revealed in the resident's assessment of the medical student?

(a) The resident, not knowing that his language was transphobic, misinterpreted the medical student's distress (e.g., shortened sentences, reduced smiling) as uncooperativeness.

(b) Evidence from emergency department literature suggests that a gender bias exists when it comes to feedback, particularly regarding issues of autonomy and assertiveness in the trainee [1]. The presence of intersectionalities (e.g., being both black and female, or, as in this example, being a masculine-presenting female) may enhance this bias further. Those in positions of power should strive to be aware of these unconscious biases when reviewing subordinates.

3. What learning opportunities were missed in this scenario?

(a) The masculine-presenting medical student missed an opportunity to learn about cardiac pathology, which was her major interest.

(b) The other medical student missed a relatively rare opportunity to learn about treating a transgender patient, which involves both medically relevant issues (e.g., considering the effects of hormone usage in the presenting complaint) and issues related to culturally sensitive care.

(c) The resident missed an opportunity to learn from the masculine-presenting medical student about the best approaches to use with gender-nonconforming colleagues.

(d) The attending missed an opportunity to teach residents and medical students about the importance of cultural humility and sensitivity in the medical care of LGBT individuals.

Cross-Cultural Tools and Skills

(a) Correct identification and clarification of the gender and preferred pronouns of a patient is an important skill for clinicians.

(b) Do not reduce an individual to their minority status and do not assume that because an individual is a member of a minority group, they wish to work with that same minority group (e.g., the medical student may be part of the LGBT community and may also have interests outside of that community).

(c) Allow trainees the opportunity to self-identify and to explain what opportunities they are hoping for in their training.

(d) Encourage trainees to engage in diverse learning opportunities, especially those that allow them to work with minority groups with which they may not have much prior knowledge or experience.

(e) Be receptive to feedback about diversity-related issues.

(f) Practice cultural humility. Even after the initial incident of referring to the patient as "it," the resident had a second opportunity to practice this skill. After the medical student advocates for her patient by asking that the patient's preferred gender be used, the resident could have acknowledged or apologized for his initially insensitive language. He could also have asked the medical student if she had noticed any other LGBT-related issues that are important to be aware of in the case of this patient.

Gender is a spectrum, not a binary construct. According to Fredrikesen-Goldsen and colleagues, "Gender refers to the behavioral, cultural, or psychological traits that a society associates with male and female sex" [2]. Thus, the term "transgender" refers to individuals who identify with a gender that is different/not congruent with their sex assigned at birth [3]. A recent nationwide study found that 0.58% of the adult US population, or almost 1.4 million individuals, identify as transgender [4]. For example, a person born with male genitalia living as a female-gendered person would be a transgender female. In contrast a person born with male genitalia who identifies as a male-gendered person would be termed a cisgender male. Gender nonconforming is a much broader category that encompasses individuals who do not ascribe to stereotypical gender norms (e.g., appearance, traditional roles, or internal experience) but who may identify with their sex assigned at birth. While there is a notable dearth of research focused on the experience of transgender individuals, recent research indicates that transgender and gender-nonconforming patients frequently feel discriminated against in the emergency room [5]. Additionally, it is likely that many of these discriminatory experiences stem from a lack of transgender/gender nonconforming training and education for providers [5].

Pearls and Pitfalls

Pearl The masculine-presenting medical student agreed to put aside her desire to see chest pain pathology in order to prioritize the needs of another patient and not disrupt patient care.

Pearl The masculine-presenting medical student respectfully and in a team-oriented manner approached the resident to discuss her concerns.

Pearl The masculine-presenting student followed up to make sure important demographic information was updated in the patient's chart.

Pitfall In acute care settings, patients will need to be seen by the next available provider, independent of commonalities that may exist between the patient and other providers.

Pitfall Providers do not usually get to pick their patients and should be given opportunities to gain experience with a diverse patient panel.

Pitfall The resident was offensive when referring to the gender of the transgender patient and most likely caused a disruption in the cohesion of the team.

Case Outcome

The resident agrees to update the patient medical record to include the appropriate patient name and gender identifier. The resident acknowledges the masculine-presenting student's concerns and apologizes for misgendering the patient. The resident joins the masculine-presenting medical student in the patient's room to continue the workup.

References

1. Mueller AS, Jenkins TM, Osborne M, Dayal A, O'Connor DM, Arora VM. Gender differences in attending physicians' feedback to residents: a qualitative analysis. J Grad Med Educ. 2017;9(5):577–85.
2. Fredriksen-Goldsen KI, Simoni JM, Kim HJ, Lehavot K, Walters KL, Yang J, Hoy-Ellis CP, Muraco A. The health equity promotion model: reconceptualization of lesbian, gay, bisexual, and transgender (LGBT) health disparities. Am J Orthopsychiatry. 2014;84(6):653.
3. Coleman E, Bockting W, Botzer M, Cohen-Kettenis P, DeCuypere G, Feldman J, Fraser L, Green J, Knudson G, Meyer WJ, Monstrey S. Standards of care for the health of transsexual, transgender, and gender-nonconforming people, version 7. Int J Transgend. 2012;13(4):165–232.
4. Gates GJ. How many people are lesbian, gay, bisexual and transgender? [Internet]. Los Angeles: The Williams Institute UCLA School of Law; 2011 [cited 2017 Nov 15]. Available from: https://williamsinstitute.law.ucla.edu/wp-content/uploads/Gates-How-Many-People-LGBT-Apr-2011.pdf.
5. Chisolm-Straker M, Jardine L, Bennouna C, Morency-Brassard N, Coy L, Egemba MO, Shearer PL. Transgender and gender nonconforming in emergency departments: a qualitative report of patient experiences. Transgend Health. 2017;2(1):8–16.

Additional Relevant Literature

Cruz TM. Assessing access to care for transgender and gender nonconforming people: a consideration of diversity in combating discrimination. Soc Sci Med. 2014;110:65–73.

Legal L, New York City Bar Association. Creating equal access to quality health care for transgender patients: transgender-affirming hospital policies. New York: Lambda Legal (US); 2016. p. 24.

McGregor AJ, Choo EK, Becker BM, editors. Sex and gender in acute care medicine. New York: Cambridge University Press; 2016. p. 256.

Chapter 39
Nurse to Nursing Student Barriers and Bias

Katherine Sullivan

Case Scenario

Karen Dunn is a 21-year-old junior baccalaureate nursing student attending her first clinical day in the emergency department (ED) of Simonville Hospital, a small community hospital located in a predominantly white upper-class town. It is a small ED with a capacity of 12 beds, each separated by curtains. There is little privacy for patients.

Karen grew up in Simonville and self-identifies as black. She is doing well in her studies, although she worries about the 30 pounds she has gained while sitting and studying over the past few years. She is excited to start learning in an active clinical setting with Jeff, a 45-year-old experienced registered nurse preceptor, who identifies as white.

Robert, an orthopedic surgeon, is 50 years old and also identifies as white. He arrives to see a 65-year-old black woman with a BMI of 42 complaining of right knee swelling, pain, and difficulty bearing weight. Jeff and Karen accompany Robert to the bedside for a knee aspiration.

After the procedure, Robert, Jeff, and Karen leave the patient together. After walking 10 feet away, Robert turns to Jeff and says, "What a big fat mama! She needs to lay off that fried chicken! These people cause their own problems, then come here and expect us to fix everything." Jeff laughs and walks away with Robert. Karen just stands there for a minute and then follows Jeff.

At the end of a busy shift, Karen says to Jeff, "Thanks so much for everything. I learned a lot today. But I have to say, I was really taken aback when the doctor called that woman in Bed 4 a fat mama, and made a comment about her eating too much fried chicken. That just did not seem right. It was a pretty racist comment. The patient could have heard us, and anyway, it just does not seem right." Jeff says,

K. Sullivan
University of Northern Colorado, Greeley, CO, USA
e-mail: Katherine.sullivan@unco.edu

© Springer International Publishing AG, part of Springer Nature 2019
M. L. Martin et al. (eds.), *Diversity and Inclusion in Quality Patient Care*,
https://doi.org/10.1007/978-3-319-92762-6_39

"That is how it is here. You can't be sensitive when you get into the real world. You have to develop a thick skin if you want to work in emergency nursing. Anyway, he is right; blacks have much higher rates of obesity than whites. You people are at high risk. Maybe he didn't say it in a politically correct way, but he is right. And he is a really good doctor."

What Was Said?

The provider said: "What a big fat mama! She needs to lay off that fried chicken! These people cause their own problems, then come here and expect us to fix everything." The nurse preceptor laughed and became complicit in a racist slur. The student was initially silent. The patient was silent but nearby; it is unclear if she heard.

Karen later attempted to bring her concerns to Jeff, who was dismissive and said, "you can't be sensitive… you have to develop a thick skin" and referred to "you people." Laughing and discounting racial slurs contribute to building and supporting a racist environment, which harms the patients and public as well as the healthcare staff. The addition of the words "you people" became, at the least, a microaggression. The preceptor labelled Karen as "the other" or "not one of us." Implicit racism may serve to keep nursing a very white profession.

What Was Done?

The student was initially silent. Given the power differentials between a student and an experienced older nurse, this would be a common reaction. The student was distressed by the remark, and this incident might impact her view of emergency nursing. She could feel marginalized, which would affect her success in the nursing program. The patient may have heard the remark and thus would feel disrespected and would not trust the care she was receiving. A lack of trust may prevent the patient from seeking future care. The preceptor failed in his role of protecting the patient from harm, by laughing and becoming complicit in a damaging comment. The preceptor also failed in his role of mentoring Karen in professional behavior. He served as a role model for unethical nursing care.

Questions for Discussion

1. Think about race, age, gender, educational level, and all the other intersecting identities that people hold. Think about the power and privileges that are associated with each identity. Do you think race is the only source of bias demonstrated in this case?

2. Less than 200 years ago, nurses were uneducated female servants working under male physician direction. Today, only about 9% of registered nurses are men [1], although 34% of physicians are women [2]. How do historical roles and identities affect patterns of unhealthy communication in the healthcare setting?

3. Karen was disturbed by the comment and spoke up twice about her discomfort. Do you think this is common? Would a young black female student, new to the clinical setting, question a racist comment with an older white male nurse preceptor or an older white professor?

4. In an emergent situation, there is a need for a hierarchy and a defined leader for communication. But in non-emergent settings, the healthiest communication occurs when team members feel empowered to have an equal voice. How can we support students in developing a professional and assertive voice to address instances of bias in the healthcare setting?

5. Karen used the word "racist." How did Jeff respond? What was the effect of Robert's comment on Karen? Which of the comments or actions were racist and which were microaggressions?

6. Knowledge about different cultures, ethnicities, races, and other identities can serve to promote stereotypes if practitioners do not think critically about that knowledge. What do you think of Jeff's comment that "you people are at high risk"? How can we gather knowledge and data about health disparities without promoting stereotypes?

Attitudes/Assumptions: The Preceptor

The preceptor assumed that it is fine to laugh at patients in the ED when among other healthcare professionals. He was oblivious that his comment and laughter were harmful to Karen, a future member of his profession. His awareness of the potential impact on the patient was completely absent. He assumed that being a "good doctor" excused Robert's damaging comments. This attitude speaks to an unhealthy workplace culture; the preceptor felt free to participate in incidents of bias, without consequences.

Attitudes/Assumptions: The Student

The student assumed that nurses would all follow the American Nurses Association (ANA) Code of Ethics, which calls for putting the patient first and treating them with respect and dignity [3]. Putting the patient first means putting the patient's interests before physician or institutional interests. Karen had assumed that all professional nurses, especially an esteemed preceptor like Jeff, should prioritize the patient's well-being by objecting to a racial slur about the patient. Karen also assumed that she was in a safe environment and that a preceptor would not insult and belittle her.

Gaps in Preceptor Knowledge

The preceptor was not conscious of the identities of others in his daily work. He did not relate nursing ethics to his daily work in the ED. He was used to focusing on tasks; he lost sight of the realization that he should, at the very least, protect his patients from harm. He was ignorant of the concept of microaggressions, as well as concepts of privilege and marginalization. He was unable to even see his own privilege. By saying "you people" to Karen, he demonstrated implicit bias. He effectively aligned himself with the other white male in the environment, marginalizing Karen and the patient. Jeff needs significant diversity training and needs to be held accountable for his behavior. Diversifying nursing is a key professional nursing goal, and Jeff needs education about his professional responsibility in supporting that goal. He needs to learn how his behavior and speech contributes to maintaining a racially homogenous nursing workforce.

Cross-Cultural Tools and Skills

The cultural conflict in this case centers on healthcare professionals acting incongruently with professional values. In many cases of cultural conflict, one culture must accommodate another and change. In this case, the change must occur in the preceptor, provider, and the ED workplace culture. The professional values are not negotiable. The process of change to a healthier ED environment, in which all are held accountable, occurs through strong leadership.

Pearls and Pitfalls

Pearl The student had the courage to speak up when she heard a racial slur. Students should be explicitly taught to speak up when harmful behaviors are observed.

Pearl The student was aware of professional standards and ethics supporting diversity and respect. The voices of all team members should be heard and respected.

Pitfall Emergency department professionals can fall into the stereotype of being tough, hard, or intolerant of non-emergent issues. Patient care suffers when uncaring behaviors are normalized.

Pitfall The preceptor felt comfortable laughing and shrugging off a racial slur, which points to an emergency department culture in which this behavior was accepted.

Pitfall When those with power (the orthopedic surgeon) promote bias, it can become widespread. Emergency department leadership needs to be proactive in promoting a culture welcoming diversity.

Pitfall A lack of diversity education among the team caused harm to both patient and student.

Case Outcome

Karen reported the incident to her trusted university nursing professor and advisor Beth, a 60-year-old white woman. Beth was responsible for clinical placement of students within the local healthcare systems, as well as teaching and advising.

Beth listened to Karen and agreed that patients should not be subjected to insults in the ED. Beth contacted the ED Nursing Director at Simonville Hospital and related what Robert had said near the patient. The Director wrote up a report of the call, stating that she was concerned the patient may have heard the comment and that this situation could generate bad publicity and a possible lawsuit. The physician was subsequently counseled about HIPAA and professional communication. The ED Director did not address Jeff's response, saying that he was a "great nurse." Beth did not want to push the issue because the university needed Jeff to precept more nursing students during the semester.

The outcome was not effective. Simonville ED continued to have a toxic workplace culture for some time. Beth failed by neglecting to use the power of her education and position to work on transforming a harmful healthcare environment. Beth could have followed up and collaborated with the ED Nursing Director in educating all staff and developing a "no tolerance" policy in this ED. Leadership sets the tone for the organizational culture.

Instead, both Beth and the ED Nursing Director failed by not managing conflict effectively. Incidences of bias need to be addressed immediately. They both focused on the physician's comment and were concerned that the patient possibly heard it. They did not acknowledge of the role of nursing in supporting a culture in which racist comments are acceptable. Either of them could have spoken to Jeff about his microaggressions and his complicity in laughing at a racist slur. Allen [4], on discussing nursing culture, stated: "The silence on racism becomes a denial of racism."

More recently, Sharma and Kuper [5] called race "the elephant in the room," as many practitioners discuss race in purely biological terms. This is exactly what Jeff did in discussing obesity. Education and training in diversity can start a much-needed discussion.

As a student, Karen displayed courage in speaking up twice about the issue: once to her nurse preceptor and once to her university instructor. Additional options for her could be:

- Report the incident to the university Diversity and Inclusion Office.
- Discuss the incident with the university Student Counseling Office.
- Contact the Dean of Students at her university.
- Call the hospital Corporate Compliance Hotline to report the incident as a violation of hospital policy or values.
- Discuss the incident with the Chair of the Nursing Program at her university.
- Report the incident to a state chapter of the American Nurses Association or Emergency Nurses Association. These organizations offer student membership and provide significant practical guidance to advocate for patient and nursing issues. The National Black Nurses Association is a smaller organization with fewer chapters; if a local chapter exists, they could also be contacted for support.

References

1. American Nurses Association. Fast facts: the nursing workforce 2014 [Internet]. Silver Springs: American Nurses Association; 2014 [cited 2017 Jul 26]. Available from: http://www.nursingworld.org/MainMenuCategories/ThePracticeofProfessionalNursing/workforce/Fast-Facts-2014-Nursing-Workforce.pdf.
2. The Henry J. Kaiser Family Foundation. Distribution of physicians by gender [Internet]. Menlo Park: Kaiser Family Foundation; 2017 [cited 2017 Jul 26]. Available from: http://www.kff.org/other/state-indicator/physicians-by-gender/?currentTimeframe=0&sortModel=%7B%22colId%22:%22Location%22,%22sort%22:%22asc%22%7D.
3. American Nurses Association. Code of ethics for nurses with interpretive statements [Internet]. Silver Springs: American Nurses Association; 2015 [cited 2017 Nov 10]. Available from: http://www.nursingworld.org/code-of-ethics.
4. Allen D. Whiteness and difference in nursing. Nurs Philos. 2006;7(2):65–78. https://doi.org/10.1111/j.1466-769X.2006.00255.x.
5. Sharma M, Kuper A. The elephant in the room: talking race in medical education. Adv in Health Sci Educ. 2017;22:761. https://doi.org/10.1007/s10459-016-9732-3.

Chapter 40
African-American Male Aspires to Become a Doctor

Marcus L. Martin, Mekbib Gemeda, Lynne Holden, and Caron Campbell

Case Scenario

Eddie Williams is an African-American male who grew up in a small, rural, Southern community with a population of 10,000. Eddie's mother completed a high school education and worked in the cafeteria at the local elementary school; his father did not complete high school and worked as a maintenance worker in the local hospital. Eddie has three older siblings, two brothers and a sister. His three siblings all completed some community college education, but they did not attend a four-year degree program. Eddie's community was racially integrated but the students in elementary, middle, and high school were predominantly African-American. Eddie's other relatives in the community included aunts, uncles, and cousins. His family attended the local African-American Baptist church.

M. L. Martin (✉)
University of Virginia, Charlottesville, VA, USA
e-mail: mlm8n@virginia.edu

M. Gemeda
Eastern Virginia Medical School, Norfolk, VA, USA
e-mail: gemedam@evms.edu

L. Holden · C. Campbell
Einstein College of Medicine, Bronx, NY, USA
e-mail: cacampbe@montefiore.org; lholden@montefiore.org

© Springer International Publishing AG, part of Springer Nature 2019
M. L. Martin et al. (eds.), *Diversity and Inclusion in Quality Patient Care*,
https://doi.org/10.1007/978-3-319-92762-6_40

K-12

Eddie was considered a "good" student in elementary and middle school and did not get into any serious trouble. He enrolled in an advanced AP Biology course in high school with the encouragement of the high school guidance counselor. He graduated in the top 10% of his class of 60 students.

Extracurricular

Eddie's family was considered low-income. He played the tenor saxophone and bass drums in the high school band for 4 years. He worked 4 h each Saturday tutoring elementary school students in reading and math at the school where his mother was employed.

Undergraduate College Years

With the encouragement and assistance of the school guidance counselor, Eddie applied to and enrolled in State University majoring in biology. His extracurricular activities while in college included pledging a fraternity, becoming a member of the premedical society, and working 10 h per week in the library. Eddie participated in a clinical enrichment program at a local medical school during the summer after his freshman year. During that time, he met an African-American physician on faculty who became his mentor. While an undergraduate, Eddie participated in research internships the summer after his sophomore and junior years. Without a prep course, Eddie took the MCAT exam after finishing his prerequisite courses junior year and did not do well the first time.

Post Undergraduate

Eddie graduated with a 2.89 science GPA and 3.1 overall GPA. He contacted a college premedical society speaker and his physician mentor from the freshman summer program for further direction. Eddie enrolled in a postbaccalaureate premedical program and did well. He retook the MCAT after utilizing test preparatory materials and taking practice exams. His MCAT score improved substantially. He began to expand his circle of mentors who helped him with the medical school application process, conducted mock interviews, and invited him to shadow them in their practices.

Medical School

Eddie was accepted to medical school and eventually received a scholarship. In medical school, Eddie experienced a number of challenges, including being one of the few black male students in the program. At times he felt out of place and like an imposter, with a curriculum lacking exploration of the social context of health disparities and perpetuating bias and stereotype.

His first year was particularly stressful. He failed two courses, anatomy in the first semester and another foundational science course in the second semester. The medical school committee established to review and make recommendations regarding the fate of students having difficulty in their courses requested Eddie meet with them. Eddie felt tremendous distress and anxiety appearing before this large group of faculty and a few student representatives. His distress was compounded by the knowledge that he was one of only two students, both minorities, meeting with the committee, and he felt that there was an implied reference to minorities generally not doing well. Eddie found himself doubting if he was really made for a medical career.

Discussion

In a recent Association of American Medical Colleges report titled *Altering the Course: Black Males in Medicine*, research found that there were less African-American male medical school matriculates in 2014 compared to 1978. "While the demographics of the nation are rapidly changing and there is a growing appreciation for diversity and inclusion as drivers of excellence in medicine, one major demographic group—black males—has reversed its progress in entering medical school. In 1978, there were 1,410 black male applicants to medical school, and in 2014, there were just 1,337. In 1978, there were 541 black male matriculates, and in 2014, we had 515. No other minority group has experienced such declines" [1].

Parents, educators, and students from low socioeconomic backgrounds identified lack of academic enrichment resources, lack of mentors, and the financial burden as three commonly perceived obstacles to attaining a health career [2]. These were clear elements for success in Eddie's journey as an African-American male. In addition to a supportive family, Eddie's story emphasizes four key components for African-American males to achieve successful admission to medical school: academics, extracurricular activities, financial aid, and mentoring.

Academics

There is a significant discrepancy in advanced math and science courses offered in US high schools with high concentrations of underrepresented minorities (URMs). For example, in 2014, one in five African-American students attended a high school that did not offer any AP courses, and one third of the high schools that have large populations of URMs do not offer chemistry [3]. Gaps in taking rigorous high school level courses contribute to a less competitive applicant to college and decreased success in college STEM courses [4]. Therefore, students graduating from college with a less competitive GPA have demonstrated better academic outcomes in medical school after successfully completing additional postbaccalaureate or Master's level coursework prior to medical school application [5, 6].

Extracurricular Activities

Studies have demonstrated that time spent in extracurricular activities positively impacts academic achievement. Students with lower socioeconomic status spend less time in such enrichment activities [7]. Students' participation in summer biomedical enrichment programs has demonstrated improved success in gaining acceptance to college and health professional school [8, 9].

Financial Considerations

The cost to attend medical school has risen substantially over the years regardless of whether the school is public or private and the student is a state resident or not. According to data from the Association of American Medical Colleges [10], the cost of tuition, fees, and health insurance for a first-year medical student who is a state resident attending a publically funded school, on average, jumped from $20,794 in 1997–1998 to $53,327 in 2017–2018. Approximately half of US medical students have come from the richest quintile of household incomes; the proportion of students from the poorest quintile has not exceeded 5.5% [11]. Due to this economic disparity, the cost of medical school is often viewed as a significant barrier for URMs and their families [12, 13]. Sources of potential funding are commonly federal dollars, local scholarship opportunities, and individual medical school-related scholarships, which can be merit or need-based [14].

One exception is the National Medical Fellowship Program (NMF), which has been providing financial resources to medical students since 1946 and has awarded $40 million to 30,000 recipients. In 1996, funding for the National Medical Fellowship Program decreased due to diminished affirmative action efforts [15]. From 1971 to 1972, NMF distributed a total of $1,687,950. From 2016 to 2017, NMF distributed a total of $899,630. The average (mean) debt for all medical students is $183,188, and for African-Americans it is $207,001 [16]. It is, therefore, important to teach financial literacy to students preparing for a medical degree along with other resources such as crowdfunding campaigns to offset the tuition.

Mentoring

Lack of confidence was the number one obstacle among URM students [2]. The confidence deficit is perpetuated by not seeing others with similar cultural backgrounds as physicians, implicit racial bias, and the imposter syndrome [3]. Multicultural mentors can alleviate inherent doubts in the African-American male during this often lonely journey. Being willing to ask for help is key to initiating the mentoring process [17]. Eddie was not afraid to seek out mentors to help him to navigate obstacles to success through joining medically related societies and pursuing outside enrichment activities such as volunteering, shadowing, research, and networking with like-minded students. The value of a mentor is strongly emphasized in opening doors of opportunity during the medical school journey. In fact, recent advances in virtual mentoring have allowed students to gain broader wisdom. The benefits of good, productive mentoring have been documented at all stages of the academic pipeline [18] and continue to be a strong force in the success of African-American male physicians.

Case Outcome

Despite the stressors, Eddie found support in the medical school Office of Diversity and Inclusion (ODI), which took him under its wing and prepared him for his progress committee meeting. The ODI also provided him with tutoring and mentoring support after the meeting and advocated for him. He also found solace and support in a learning community of mentors and advisors of color organized by the office that included students, residents, and physicians of color in the community. Eddie graduated on time with his medical school class and matched in an Internal Medicine residency not far from his hometown.

References

1. Association of American Medical Colleges. Altering the course: black males in medicine. Washington: Association of American Medical Colleges; 2015. p. 49. Available from: https://members.aamc.org/eweb/upload/Black_Males_in_Medicine_Report_WEB.pdf.
2. Holden L, Rumala B, Carson P, Siegel E. Promoting careers in health care for urban youth: what students, parents and educators can teach us. Inf Serv Use. 2014;34(3–4):355–66. https://doi.org/10.3233/ISU-140761.
3. Staats C, Capatosto K, Wright RA, Jackson VW. State of the science: implicit bias review. 2016 ed. Columbus: Kirwan Institute for the Study of Race and Ethnicity; 2016. p. 108.
4. Lahmon C. Dear colleague letter: resource comparability [Internet]. Washington: U.S. Department of Education Office for Civil Rights; 2014 [cited 2017 Nov 29]. Available from: https://www2.ed.gov/about/offices/list/ocr/letters/colleague-resourcecomp-201410.pdf.

5. Bottia MC, Stearns E, Mickelson RA, Moller S, Parker AD. The relationships among high school STEM learning experiences and students' intent to declare and declaration of a STEM major in college. Teach Coll Rec. 2015;17(3):1–46.
6. Lipscomb WD, Mavis B, Fowler LV, Green WD, Brooks GL. The effectiveness of a post-baccalaureate program for students from disadvantaged backgrounds. J Assoc Am Med Coll. 2009;84(10 Suppl):S42–5. https://doi.org/10.1097/ACM.0b013e3181b37bd0.
7. McDougle L, Way DP, Lee WK, Morfin JA, Mavis BE, Matthews D, Latham-Sadler BA, Clinchot DM. A national long-term outcomes evaluation of U.S. premedical postbaccalaureate programs designed to promote healthcare access and workforce diversity. J Health Care Poor Underserved. 2015;26(3):631–47. https://doi.org/10.1353/hpu.2015.0088.
8. Bean N, Gnadt A, Maupin N, White SA, Andersen L. Mind the gap: student researchers use secondary data to explore disparities in STEM education. Prairie J Educ Res. 2016;1(1):32–54. https://doi.org/10.4148/2373-0994.1002.
9. Cregler LL. Enrichment programs to create a pipeline to biomedical science careers. J Assoc Acad Minor Phys. 1993;4(4):127–31.
10. Tuition and student fees report. Washington: Association of American Medical Colleges; 2017 [cited 2017 Dec 12]. Available from https://www.aamc.org/data/tuitionandstudentfees/.
11. Jolly P. Diversity of U.S. medical students by parental income [Internet]. Washington: AAMC; 2008 [cited 2017 Nov 29]. Available from: https://www.aamc.org/download/102338/data/aib-vol8no1.pdf.
12. Kowarski I. How to attend medical school for free [Internet]. New York: U.S. News & World Report; 2017 [cited 2017 Nov 29]. Available from: https://www.usnews.com/education/best-graduate-schools/top-medical-schools/articles/2017-07-13/how-to-attend-medical-school-for-free.
13. Greyson SR, Chen C, Mullan F. A history of medical school debt: observations and implications for the future of medical education. Acad Med. 2011;86(7):840–5.
14. Marcu MI, Kellermann AL, Hunter C, Curtis J, Rice C, Wilensky GR. Borrow or serve? An economic analysis of options for financing medical school education. J Assoc Am Med Coll. 2017;92(7):966–75. https://doi.org/10.1097/ACM.0000000000001572.
15. Johnson L. Minorities in medical school and National Medical Fellowships, Inc.: 50 years and counting. Acad Med. 1998;73:1044–51.
16. Diversity in medical education: facts and figures 2016. Washington: Association of American Medical Colleges; 2016 [cited 2017 Dec 12]. Available from http://www.aamcdiversityfactsandfigures2016.org/report-section/section-1/.
17. Syed M, Azmitia M, Cooper CR. Identity and academic success among underrepresented ethnic minorities: an interdisciplinary review and integration. J Soc Psychol Study Soc Issues. 2011;67:442–68. https://doi.org/10.1111/j.1540-4560.2011.01709.
18. McLaughlin C. Mentoring: what is it? How do we do it and how do we get more of it? Health Serv Res. 2010;45(3):871–84.

Part IV
Resident Physician Cases

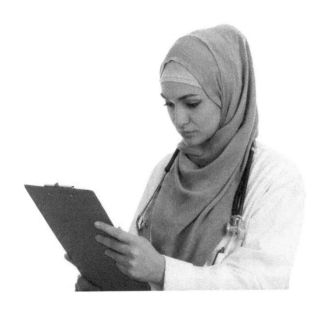

Chapter 41
Colored Resident

Vanessa Cousins and Erika Phindile Chowa

Case Scenario

A 67-year-old immunocompromised white female presents to an academic emergency department with altered mental status and fever. She was last seen normal by her family 2 days ago. The patient is brought to the emergency department by her two children.

Review of Symptoms

Unable to obtain from patient secondary to altered mental status.

Past Medical History

Hypertension, rheumatoid arthritis, and diabetes.

Medication Rituximab weekly, Prednisone 20 daily, Insulin Lantus 40 units daily, Lisinopril 20 mg daily.

V. Cousins (✉) · E. P. Chowa
Department of Emergency Medicine, Emory University, Atlanta, GA, USA
e-mail: vcousin@emory.edu; Erika.phindile.chowa@emory.edu

Family History

Noncontributory.

Social History

Retired, single, and lives at home alone.

Physical Exam

Vital Signs T 39 C, BP 140/90, pulse 120, O_2 Sat 95%, RA RR 16.

General The patient is lethargic and disoriented to person, place, and time.

Skin Skin is clear without any rashes.

HEENT Dry mucous membranes, posterior oropharynx clear, no lymphadenopathy.

Cardiovascular Heart sounds are normal. Tachycardia, no murmurs.

Respiratory Lungs clear to auscultation bilaterally.

Abdomen Abdomen is soft and non-tender with normal bowel sounds.

MSK No edema.

Neuro Normal motor, normal sensory, patient with gait ataxia.

What Was Said?

After examining the patient, the emergency medicine resident briefly speaks with the patient's children to obtain collateral history and then steps out to report her findings to the attending physician. Given the patient's altered mental status and fever, the resident initiates a sepsis workup, which includes chest X-ray, cbc, comprehensive metabolic panel, urinalysis, blood, and urine cultures. She starts antibiotics immediately. Urinalysis and chest X-ray come back negative for infection. The patient has a leukocytosis of 20. The resident is now concerned for meningitis. Realizing that this patient will need a further workup, including a lumbar puncture, the resident orders a head CT and approaches the family for informed consent. She attempts to update the family and explain next steps. After discussing the care of the patient with the family and addressing their questions and concerns, the resident walks out of the room to prepare for a lumbar puncture. The attending physician enters the room to introduce himself to the family and ask if their concerns have been addressed. The family approaches the attending and reports, "The resident has explained everything to us. She is kind; however, we are not comfortable with a colored doctor in training taking care of our mother. We would prefer you perform the procedure and take care of her from this point forward."

What Was Done?

The attending, a white male physician, responds with a gentle voice and a calm demeanor stating, "This resident is the only resident available in the emergency department right now and is she is one of the most qualified physicians I know who can perform this lumbar puncture. I have done several lumbar punctures in my training, however the residents here often perform all of the procedures and have a depth of experience. You are in good hands." The family heard the attending but still refused to agree to the resident caring for their mother. The attending then responds, "You are free to decline this procedure against medical advice, and seek care elsewhere, but your mother is very sick and needs prompt care. I highly recommend that you allow us to take the best possible care of your mother at this time."

Question for Discussion

1. What attitudes and assumptions exist?

Attitudes/Assumptions: The Attending Physician

The attending physician ultimately disregards the patient's family's wishes to have another provider perform the procedure and passive aggressively forces them to choose between having the resident perform the procedure and seeking care elsewhere. The attending assumes the motive is that the family lacks confidence in the resident's abilities. The family's reasoning, however, is unclear.

Attitudes/Assumptions: The Patient

The patient's family is uncomfortable with the "colored doctor" in training caring for their mother, assuming the care provided by this resident may somehow be inferior.

Gaps in Provider Knowledge

The attending physician was not well equipped to navigate this racially tense situation with the patient's family members. His communication skills were lacking [1]. He did not utilize or take advantage of any hospital tools (such as an ethics committee), and he did not take the time to better understand their wishes or explain his perspective.

Cross-Cultural Tools and Skills

In this scenario, there are a few different approaches that can be utilized to defuse certain tensions and allow all parties to gain a better understanding. They all require the physician to display a cultural competence that enables him to sensitively address the family's concerns while further educating them [1]. First, the attending physician should explore and learn more about the family's beliefs. After listening carefully, he should then take the time to respectfully explain the hospital's policy and stand on racism, without forgetting to acknowledge how they feel. At this point, discussion and negotiation may take place [1].

Pearls and Pitfalls

Pitfall The attending did not use the interaction as an opportunity to educate the family about his stance on racism as well as the hospital/emergency department's stance. The family was inappropriate in their use of the word "colored" [2].

Pitfall The attending physician did not explore the patient's family's wishes further (why they didn't want the "colored resident" taking care of their mother) before dismissing them [2].

Pearl The physician maintains a calm demeanor while expressing and assuring confidence in the resident's capabilities [1].

Pitfall Realizing the gravity of the patient's prognosis without immediate treatment, the attending should not have discussed seeking care elsewhere with the patient's family at that time. The attending physician was also capable of performing the procedure and taking care of the patient without the resident [3].

Pitfall The attending and resident did not debrief about this case. A conversation following this patient encounter would help address the microaggressions the resident may have felt. The resident needs to know that her feelings are validated and that her attending supports her [4].

Case Outcome

After much debate among themselves, the family agrees to allow the resident to resume care of their mother and perform the lumbar puncture. The procedure is done without complication, and the patient is admitted to the hospital for further treatment.

References

1. Selby M, Neuberger J, Easmon C, Gough P. Education and debate: dealing with racist patients: doctors are people too: commentary: a role for personal values and management: commentary: isolate the problem: commentary: courteous containment is not enough. BMJ. 1999;318:1129–31.
2. Reynolds KL, Cowden JD, Brosco JP, Lantos JD. When a family requests a white doctor. J Pediatr. 2015;136(38):1–6.
3. Singh K, Sivasubramaniam P, Ghuman S, Mir HR. The dilemma of the racist patient. Am J Orthop (Belle Mead NJ). 2015;44(12):E477–9.
4. Epner DE, Baile WF. Patient-centered care: the key to cultural competence. Ann Oncol. 2012;23(Suppl 3):33–42.

Chapter 42
Muslim Resident Cases

Aasim I. Padela, Munzareen Padela, and Altaf Saadi

Case 1. "I Don't Want Her Taking Care of Me"

Case Scenario A 55-year-old white man presents to an outpatient clinic for a specialty ophthalmology appointment. He is greeted by the white male ophthalmology resident accompanied by a female, Muslim medical student wearing a ḥijāb.[1] The resident introduces himself and the medical student to the patient. The patient gives a disapproving look and asks the medical student a barrage of questions: "Where are you from? You're one of those Muslim types right? You probably can't even touch me because I'm Christian. Are you even a citizen? I don't want her taking care of me." Sensing the growing tension in the air with each subsequent question, the resident attempts to reorient the patient back to the clinical encounter, stating, "She's just here to observe, I will be the one taking care of you."

---

[1] The Arabic word ḥijāb comes from a root verb meaning to cover and refers to a headscarf some Muslim women wear as a religious observance and sign of their religious identity.

A. I. Padela (✉)
MacLean Center for Clinical Medical Ethics, The University of Chicago, Chicago, IL, USA
e-mail: apadela@medicine.bsd.uchicago.edu

M. Padela
The University of Chicago, Chicago, IL, USA
e-mail: mpadela@uchicago.edu

A. Saadi
University of California Los Angeles National Clinical Scholars Program,
Los Angeles, CA, USA
e-mail: asaadi@mednet.ucla.edu

© Springer International Publishing AG, part of Springer Nature 2019
M. L. Martin et al. (eds.), *Diversity and Inclusion in Quality Patient Care*,
https://doi.org/10.1007/978-3-319-92762-6_42

Review of Symptoms

The patient complains of double vision in his right eye, which he first noticed about 1 week prior to his visit. His vision has gotten slightly worse since symptom onset. He reports a headache that has been present over the course of the last 3 weeks, mild to moderate in severity. He has some aching in his jaw and tongue during meals during that time frame.

Past Medical History

Hypercholesterolemia, hypertension on medications.

Family History

Noncontributory.

Social History

Smokes half a pack of cigarettes daily for 15 years; no alcohol or other recreational drugs.

Physical Exam

Vitals Signs Normal temperature, blood pressure 148/85, pulse 85.

HEENT Visual acuity is decreased in the right eye. Pupils are equal, round and reactive to light. There is a trace afferent pupillary defect on the right. Extraocular movements are full. There is no nystagmus. Visual fields reveal a unilateral visual field defect, with a superior altitudinal hemianopsia. Dilated fundoscopic exam reveals optic disc edema. There are no carotid bruits.

What Was Said?

The medical student responds that she is from New York, but this does not appease the patient who continues to question her background and "otherness."

What Was Done?

The resident attempts to alleviate the tension in the room by redirecting the attention away from the medical student and back to the patient; however, he does not actually address the patient's concerns nor the student's discomfort in that unsafe learning environment. The resident completes the examination and reports the clinical aspects of the case to the attending. The medical student is not involved in the case beyond observation. The attending returns later, reexamines the patient, recommends diagnostic testing to confirm giant cell arteritis (inflammatory markers and a temporal artery biopsy), and initiates steroid therapy. The patient understands the clinical plan and need for close follow-up. The encounter remains profoundly disconcerting for the medical student, but she felt uneasy in discussing her experience with the clinical care team.

Questions for Discussion

1. What attitudes or assumptions are present?

Attitudes/Assumptions: The Patient

(a) Assumption of foreignness simply because of medical student's appearance. Even before asking whether she was a citizen, inherent in the question "Where are you from?" was an assumption that she is not from "here."
(b) Assumption that her Muslim faith precluded her from touching him as a patient and that she would treat him differently based on his faith. The medical student was not empowered in this encounter to address these incorrect assumptions.

2. What are the potential consequences of the resident not addressing what was said?

(a) By not addressing the misconceptions or prejudice behind the patient's line of questioning, the resident left the door open for clinicians in the future to be subjected to suspicion and prejudicial treatment by this patient.
(b) At the same time, the student trainee was also left without the knowledge, tools, and/or practical approach by which to redress stereotyping and prejudice in clinical encounters.

Cross-Cultural Tools and Skills

An alternative approach would have been to allay the patient's concerns while acknowledging that the medical student was a qualified and valuable member of the healthcare team. For example, one might have said something like, "I understand it may be overwhelming to meet multiple members of the care team, but I can assure you that [medical student] is excellent, qualified, and has been helpful on our medical team taking care of diverse patients from all backgrounds and faiths." Such a statement may have diffused some of the tension while simultaneously acknowledging the patient's ability to choose providers, allayed concerns about the trainee's clinical abilities, and maintained the medical student's dignity by voicing support for her presence. While this brief, and potentially one-time, clinical encounter might not be the appropriate circumstance during which to address the patient's biased views, such an approach could have set the stage for addressing the patient's knowledge gaps and the medical trainee's practice gaps.

Pearls and Pitfalls

Pearl The resident redirects the patient toward a clinical question in order to focus on patient care, keeps the student in the room, and continues to observe.

Pitfall Addressing the patient's concerns and affirmatively supporting the student may have allowed for an improved educational opportunity for the medical student and a teaching moment for the patient.

Pitfall Not discussing directly with the medical student or the attending to validate the medical student's discomfort and to nurture a psychologically safe learning environment.

Case Outcome

The medical student silently observes the entire interaction, while the resident conducts the history taking, physical examination, and management. The patient receives the appropriate evaluation and care for giant cell arteritis.

Case 2. Muslim Patient Encounter in the Emergency Department[2]

Case Scenario A 67-year-old South Asian female presents to the emergency department (ED) anxious, in moderate respiratory distress, and having choreic movements of her upper torso. Her son identifies a South Asian male resident in the ED and asks him, "My mother saw that you are working, can you take care of her?"

---

[2]This case is developed from Padela A. Can you take care of my mother? Reflections on cultural competence and clinical accommodation. Acad Emerg Med 2007;14(3):275–7.

The resident answers affirmatively, understanding the implication of the son's question to mean that perhaps a shared background between the patient and provider would facilitate cultural understanding in the clinical encounter.

The patient's history is notable for her not having been able to urinate or defecate since she fell on her back 24 h prior. She also describes shooting pains from her lumbar region and difficulty ambulating. An hour prior to her presentation, she felt sudden onset substernal chest pressure with dyspnea, finally prompting her to come to the ED. The patient is reluctant to be examined by a male doctor. After much coaxing, the resident is able to perform the physical exam; however, the patient adamantly refuses a rectal examination.

Review of Symptoms

There are no fevers, chills, or recent sick exposures. She did not lose consciousness with the fall and there was no head strike. She has not had any burning with urination or foul odor to her urine prior to the past 24 h.

Past Medical History

Parkinson's disease on medications, constipation, hypertension.

Family History

Noncontributory.

Social History

She lives with her son and his family. She is married with three children. She does not smoke, drink alcohol, or use recreational drugs.

Physical Exam

General Anxious appearing.

Respiratory Clear to auscultation; no accessory muscle usage.

Cardiovascular Regular rate and rhythm without murmurs.

Back Spinal tenderness in the lumbar region; no costovertebral angle tenderness (examined with gloves, thereby avoiding direct skin-to-skin contact).

Questions for Discussion

1. Why was the Muslim woman reluctant to engage in parts of the physical exam?

Attitudes/Assumptions: The Muslim Patient and Her Son

(a) The patient felt that the provider would understand her need for maintaining modesty, an overarching Islamic ethic pertaining to interaction between the sexes that applies to both men and women. For many Muslim women (whether or not they wear the headscarf), covering up the body is important particularly when they are in the company of males who they are not related to by blood or marriage.

(b) The encounter began with a request for a resident who appeared to share a similar background, rooted in the patient's hope that this cultural and religious similarity would improve the clinical encounter in a time of emotional and physical vulnerability.

Attitudes/Assumptions: The Resident

(a) There is significant variation in practice among Muslims, including observant Muslim women. The resident asked the patient to participate in all components of the exam without making assumptions about her beliefs and practices.

(b) Although he explained the recommendation and clinical need for a rectal exam, he understood the patient's refusal based on her religious and cultural mores. Furthermore, given the imaging diagnostics that were going to be performed, he felt that forgoing the rectal was justified both medically and ethically. Nonetheless, his attending physician chastised him for missing this crucial part of the examination, as it was not "standard" practice.

Attitudes/Assumptions: The Attending Physician

(a) During acute and critical healthcare encounters, e.g., in the emergency room setting, it is often difficult to provide culturally responsive, patient-centered healthcare. Protocols and convention assist in providing high-quality care when time and resource limitations can constrain fully accommodating patient preferences and values. In this case, spinal cord compression was a possible diagnosis, and a rectal exam to assess for muscle strength would have helped delineate the possibility and urgency of such a condition.

2. What could have been done differently?

(a) If a female provider were present and available, she could have been asked to perform the rectal examination, provided the patient would have accepted the exam from that provider.
(b) The attending physician could have interpreted the deferral of the rectal exam as an appropriate cultural accommodation based on patient values. The patient appeared to make an informed decision, and diagnostic imaging would have been performed regardless of the rectal exam's results.

Case Outcome

Diagnosis Degenerative disc disease, low back pain, and worsening constipation in setting of progressive Parkinson's disease.

Disposition Home with physical therapy services.

Soon after the completion of the physical examination, the patient has a bowel movement, reassuring concerns about spinal cord compression. However, given her fall, an MRI of the lumbosacral spine is completed and reveals significant degenerative disc disease at multiple lumbar levels. A CT-PE protocol is also completed and is negative for pulmonary embolism. Her troponins are negative, and there are no EKG changes to raise concern for unstable angina or myocardial infarction. A discussion with the patient's outpatient neurologist raises the potential need for adjusting Parkinson's medications given worsening constipation, as well as slowed movement and gait disturbance contributing to worsening back pain symptoms. The plan is for her to see her neurologist in the clinic to discuss further medication changes.

Cases 3 and 4. "I Don't Want a Terrorist Taking Care of Me"

Case Scenario 3 A middle-aged Caucasian male patient presents to a university-based emergency department (ED) complaining of abdominal pain, with vital signs that are within normal limits. After the nurse's evaluation, he is placed into a patient room awaiting evaluation by a resident physician.

A bearded, South Asian physician enters the room to begin the evaluation and the patient says, "I want to see a different doctor. I don't want a terrorist taking care of me." The resident physician is left speechless but notes that the patient does not have abnormal vital signs, does not appear to be in distress, and was firm in his request. He leaves the room to consult with the attending physician.

Case Scenario 4 A college-aged Caucasian male patient presents to a university-based ED complaining of back pain. On triage evaluation, the nursing staff reports vital signs that are within normal limits and no bony tenderness of the spine. The patient is placed in a room awaiting evaluation by a resident physician.

A bearded, South Asian physician performs a focused patient history and physical examination. The patient reports having been playing tackle football with his friends the day prior and waking up today with lower back pain.

Review of Symptoms

The patient denies fevers or chills, muscular weakness, or numbness and tingling.

Past Medical History

None.

Family History

Noncontributory.

Social History

The patient is a sophomore in college and lives in a dorm. He reports socially drinking alcohol on weekends but denies any recreational drug use or smoking.

Physical Exam

General Comfortable and conversant, does not appear to be inebriated.

Respiratory Clear to auscultation.

Cardiovascular Regular rate and rhythm without murmurs, strong dorsalis pedis pulses bilaterally.

Back No spinal tenderness in the cervical, thoracic, or lumbar region; no step-offs; no costovertebral angle tenderness; small discrete <2 inch circumference bruises with yellowish hue in the paraspinal L2 region on the right.

Neuromuscular 5/5 strength in hip flexion and knee extension bilaterally without back pain. The patient is able to ambulate with normal gait, no weakness in plantar and dorsiflexion of feet bilaterally.

The resident physician tells the patient that he likely has back pain of musculoskeletal origin and will order some pain medication in the ED and have his supervising physician come in to confer. As the nurse comes to administer ibuprofen, the patient tells her that he "does not want a terrorist" as a doctor and wants to see another doctor. The nurse tells the patient that the resident physician is highly capable and is the only resident doctor in that part of the ED. The patient responds, "It is my right to choose my doctor, and I want someone else." The nurse conveys the patient's request to the attending physician out of earshot of the resident, who is in another patient's room.

Questions for Discussion

1. Are patients within their "rights" to choose their healthcare providers? What ethical values and principles are at stake?
2. What are the limits or constraints on patient choice in the clinical encounter?
3. How should the attending respond to these requests? Are the two scenarios different in any way that would change the response?
4. Do some healthcare disparities reflect patient preferences like these?

Attitudes/Assumptions: The Patients

(a) Given the sociopolitical climate, stereotyping Muslims as unethical, irrational, and "bad" individuals is a norm. This caricature creeps into all social spheres including the healthcare environment. It is hard to assess the underlying rationale for the patient's request, but fear, misunderstanding, and overt prejudice could all play roles. Nonetheless, it is clear that the patients do not feel comfortable with the resident physician and have voiced their preferences to have another care provider.

Case Outcomes

Case Scenario 3 The attending physician listens to the resident's report and asks whether the patient is "dying" or appears intoxicated. The resident replies in the negative to each. Then the attending apologetically says, "I know this must rub you the wrong way, but the patient comes first." The attending explains that patients are within their rights to choose their physicians and offers the analogy of stable patients being allowed to choose not to be seen by medical students and trainees. She further states that all patients who come to the ED are stressed and vulnerable, and as healthcare providers, we should try to make them as comfortable as possible. The attending tells the resident to give the case to another resident and "move on."

Case Scenario 4 The attending physician finds the resident in another patient's room and asks him to step out and present the "back pain" case. After listening to the patient history, physical examination, and the resident's assessment and plan, he tells the resident to continue seeing other patients and that he, the attending, will discharge the patient. Upon entering the patient room, the attending physician conveys the diagnosis and discharge plan and asks the patient why he did not want to be seen by a Muslim doctor. The patient offers, "I do not trust them nor like them, and I am within my rights to choose." The attending responds by saying, "This is not Burger King. You cannot have it your way. This is the ED and we *all* provide the best care we can to whoever walks through that door." He then hands the patient the discharge paperwork and says, "If you do not like the doctors here then take your bigoted self elsewhere."

Questions for Discussion

1. The two attendings took vastly different approaches to the patient requests. Which do you align with and why?
2. How do you think the future healthcare-seeking behavior of the patients in the two scenarios would be influenced by their particular ED encounters?
3. Should the ED be a place where we can educate patients about tolerance and trust?

Chapter 43
Female Resident

R. Lane Coffee Jr., Susan Sawning, and Cherri D. Hobgood

Case Scenario

A 60-year-old male presents to the emergency department with a chief complaint of chest pain and shortness of breath (SOB) for 2 h.

Review of Symptoms

The 2 h of SOB is associated with diaphoresis and central chest pain that radiates to the back. The patient states the pain is dull and unrelenting. He reports nausea – one attempt to vomit which was unsuccessful. The patient has experienced pain like this before while working, but it has always resolved with rest.

Past Medical History

Type II diabetes mellitus (DM), hypertension.

R. L. Coffee Jr. (✉) · C. D. Hobgood
Department of Emergency Medicine, Indiana University School of Medicine, Indianapolis, IN, USA
e-mail: rlcoffee@iu.edu; chobgood@iu.edu

S. Sawning
University of Louisville School of Medicine, Louisville, KY, USA
e-mail: susan.sawning@louisville.edu

Family History

Father died in his 40s suddenly, unknown cause. Mother is still alive in her 80s with congestive heart failure (CHF) and DM. Brother had a "heart attack" at 55 and now has a pacemaker.

Social History

40 years of tobacco abuse, one pack per day; occasional alcohol; lives with spouse; has two adult children who live outside the home; high school education and works in a factory.

Physical Exam

Vital Signs P 102, R 22, BP 175/ 98, O_2 saturation 94% RA, pain scale 8/10.

General Moderately obese male who appears anxious and diaphoretic.

Neuro Alert and oriented × 3, CN 2–12 intact, normal motor 5/5 upper and lower extremities.

Psych Normal affect and orientation.

What Was Said?

The female resident physician, Dr. Allison, enters the room, wearing scrubs with her name embroidered on the pocket of the scrub top. She asks the patient how he would like to be addressed and introduces herself as the physician. The patient responds pleasantly and provides the history of present illness and past medical history in response to the physician's questions. He then proceeds to comment, "Nurse, I'm really tired, and I've gone over this information twice now. When will I see the doctor?" The resident physician responds by saying, "I am the doctor and I'd like to examine you now." The patient looks a bit confused and says, "I thought you were the nurse." The resident physician states, "No, I'm the doctor, let's get the examination done so I can order tests and get your workup moving." The patient says, "I'm not sure I trust a woman to take care of me. I don't mean to be offensive, sweetheart, and you might be fine to take care of babies, but I need a real doctor to take care of me."

What Was Done?

The resident physician firmly and pleasantly informs the patient of her credentials and capacity and offers options, but does not offer the option of another provider in the emergency department. "I realize this might be a change for you; however, I am an emergency physician and am well qualified to take care of your condition and will be working in partnership with my boss, who is the attending physician. If you choose not to have me as a provider, I will be happy to arrange another option; however, I believe your condition is serious, and you require immediate attention." The resident explains the situation to the attending physician. They go back into the room together. The attending introduces him/herself and states, "Hi Mr. Smith, I'm Dr. Sullivan. I'm working with Dr. Allison today and she told me of your concerns. We do understand that patients have a choice in where they seek care but in an emergency situation, who provides that care is based on the providers present at the time. We are a teaching hospital, and Dr. Allison is one of our top residents and she will be providing care to you today under my supervision. However, if you choose not to receive care here, you are free to leave, or I will be happy to transfer you to another facility, but I want to assure you that if you choose to stay, Dr. Allison will provide your care and it will be of the highest quality."

Questions for Discussion

1. What are other possible strategies for the resident physician to deploy in order to mitigate the assumption that she is not a qualified provider?
2. What are other possible strategies for the attending physician to deploy in order to provide education to the patient and support of the resident physician?
3. What are some attitudes/assumptions displayed in this case?

Attitudes/Assumptions: The Patient

Despite the resident physician introducing herself properly and having correct identification, the patient automatically assumes the resident physician is the nurse based on gender [1]. Further, the patient assumes that the female physician is of lesser stature than a male physician and in fact is not a qualified provider or a "real doctor."

Attitudes/Assumptions: The Physician

The resident physician assumes that the patient is uninformed about women physicians and explains her training. She has a duty to provide care in a professional and compassionate manner.

Gaps in Provider Knowledge

The resident may benefit from further understanding the underlying reasons that a patient may request gender-concordant care outside of a perceived lack of competence. Many patients feel that shared gender-life experiences help facilitate trust and communication with their providers [1, 2]. The resident physician does acknowledge that the patient is feeling uncomfortable ("I realize this might be a change for you"); however, further validation of the patient's feelings may be needed to gain a deeper sense of trust. For example, the physician may want to lead with: "I understand that you may feel uncomfortable with a physician who is not a male like you. I validate your feelings of concern and understand that you feel unsure if you can trust a woman to take care of you." Acknowledging and validating this up-front may help the patient hear the discussion around competency. Additionally, the attending might want to reemphasize the resident's discussion about timeliness being of utmost importance. This patient's health could be compromised by the delay in care, and reemphasizing this to the patient is an important step for the attending.

Cross-Cultural Tools and Skills

It is very important for providers to use open-ended language when navigating patient requests for gender-concordant care and steer away from personalizing the request or becoming defensive during the discussion (e.g., "Can you tell me more about why you would like to see a male physician today instead of Dr. Allison?"). Using open-ended language can help the provider understand the patient's perspective more and address specific concerns. It is also important for providers to remember that there are multiple reasons that patients might request a physician of another gender. For example, some patients have religious belief systems that frown upon patients being cared for by a physician of another gender. Asking questions using open-ended language and keeping the dialogue going can help physicians and patients build trust and understanding in the clinical relationship.

Pearls and Pitfalls

Pearl The attending physician supported the female resident to provide care to the patient [3].

Pearl The female resident maintained a positive attitude.

Pitfall It would be a pitfall if the resident physician fell victim to the emotions of anger and resentment. When your validity as a professional is questioned, you can easily become angry and push the encounter into a hostile confrontation. This results in loss of professionalism and control of the situation. You begin to resent the patient and belittle their intelligence. This may unknowingly result in a lower standard of care being delivered because you limit resources or do not reassess as often secondary to "bad" feelings.

Pitfall It would be a pitfall if the attending did not support the resident in the provision of care. This would have undermined her credibility and limited her capacity to be effective in the future.

Pitfall It would be a pitfall if the resident chose not to inform the attending and simply traded the case to a male colleague. This would also undermine her credibility with her colleagues and limit her capacity to be seen as an effective resident who could manage her own caseload and difficult patient encounters.

Case Outcome

The patient decided that the female resident physician was confident and capable of providing care. He proceeded with the examination and was admitted to the inpatient team for cardiac assessment.

References

1. Whitgob EE, Blankenburg RL, Bogetz AL. The discriminatory patient and family: strategies to address discrimination toward trainees. Acad Med. 2016;91(11):S64–6.
2. Peek M, Lo B, Fernandez A. How should physicians respond when patients distrust them because of their gender? AMA J Ethics. 2017;19(4):332–9.
3. Vassar L. How medical specialties vary by gender [Internet]. Chicago: AMA Wire. 2015 [cited 2017 Nov 6]. Available from: https://wire.ama-assn.org/education/how-medical-specialties-vary-gender.

Chapter 44
Female Resident Referred to as a Nurse

Jeffrey Druck and Shanta Zimmer

Case Scenario

A 73-year-old grandmother is brought in by ambulance with a chief complaint of confusion. She is febrile to 103.1 °F and confused but is alert and oriented times two. She is accompanied by her adult children, a 40-year-old daughter and a 38-year-old son. In the patient treatment area, the resident, a young white woman, arrives at the bedside to examine the patient. The history is contributory for a productive cough and a history of diabetes and hypertension; on exam, the physical exam reveals rales at the right base and no neurologic deficits. After completing the history and physical exam, the family asks when the doctor is coming in. The resident explains that she is the patient's doctor; the family states they understand, but then ask again when the doctor is coming in. The resident leaves without any further discussion.

Review of Symptoms

Increased cough for 4 days, with yellow sputum; acting normally yesterday, but upon waking today, the patient misidentified family members.

Past Medical History

Diabetes, controlled with diet, and hypertension, controlled with an ACE inhibitor.

J. Druck, MD (✉) · S. Zimmer, MD
University of Colorado School of Medicine, Aurora, CO, USA
e-mail: Jeffrey.Druck@UCDenver.edu; Shanta.Zimmer@UCDenver.edu

© Springer International Publishing AG, part of Springer Nature 2019   321
M. L. Martin et al. (eds.), *Diversity and Inclusion in Quality Patient Care*,
https://doi.org/10.1007/978-3-319-92762-6_44

Family History

Diabetes only.

Social History

The patient lives at home with her two adult children. She occasionally imbibes alcohol but does not smoke or use drugs.

Physical Exam

Vital Signs Temp, 103.1 °F; pulse, 120; BP, 95/65; respirations, 22, O_2 Sat 94% on room air.

General Frail, elderly female, mildly confused, attended at bedside by her two adult children.

Eyes Pupils equal, round, reactive to light, sclerae anicteric, normal lids.

Cardiovascular Tachycardia with no murmurs, gallops, or rubs.

Respiratory No use of accessory muscles, rales at the right base.

ENT Oropharynx clear, no erythema, uvula midline.

Abdomen Non-distended, non-tender with normal bowel sounds, no hepatosplenomegaly.

Extremities No clubbing, cyanosis, or edema.

Skin No rashes or lesions.

Neuro Grossly intact, CNII-XII intact, moves all four extremities, no obvious sign of deficit.

Neck Supple, non-tender, no adenopathy, no meningismus.

Questions for Discussion

1. Why did the family members keep asking when the doctor was coming in?

Attitudes/Assumptions: The Family

(a) Possible assumptions around who can be a physician
(b) Possible gender assumptions around power and control
(c) Desire for the best care for their mother
(d) Possible assumptions about age and competence

Attitudes/Assumptions: The Physician

(a) I've spent 4 years in medical school and 3 years in residency, and I am still not seen as a doctor.
(b) It is most likely due to my gender that they assume I am not a doctor.
(c) Why don't they listen to me?

Gaps in Provider Knowledge

(a) Lack of certainty around why the family continues not to acknowledge her position
(b) Concern for how this issue may affect her ability to care for this patient
(c) Lack of knowledge of how to appropriately respond to what she sees as a microaggression

2. What actions could have been taken by the doctor to respond to this issue?

Cross-Cultural Tools and Skills

(a) Approach the family directly.
(b) Inquire about the conflict and expectations.
    (i) Reflect on commentary.
    (ii) Reframe the question.
(c) Ask for assistance from a more senior team member.
(d) Look for support from other team members.
(e) Debrief with team members.
(f) Consider focusing on medical care.

3. What medical issues concern you about this case?

(a) The resident should discuss the plan for evaluation and possible admission and clarify other team members' and familial expectations. There is no question gender bias exists in medicine, and this gender bias can affect feelings of trustworthiness [1, 2]. An open and honest discussion may result in elucidating a difference of expectations [3].

(b) The family may be concerned about trust of the female resident's opinion, limiting the therapeutic relationship [4]. This will affect medical decision-making going forward.

4. Which components of the Emergency Medicine Milestones of the ACGME competencies are incorporated in the case?

(a) Patient-centered communication: Demonstrates interpersonal and communication skills that result in the effective exchange of information and collaboration with the patient

(b) Professional values: Demonstrates compassion, integrity, and respect for others as well as adherence to the ethical principles relevant to the practice of medicine [5]

Case Outcome

Diagnosis Pneumonia

Disposition Admission

After an appropriate history is obtained utilizing the principles above, the patient is treated for her fever and given antibiotics for a pneumonia diagnosed on chest X-ray. A discussion occurs between the resident and the patient's family clarifying her role in their mother's care and how the decision to provide the best possible care is being implemented based upon the resident's decisions. In addition, the resident speaks directly about the family's confusion about her role, so other providers who care for this patient do not experience the same issues. The family was given time to ask additional questions and was instructed to vocalize any further issues they had. The faculty in the emergency department debriefed with the resident, echoing ongoing support for her competence and autonomy at the bedside.

References

1. Coombs AA, King RK. Workplace discrimination: experiences of practicing physicians. J Natl Med Assoc. 2005;97(4):467–77.
2. Robinson GE. Stresses on women physicians: consequences and coping techniques. Depress Anxiety. 2003;17(3):180–9.
3. Sue DW, et al. Racial microaggressions and the power to define reality. Am Psychol. 2008;63(4):277–9.
4. Ladha M, et al. The effect of white coats and gender on medical students' perceptions of physicians. BMC Med Educ. 2017;17(1):93.
5. The Emergency Medicine Milestone Project [Internet]. Chicago: The Accreditation Council for Graduate Medical Education; 2012 [cited 2014 5 Aug]. Available from: http://www.acgme.org/acgmeweb/Portals/0/PDFs/Milestones/EmergencyMedicineMilestones.pdf. Joint publication with the American Board for Emergency Medicine.

Chapter 45
Black Lesbian Female Resident

Ava Pierce and Marquita Hicks

Case Scenario

The Medical Intensive Care Unit (MICU) team arrives at the emergency department (ED) to evaluate several patients who were assigned to their team for admission. The patients have not been assigned inpatient hospital beds yet, but they have been closely monitored by residents in the ED. The team enters the room of the first patient, and the ED resident who is rotating on the MICU service presents the case to the attending. The attending asks the resident a series of questions during the presentation, including several that no one on the resident team can answer.

The team moves to the next patient's room, and the next resident presents his patient to the attending and team. The attending asks him one simple question that everyone knows the answer to. The team moves to the next room to evaluate another patient who was evaluated by the off-service ED resident. During this presentation, the attending again asks the resident one simple question but then asks several questions in the presence of the patient that none of the residents know the answer to.

When the MICU team arrives at the MICU, the upper-level medicine resident states that the ED resident had trouble placing an ultrasound-guided IJ central line during the night. When the next patient needed a central line, rather than helping the ED resident place the central line, the attending told the ED resident that she will not be allowed to attempt this line because the patient is critical, and she will get a chance to attempt central venous access procedures later.

A. Pierce (✉)
UT Southwestern Medical Center, Dallas, TX, USA
e-mail: Ava.pierce@utsouthwestern.edu

M. Hicks
The University of Alabama at Birmingham, Birmingham, AL, USA
e-mail: Mnhicks@uabmc.edu

© Springer International Publishing AG, part of Springer Nature 2019
M. L. Martin et al. (eds.), *Diversity and Inclusion in Quality Patient Care*,
https://doi.org/10.1007/978-3-319-92762-6_45

Over the next couple of weeks, the ED resident notices that she is not offered the same number of procedures as the other team members. This pattern of behavior continues for the next 4 weeks of the rotation. At the end of the rotation, the ED resident's evaluation states that her clinical knowledge base and procedural skills are significantly lower than the remainder of the residents with the same level of training. The attending is a white male, the resident is a black lesbian female, and the remainder of the team consists of white male residents.

What Was Said?

During the rotation, the attending spoke with the resident privately and expressed concern for her ability to succeed on the rotation. He stated, "I know sometimes you all have difficulties on the MICU rotation due to the severity of the patients' conditions." Throughout the rotation, the other residents received ample opportunities to perform procedures. When procedures were indicated on the female resident's patients, the attending would explicitly advise the MICU fellow to "supervise closely." During the rotation, the resident asks the attending if there are certain journals or texts she can read to be better prepared and increase her knowledge during the next 4 weeks of the rotation. She also asks for recommendations on how she can improve her procedural skills.

What Was Done?

The attending uses a condescending tone based on his assumptions that the underrepresented in medicine resident lacks the intellectual capacity to succeed. During interactions with patient and families, the resident is interrupted consistently by the attending when she is providing explanations and plans of care. The attending tells the resident she needs to read more but does not give examples of the journals and texts that would be helpful. The attending also states that the resident just needs to do more procedures to improve her procedural skills. There is a constant critique of the resident, but there is never any constructive guidance or specific instructions that will lead to a plan for improvement.

Questions for Discussion

1. What could be the basis for treating this resident differently than the others?

Attitudes/Assumptions: The Resident

(a) The attending is biased against me because I am black and gay. He thinks that I do not have the intellectual ability to be successful on this rotation.

Attitudes/Assumptions: The Attending

(a) The underrepresented in medicine resident lacks the intellectual capacity to succeed. Her lifestyle contradicts my Christian beliefs.

Gaps in Provider Knowledge

The provider is untrained and oblivious to the problem. He does not understand the level of implicit bias that he brings into his interactions with underrepresented in medicine residents. Bias is deeply engrained in our society. It is difficult to adequately educate an individual if the educator is subliminally fixated on the individual's perceived inferior intellect. Bias can be a tremendous educational barrier because it places limited expectations on the students [1]. To reduce these gaps in learning, attendings should sincerely educate themselves about issues of diversity and inclusion. Medical practitioners must endeavor to respect the oath: "Do no harm." Medical educators should do no harm to their residents by not allowing bias to inhibit the resident's acquisition of knowledge.

2. How could this interaction be improved?

Cross-Cultural Tools and Skills

Professional development activities, such as cultural sensitivity and implicit bias training and emotional intelligence classes, would alleviate the social bias in medical education. In medical education, racially biased decisions often go unnoticed. This implicit racial bias can contribute to the failure to achieve greater inclusion of underrepresented students in medical education [2].

Pearls and Pitfalls

Pearl Diversity dynamics include both interpersonal and intrapersonal factors that impact organizational culture [3].

Pearl Microaggressions are brief and commonplace daily verbal, behavioral, and environmental indignities, whether intentional or unintentional, that communicate hostile, derogatory, or negative racial, gender, religious, or sexual orientation insults and slights to the target person or group [3–5].

Pearl Microaggressions cause psychological distress and create disparities in health care, education, and employment [4].

Pearl We must work to end microaggressions and negative stereotyping in the healthcare setting [3].

Pitfall If there are interpersonal power differentials, such as those between an attending and a resident, the resident often will not confront the bias they have encountered due to fear of the consequences of addressing the microaggressions [3, 4].

Pitfall The resident had response indecision and did not know the best way to respond to this bias, so she did not respond at all [3].

Pitfall Historically, society's emphasis on resilience has placed responsibility on the individual who is struggling to find inner strength and resources for success, basically excusing the cultural and social framework that creates toxic stress [6].

Case Outcome

The resident did not report her concerns about this attending. She stated that she feared further retribution if she discussed her concerns. She did not disclose this incident until she had been an attending for several years. She is currently an ED attending at an institution that has a Chief Diversity Officer and Dean for Diversity, Inclusion, and Student Affairs. She realizes that if she had a similar resource in her training institution, she may not have stayed silent. Additional resources that may have been beneficial to her were her program director, ED chair, or the hospital GME Director.

References

1. Hall J, Fields B. Continuing the conversation in nursing on race and racism. Nurs Outlook. 2013;61(3):164–73.
2. Ansell DA, McDonald EK. Bias, black lives, and academic medicine. N Engl J Med. 2015;372(12):1087–9. https://doi.org/10.1056/NEJMp1500832.

3. Brody A, Farley J, Gillespie G, Hickman R, Hodges E, Lyder C, et al. Diversity dynamics: the experience of male Robert Wood Johnson Foundation nurse faculty scholars. Nurs Outlook. 2017;65(3):278–88.
4. Sue DW. Microaggressions in everyday life: race, gender, and sexual orientation. New York: Wiley; 2010. 352 p.
5. Bleich M. Microaggression and its relevance in health care. J Contin Educ Nurs. 2015;46(11):487–8.
6. Ulloa JG, Talamantes E, Moreno G. Microaggressions during medical training. JAMA. 2016;316(10):1113–4.

Chapter 46
Attending to Resident: Gender Bias

Georges Ramalanjaona and Benjamin Ramalanjaona

Case Scenario

A 50-year-old white male attending physician, an eastern European native, made an insensitive remark publicly toward a female off-service resident regarding her procedural skills. The attending physician asked the resident to get a central line access to an unstable patient in order to draw blood and give IV fluids. Several attempts at the central line placement were unsuccessful. The attending physician yelled at the resident publicly in front of her peers, stating that her procedural skills were poor in spite of his teaching her the proper technique previously. The resident became tearful and felt that she was targeted because of her gender.

What Was Done?

Although the intent of teaching was laudable, the manner in which it was performed was inappropriate and resulted in public humiliation of the female resident. It was therefore unacceptable behavior. In doing this, the faculty member breached the rule of confidentiality of the resident's evaluation as stipulated in the Residents' Handbook. The resident filed a written complaint against the faculty member to the Director of Medical Education (DME).

G. Ramalanjaona (✉)
Essen Medical Associate, Bronx, NY, USA

B. Ramalanjaona
State University of New York Downstate Medical Center, Brooklyn, NY, USA

© Springer International Publishing AG, part of Springer Nature 2019
M. L. Martin et al. (eds.), *Diversity and Inclusion in Quality Patient Care*,
https://doi.org/10.1007/978-3-319-92762-6_46

Questions for Discussion

1. What assumptions or gaps in knowledge led to this encounter?

Attitudes/Assumptions: The European Male Attending

(a) The sense that his authority allowed him to yell at the resident.
(b) A display of impatience in the teaching role is okay in critical cases.

Gaps in Provider Knowledge

(a) The attending's understanding of the teacher/student relationship is lacking.
(b) The attending's communication timing was poor regarding procedural technique feedback.
(c) The attending displayed lack of a empathy for the junior learner.

Attitudes/Assumptions: The Female Resident

(a) The resident lacked recognition of insufficient technical skills on complicated procedures.
(b) The resident lacked progress on advanced procedures in previous training sessions.
(c) The resident lacked judgment on getting assistance from other senior peers/attendings to complete a procedure.
(d) The resident assumed she was targeted because of her gender.

2. How could this encounter have gone differently?

(a) The attending could have dealt with the resident's poor performance in a private setting.
(b) The resident could have been more assertive in communicating with the attending to obtain assistance in completing the procedure on this unstable patient.

Cross-Cultural Tools and Skills

(a) Improve cross-cultural skills by integrating curricula in clinical practice and medical education as published by the ACGME/ABEM [1].

(b) Incorporate elements of the Emergency Medicine milestones of ACGME components [2] as part of the faculty development. It includes professional values, interpersonal and communication skills, respect of others, as well as adherence to the ethical principles relevant to the practice of medicine.
(c) Embrace dual faculty role as teacher and role model for a diverse population of medical learners [3, 4].
(d) Attend regular meetings with the DME to evaluate progress/behavior during the academic period.

Pearls and Pitfalls

Pearl The attending provided the resident an opportunity to perform a complicated procedure.

Pitfall The faculty member may not be aware of his own cultural bias toward female subordinates as he was raised in a culture of male dominance.

Pitfall Lack of knowledge of confidentiality when dealing with residents' performances.

Pitfall Lack of communicating with residents in a professional manner.

Pitfall Although the attending's intent to teach the resident was laudable, his insensitive remark in a public forum was unacceptable and did not achieve the intended goal of improving skills, but rather resulted in a formal complaint and disciplinary action toward him.

Case Outcome

The resident filed a formal disciplinary complaint against the faculty member according to the rules of the institution's residency guidelines. The event was witnessed by other residents during that rotation period. The disciplinary process was followed and included:

1. Formal notification of the involved faculty member by the DME within 15 days of receipt of the written complaint with request for a meeting with faculty
2. Regular meeting with the DME within 30 days to assess the faculty member's progress in dealing with diversity/inclusion issues
3. A reading assignment for the involved faculty member on diversity/inclusion with questions and answers and requests to follow up with DME

Once approved by the Faculty Development Committee, the corrective action plan was allowed to proceed. Resident witnesses were helpful in the testimony. In this case, the faculty member successfully complied with all the required elements of the plan without any negative impact on promotion and appointment. The resident successfully completed formal instruction on advanced procedural skills and was allowed to advance to the next level of training.

References

1. Accreditation Standards [Internet]. Washington: Liaison Committee on Medical Education; c2017 [cited 2017 Nov 8]. Available from: http://lcme.org/publications/#Standards.
2. The Emergency Medicine Milestone Project [Internet]. Chicago: The Accreditation Council for Graduate Medical Education; 2015 [cited 2017 Nov 8]. Available from: http://www.acgme. org/acgmeweb/portals/0/PDFs/Milestones/EmergencyMedicineMilestones.pdf. Joint publication with the American Board of Emergency Medicine.
3. Wright SM, Carrese JA. Serving as a physician role model for a diverse population of medical learners. Acad Med. 2000;78:623–8.
4. Wright SM, et al. Attributes of excellent attending physician role models. NEJM. 1998;339:1986–93.

Chapter 47
Resident Toward Intern Barriers and Bias

Marcee Wilder and Lynne D. Richardson

Case Scenario

On three separate occasions, a white senior resident made disparaging remarks to a black intern. On the first occasion, during morning report, the intern suggested a possible differential diagnosis. The senior resident looked at her and sarcastically said, "Where did you go to medical school?" The intern did not answer. On another occasion, when the intern was presenting one of her cases at morning report, the same senior resident remarked, "I can't believe it took you that long to make the diagnosis." Again, the intern said nothing. During a clinical shift in the department, the black intern and her white co-intern were alternating supervised intubations by the white senior resident. When it was the black intern's turn in the rotation to intubate a patient in the resuscitation bay, the white senior resident asked her co-intern to intubate the patient instead. He then told her, "I think that would've been a difficult airway for you; I'll give you the next one." After this interaction, the black intern was visibly upset. Immediately after the clinical shift, the black intern was approached by her co-intern, who asked what the senior resident had against her. The black intern replied, "He thinks I don't belong in this residency because I am black." The co-intern was shocked and said, "Oh no, I'm sure you are wrong."

M. Wilder
Department of Emergency Medicine, Icahn School of Medicine at Mount Sinai,
New York, NY, USA

L. D. Richardson (✉)
Department of Emergency Medicine, Department of Population Health Science and Policy,
Icahn School of Medicine at Mount Sinai, New York, NY, USA
e-mail: Lynne.Richardson@mssm.edu

© Springer International Publishing AG, part of Springer Nature 2019
M. L. Martin et al. (eds.), *Diversity and Inclusion in Quality Patient Care*,
https://doi.org/10.1007/978-3-319-92762-6_47

What Was Said?

The white senior resident said to the black intern, "Where did you go to medical school?", "I can't believe it took you that long to make the diagnosis," and "I think that would've been a difficult airway for you."

The black intern said to the white co-intern, "He thinks I don't belong in this residency because I am black."

The white co-intern said, "Oh no, I'm sure you are wrong."

What Was Done?

The black intern spoke with her faculty advisor, who encouraged her to speak with the residency leadership. She did this and was told that the program did not condone the senior resident's condescending attitude. They subsequently told her that they had spoken to the senior resident and the co-intern. They assured her there was no racial bias involved.

The black intern was dissatisfied and spoke again to her faculty advisor. She was informed that she could file a formal complaint with the institution but decided not to do that. Since the residency leadership did not believe her, she thought reporting it outside the department would adversely affect her treatment by the residency leadership and the other residents in the program.

Question for Discussion

1. What underlying assumptions are present?

Attitudes/Assumptions: The Resident

The white senior resident publicly ridicules the intern's knowledge and clinical skills. He also causes her to miss an opportunity for a procedure during a clinical shift. Does he do it to deliberately hurt her? Does he do it to make himself feel superior? Is this resident exhibiting implicit bias toward the black intern? Is this resident exhibiting explicit racial bias against the black intern? Does he have insight into his own bias? Is it possible that this resident exhibits bias toward black patients?

Attitudes/Assumptions: The Interns

The black intern felt disliked and disrespected by the white senior resident and believes him to be racist. She felt humiliated and angry when he treated her as though she was inferior in front of others. She felt like he abused his power as a senior resident by taking an intubation procedure from her. Does it make her doubt her ability to become an emergency physician? Does it interfere with her ability to learn and ask appropriate questions? Does the co-intern's reaction make her feel isolated or misunderstood?

The white co-intern noticed the way the senior resident spoke to and treated the black intern. He then expressed incredulity that it could have been due to racism. Why does he doubt that his senior resident might be racist? Does he think his co-intern is overreacting? Paranoid? Does the suggestion make him uncomfortable because he does not want to believe one of his fellow residents is racist? Is he exhibiting implicit bias?

Pearls and Pitfalls

Pearl Implicit bias refers to attitudes or stereotypes that affect our understanding, decision-making, and behavior, without our even realizing it. Strategies to raise awareness of unconscious assumptions and their influence on evaluation should be employed in residency training programs [1, 2].

Pearl Explicit bias results from consciously held beliefs that members of one group are inferior to members of another group. Those in leadership roles should be vigilant in confronting anyone who makes, or allows others to make, remarks that label or denigrate other staff members. Whether openly prejudicial or subtly stereotypical, such comments should not be tolerated. Failure to act may result in a work environment that is hostile to members of the affected group [3–5].

Pitfall Individuals who are the target of implicit or explicit bias experience damaging emotional consequences: a lack of confidence in professional roles, feelings of being on guard at all times, self-doubt, and frustration with the system in which they work [4].

Pearl Racial bias is contagious. Just observing a biased person express subtle negative bias toward a black person may shift another individual's attitude.

Pitfall Programs that fail to ensure that residents learn to give evaluation and feedback that is fair and free from racial bias have failed to meet important resident competencies in the areas of Professionalism, and Interpersonal and Communication Skills [6, 7].

Case Outcome

The black intern completed the residency but was angry and resentful toward the program. She warned black applicants to the residency to stay away because they would not be supported in this program. The white senior resident continued to treat black staff members and patients in a disrespectful manner.

References

1. AAMC diversity portfolios [Internet]. Washington: Association of American Medical Colleges; 2017 [cited 2017 Nov 29]. Available from: https://www.aamc.org/initiatives/diversity/portfolios/.
2. Sabin JA. Implicit bias: implications for health and healthcare [Internet]. Seattle: University of Washington. 2017 [cited 2017 Nov 29]. Available from: http://healthequity.wa.gov/Portals/9/Doc/Meetings/2017/09-13/Tab05a-ImplicitBiasPresentation.pdf.
3. Betancourt JR, Corbett J, Bondaryk MR. Addressing disparities and achieving equity: cultural competence, ethics, and health-care transformation. Chest. 2014;145(1):143–8.
4. Liebschutz JM, Darko GO, Finley EP, Cawse JM, Bharel M, Orlander JD. In the minority: black physicians in residency and their experiences. J Natl Med Assoc. 2006;98(9):1441–8.
5. Markakis KM, Beckman HB, Suchman AL, Frankel RM. The path to professionalism: cultivating humanistic values and attitudes in residency training. Acad Med. 2000;75:141–50.
6. Nivet MA. Diversity 3.0: a necessary systems upgrade. Acad Med. 2011;86:1487–9.
7. The Emergency Medicine Milestone Project [Internet]. Chicago: The Accreditation Council for Graduate Medical Education and the American Board for Emergency Medicine; c2012 [cited 2014 Aug 5]. Available from: http://www.acgme.org/acgmeweb/Portals/0/PDFs/Milestones/EmergencyMedicineMilestones.pdf.

Chapter 48
The Trojan Letter of Recommendation

Mikhail C. S. S. Higgins

Case Scenario

A Latina female third-year anesthesiology resident is approached by a prominent anesthesiology attending who excitingly expressed interest in writing a letter of support for her application to a competitive fellowship in pain management. The resident is elated by the attending's expression of genuine interest to help advance her career. However, while the older white male attending had proctored her in numerous cases, she reflected that her prior interactions never strongly suggested that the attending cared that much about her progress as a resident. While he was always willing to teach her over the prior 3 years, he made minimal eye contact with her, and although he was always very professional, he treated her with a subtle but distant air compared to her co-residents. Despite that, she was excited to have a prestigious full professor faculty member offer to write a letter of support on her behalf.

She fielded her application to six programs, supported by four faculty letters of recommendation. She received an early invitation to interview at a nearby program. During that interview, the female African-American program director explained to the candidate that while the selection committee invited her there to consider her for the position, they were concerned enough to notify her that she may have been a potential target of slander. They had a strong sense that this was the case considering that three of her letters strongly touted her exceptional clinical competency, professionalism, and work ethic, while one of the letters was an outlier and tactfully argued the opposite. The program director explained that while their confidential and unconventional disclosure of this to her was completely outside of standard operating procedures, they thought it necessary to offer her an opportunity to regroup and resubmit a revised application.

M. C. S. S. Higgins, MD, MPH
Boston University School of Medicine, Boston, MA, USA
e-mail: Mikhail.Higgins@bmc.org

© Springer International Publishing AG, part of Springer Nature 2019
M. L. Martin et al. (eds.), *Diversity and Inclusion in Quality Patient Care*,
https://doi.org/10.1007/978-3-319-92762-6_48

Presuming that the letter was from the attending that had strangely offered to submit one on her behalf, she resubmitted her application to five other programs, swapping his letter out for that of a junior faculty attending with whom she had a better professional relationship. She received no additional interviews from the first batch of six programs to which she applied. However, she received invitations to interview at all programs to which she submitted her revised application. Ultimately, she matriculated into her top fellowship choice, incidentally becoming the first Latina female anesthesiology pain fellow to graduate from that prestigious program.

What Was Done?

A senior male attending offers to write a letter of recommendation to support a resident applying for a competitive anesthesiology fellowship. Unbeknownst to the resident, the letter denigrates her clinical proficiency and professional achievements, implicitly seeking to sabotage her candidacy for a competitive fellowship position.

No report of the alleged slander was executed. However, the interviewing program director informed the resident of the suspicions of the screening committee. Once informed, the resident did not share the suspicion with anyone.

No institutional support or disciplinary action was sought or incurred. The resident may have been uncertain as to where she should seek support, recourse, or disciplinary action. Perhaps given the third-party program's confidential and unconventional disclosure to the resident, which was outside of standard operating procedures, the resident chose not to seek support from her home institution or independent counsel. She may have been similarly uncertain as to the risks of jeopardizing the benevolent program. Finally, the resident may have also been concerned about potential retribution by the full professor faculty member or the potential professional backlash if disciplinary action was sought.

Questions for Discussion

1. What underlying attitudes or assumptions contributed to this situation?

Attitudes/Assumptions: The Attending

(a) The resident's attending who wrote the letter of recommendation acted malevolently. Whether his macroaggression was secondary to his perception of justified professional disfavor, or was a gender or ethnicity provoked discrimination, is unknown.

Attitudes/Assumptions: The Resident

(a) The resident was innocent and potentially naïve to the possibility and presence of such a slanderous macroaggression by a trusted attending offering to write a letter of recommendation.

(b) Once notified by the African-American residency program director, the Latina resident was grateful, respectful, and reacted with poise. Her decision to not instigate the situation further reflects maturity and decisiveness.

2. What specific gaps in the resident's knowledge may have contributed to this situation?

Gaps in Provider Knowledge: The Resident

(a) The resident may have lacked particular soft emotional skills that may have detected subtle undertones or microaggressions in past professional interactions, appropriately clueing her into the attending's attitude toward her.

(b) Provided that microaggressions were previously perceived and recognized, they could have been addressed in advance, possibly by identifying a professional mentor in a position of authority with whom to discuss the situation and determine the best course of action [1].

(c) Moreover, such prior knowledge would have likely resulted in her not accepting the disingenuous offer to write her a letter of recommendation.

3. What specific cross-cultural tools and skills are called into question in the cited narrative?

Cross-Cultural Tools and Skills

(a) Bridging real or perceived gaps across cultures, ethnicities, and races that occur between colleagues, patients and providers, or trainees and attendings is challenging but necessary [1].

(b) Empathy and respect, informed by open, diligent communication and an inclination to seek first to understand and then be understood, are priceless tools of the professional healthcare provider.

Pearls and Pitfalls

Pearl The interviewing program director (female, African-American) assumed compassion, empathy, and courage, which are critical characteristics of clinical excellence and leadership by sharing with the unaware resident that she was a potential victim of slander [2].

Pitfall While not consistent with standard operating procedures for fellowship applications, another program director in this situation may have understandably chosen not to become "involved" and alert the candidate of the suspected ill-conceived letter. However, the failure to act would likely have resulted in the resident's career being unknowingly compromised in the process.

Pearl The resident requested a new letter by a junior faculty member with whom she had a well-cultivated professional relationship and who had been visibly supportive of her performance and career advancement.

Pearl Armed with information to fuel a potentially injurious charge to the faculty member, the resident chose not to confront the attending at her home institution or seek disciplinary action through a third party. Instead, she focused on the most important task at hand of revising her application and securing her desired fellowship.

Pitfall The most prestigious faculty members are often sought for letters of recommendation, even in cases where a candidate shares a questionable professional rapport with the faculty member. The most valued letters tend to be written by those truly familiar with the candidate's proficiency, who can speak specifically to their deservedness of the desired position.

Pitfall In the face of microaggressions and macroaggressions that may be fueled by dynamic power differentials or implicit biases related to gender, race, culture, or religion, an emotional response often arises. Unfortunately, the retribution or punitive/disciplinary action that is often reactively sought may result in compromising the ultimate end the trainees seek. Focusing on the task at hand, seeking forgiveness, and pressing on is often the wiser, higher road [1, 2].

Case Outcome

The candidate accurately assessed her situation and deduced that the anomalous letter of concern, flagged by the program director acting as a Good Samaritan, was from the attending that made an unsolicited offer to write a letter of recommendation on her behalf. She did not approach the attending or attempt to influence the decision of the programs that had already processed her application, which was tainted by the maligning letter of recommendation. She requested a new letter by a junior faculty with whom she had a solid professional rapport and who had demonstrated support for her advancement. She resubmitted her revised application to new programs and ultimately accepted a position at her top choice.

References

1. Acker J. Inequality regimes: gender, class, and race in organizations. Gend Soc. 2006;20(4):441–64.
2. Piderit SK, Ashford SJ. Breaking silence: tactical choices women managers make in speaking up about gender-equity issues. J Manage Stud. 2003;40(6):1477–502.

Chapter 49
When Sisterhood Alone Just Isn't Enough

Aisha Liferidge and Reem Alhawas

Case Scenario

A 45-year-old white female presents to a level 1 quaternary academic center emergency department in an urban city with the chief complaint of "I need a second opinion."

She asks to have a previously diagnosed thyroid nodule reassessed and managed. The patient reports having a left-sided thyroid nodule diagnosed by ultrasound 1 year prior. At that time, she was offered a biopsy of the nodule to determine its pathological makeup, but declined as she was not convinced that there was actually a nodule there. Incidentally, an area of slight protrusion on the patient's neck had been discovered during a routine annual examination by her primary care provider. When initially discovered, she had no associated symptoms, but now reports noting that the protrusion seems more apparent than before and is occasionally slightly tender to the touch. She also reports experiencing insomnia, irritability, and exertional intolerance. Additionally, she reports being concerned that she may be "going through the change" given that she often finds herself feeling very hot and sweaty. She denies any chest pain, shortness of breath, lower extremity edema, weight changes, cold symptoms, or rash.

A. Liferidge (✉)
George Washington University School of Medicine and Health Sciences,
Washington, DC, USA
e-mail: aliferidge@mfa.gwu.edu

R. Alhawas
George Washington University School of Medicine and Health Sciences,
Washington, DC, USA

Imam Abdulrahman Bin Faisal University School of Medicine, Dammam, Saudi Arabia
e-mail: rahawas@email.gwu.edu

© Springer International Publishing AG, part of Springer Nature 2019
M. L. Martin et al. (eds.), *Diversity and Inclusion in Quality Patient Care*,
https://doi.org/10.1007/978-3-319-92762-6_49

Review of Symptoms

Bowel movements are recently looser than normal; increased feelings of anxiety and loneliness lately.

Past Medical History

Well-controlled asthma, no history of intubations, uses albuterol inhaler rarely for mild flares; depression, stopped taking prescribed fluoxetine 2 years ago due to feeling that it caused her to gain weight.

Family History

Mother living, with hypertension; father died 20 years ago from complications of alcoholism.

Social History

Smokes 10 cigarettes a day for the past 20 years; never drinks alcohol; has never used illicit drugs; works for cleaning company; lives alone in an apartment in a suburb of the city; has pet cat.

Physical Exam

Vital Signs Temperature 99.0 F, blood pressure 133/75, pulse 97, respiratory rate 12.

General Appears well and in no acute distress, airway intact.

Head and Neck Normocephalic and atraumatic; subtle fullness to left side of anterior neck.

Neuro Moving all extremities.

What Was Said?

An African-American female attending physician, dressed in casual business attire and a long white coat, and her Saudi Arabian female senior emergency medicine resident physician, dressed in a pair of scrubs with no head attire, enter the examination room to see the patient. The attending first introduces herself as the "supervising physician" and her accompanying resident as the "senior resident physician." The attending physician then asks the patient, "What brings you in today? What can we do for you?" The patient appears a bit apprehensive, but proceeds to explain that she is there because of a mass in her neck which was diagnosed a year ago; she says she is not convinced that she actually has a neck mass and wants a second opinion.

Before the attending physician has the opportunity to proceed and ask more questions as a part of a focused history, the patient abruptly interrupts her and angrily says, "Wait! I need to see a doctor! Where is the doctor?!" Caught a bit off guard, the attending physician pauses and then calmly reintroduces herself and her resident physician as the doctors who will be taking care of her. Referring to the resident physician with an eye glance, the patient proceeds to only address the attending physician, saying, "But she can't be a doctor, she's Mexican! She must be a nurse!"

At that point, both the attending and resident physician look at each other perplexed. They both wonder if the patient is seriously confused about their roles or if she somehow lacks the mental capacity to comprehend the reality of the situation. The attending physician tries again, saying, "Ma'am, we are both doctors. She is not a nurse, nor is she Mexican." The resident attempts to further reassure the patient by saying, "Ma'am, I'm one of the physicians here. Take a look at my ID badge." The patient then begins to shuffle through her personal belongings saying that she needs her glasses in order to clearly see the resident physician's name badge. She says that she needs to make sure that the resident physician is not a nurse. As the patient anxiously goes through her bag to find her glasses, the attending and resident physicians just stand there waiting patiently for her to find her glasses, feeling rather shocked and not sure of what to do next.

Once the patient finds her glasses, the resident physician says, "Ma'am, I am a doctor," and hesitantly extends her name badge within less than a foot from the patient's eyes so that she can clearly see that it reads "Physician." The resident physician is humiliated and in disbelief that her credentials were questioned to this extent. In her mind, she tries to understand what is happening by processing whether the issue is that the patient lacked mental capacity or was simply ignorant and being rude. The attending physician feels embarrassed for her resident physician and begins to feel annoyed by the patient's behavior. Despite being shown the resident physician's name badge, the patient still insists, "No! She's just a Mexican—a Mexican nurse. A resident physician-what does it even mean?! I'm leaving!" The attending physician, becoming impatient with the blatant disrespect, says to the patient, "Ma'am, we are happy to care for you, but you are welcome to seek care elsewhere. We are the physicians who would manage your care, but you have the right to leave, knowing the risks associated with leaving." The patient then angrily says, "I don't trust you. I don't trust you to take care of me. I want to leave and will go to another hospital." As the patient gathers her things and makes ready to leave the room, the attending physician exits the room, saying to the resident physician, "Sign her out AMA." The resident physician then exits the room after the attending physician. The patient rushes out of the emergency department, refusing to wait for her discharge paperwork.

What Was Done?

In this case, the patient's blatant bias against Mexican people, apparent ignorance by thinking that the Saudi Arabian resident physician was Mexican, and sexism by assuming that the resident physician was a nurse–a role traditionally held by females–rather than a physician, precluded there being any meaningful clinical interaction. Prior to having the opportunity to take an adequate history and perform a full physical examination, the patient's erroneous and accusatory outbursts resulted in almost immediate cessation of the encounter. The fact that the patient was also apparently not satisfied with being cared for by the African-American female attending physician (although she never verbalized this)–who was dressed in more traditionally authoritative physician attire–raises concern for the possibility that the patient was biased against Mexicans and African Americans, and perhaps females of color or just females in general. Somehow, the resident physician seemed to be an easier target, perhaps because of her more casual clinical attire and/or the Arabic accent of her speech.

Once outside of the patient room and back at the doctors' workstation, the attending physician profusely apologizes to the resident physician for having to endure such disrespect and disregard. She asks the resident physician if she has ever experienced such treatment. The resident physician responds with a nervous smile, "No. Never so blatantly! I'm used to being perceived as a nurse just because of my gender, from both male and female patients equally, but never faced anything like that." The attending physician then reassures the resident physician that she, too, has never experienced that degree of overt racism and sexism; she reminds her that she is in fact an excellent physician and to try not to be overly bothered by the incident.

No official reports are made, and the day in the emergency department continues as per usual for both the attending and resident physician.

This case illustrates the effects of patient-initiated bias toward healthcare providers and how it can impede access to care while traumatizing the clinician [1–3]. The bias in this case was based on race, gender, and linguistic accent. It also illustrates that there may be a link between mental illness and bias or, at least, distrust of healthcare providers. This patient had a known history of anxiety and depression, which played a role in this encounter and likely influenced a repetitive cycle of emotional and impulsive behavior that led to her suboptimal utilization of and access to health care.

Questions for Discussion

1. Which is more commonly encountered in the clinical setting: overt racism or sexism?

   In 1961, John F. Kennedy introduced affirmative action policies in order to level the playing ground for people of color. In 1967, President Johnson recognized the need to broaden the definition of groups discriminated against and added gender to the affirmative action eligibility list. Nearly a half a century later in 2016, Secretary of State Hillary Clinton ran for President of the United States as the first serious female contender. She surprisingly lost to Donald Trump, a businessman with no political experience who was projected to lose by wide margins. This highlights the idea that perhaps sexism is more prevalent than racism given that America elected its first African-American President for two terms just prior the 2016 Presidential election, yet an experienced politician like Hillary Clinton lost to an inexperienced man [4]. In the clinical context, while there is significant data that supports the negative effects of sexism on female patient outcomes and policies that condemn gender-based discrimination in medicine [5], there is a paucity of data on the existence of and effects of patient-initiated sexism toward female providers. Future studies should explore this issue.

2. How common is it for perpetrators of sexism against females to themselves be of the female gender?

   While there are studies that purport that female perpetrators of sexism against other females in criminal acts tend to be viewed as less common and dangerous, little data exists within the medical literature that quantifies the extent of female-on-female patient-initiated bias. There is literature, however, which describes a more primitive phenomenon of competition among females that relates to using beauty as a resource for securing a male to provide offspring and sustenance; some believe that this sentiment still prevails, even if subconsciously, and manifests itself in various ways today. In fact, Fretté asserts, "In general, modern women do not possess the solidarity you might hope for or even expect in a world that is supposedly heading toward gender equality." She goes on to say, "When women can finally relegate beauty to a fun life expression, rather than a prerequisite of success, it might be safe to say that we will see less tension between our sisters [6]." Future studies should explore this issue.

3. Does ACGME require that racist and/or sexist incidents against medical residents be formally reported and managed post-incident?

   In February 2017, the Chief Executive Officer of the Accreditation Council of Graduate Medical Education, Dr. Thomas Nasca, wrote a letter to the graduate medical education community in response to the executive order "Protecting the Nation from Foreign Terrorist Entry into the United States." He proclaimed, "Discrimination on the basis of race, gender, religious beliefs, sexual orientation, or other factors is a violation of our personal and professional values. To this end, we have worked with the AAMC and others to co-author a letter to President Trump representing the values of the profession, and concerns over these actions" [7]. Additionally, the ACGME has an official policy on diversity, inclusion, and equity, but there does not appear to be any official reporting mandate.

4. What percentage of hospital institutions and/or departments have policy that speaks to employee-targeted racism and/or sexism, particularly patient-initiated, and its management?

   While the American Hospital Association has an initiative around "Equity of Care," which seeks to alleviate health disparities, and has even published toolkits about increasing provider diversity within health care, little official policy focuses on the provider as the victim of discrimination. This is similarly the case among medical specialty societies, many of whom have policy that speaks to workplace violence against providers [8], but not to nonphysical violations such as discriminatory treatment by patients. Traditionally, the focus has been to protect and advocate for patients and their rights. Yet the negative effects of provider-targeted discrimination, such as decreased workforce diversity and associated health disparities, warrant the need to set boundaries in order to protect the provider.

5. Is there an association between mental illness and racist and/or discriminatory ideology and/or behavior, and does such bias place the mentally ill at a disproportionate disadvantage related to access to care and health outcomes?

   Some psychiatrists argue that racism is a mental illness. In the 1960s, Harvard psychiatrist Dr. Alvin Poussaint and his colleagues made this assertion and even petitioned the American Psychiatric Association (APA) to add extreme racism as an official *Diagnostic and Statistical Manual of Disorders* (DSM) condition as a delusional disorder. When one considers that racism is essentially the belief that–based solely on skin color and ethnicity–one group of humans is inherently inferior to another despite an abundance of scientific proof that genetically says otherwise, indeed the idea of there being delusional thoughts involved is a reasonable assertion. Therefore, one hypothesis might be that individuals who are racist carry some degree of delusional beliefs, which results in mistrust, and, thus, disadvantage related to their ability to optimally access and utilize the healthcare system.

6. How does a provider's linguistic accent affect their patients' perceptions of and biases towards them?

   One's linguistic accent often influences others' perceptions of that person leading to conscious and unconscious biases. A 2015 German and UK study used speech samples of strong German accents to test the idea of whether individuals choose to compete against or cooperate with people who have different and strong linguistic accents. The study found that in fact people are more likely to compete with others who speak differently. This was interpreted as discrimination because the judgment was not based on performance but rather perception related to the speech samples [9].

   In an emergency department clinical setting such as the one from this case, there is limited opportunity for the provider and patient to get to know each other; therefore, patients might use audible and visual characteristics such as linguistic accent, race, and gender as surrogates to "knowing" their provider, sometimes resulting in unfair judgements and erroneous distrust.

Attitudes/Assumptions: The Provider

(a) Associating patient's racist and sexist comments with her chronic mental illness

Assumptions/Attitudes of the Patient

(a) Associating darker skin color with being Mexican
(b) Associating Mexican race with incompetence/inferiority
(c) Associating female gender with being a nurse and not a physician
(d) Associating the nursing profession with incompetence/inferiority
(e) Associating linguistic accents with incompetence/inferiority

Gaps in Provider Knowledge

(a) Understanding of patient's past medical history
(b) Understanding of patient's past experiences with the healthcare system
(c) Understanding of patient's past experiences with people and providers of color
(d) Understanding of patient's past experiences with people and providers of female gender

Pearls and Pitfalls

Pearls In this case, the physicians successfully managed the situation by choosing to remain calm, not become irritated, and give the patient the benefit of the doubt. Taking the patient's concerns seriously and allowing her time to visualize the resident physician's name badge in order that she might feel most comfortable illustrated maturity, patience, and humility on the physicians' parts. It is important to maintain an open mind and understand that human behavior, even if inappropriate, is the result of preceding incidents, the details of which a stranger might not know or understand [1–3].

Pitfalls A potential pitfall would have been the physician allowing emotions to hinder her ability to be objective and maintain the patient's best interests as a priority. Always consider whether the patient has adequate capacity to make decisions. Ensure that the patient is always aware of potential risks associated with aborting care against medical advice [3]. This case was handled well and its ultimate outcome was unfortunate, but appropriate [3].

Case Outcome

The patient left the emergency department of her own accord immediately after the attending and resident physicians left the patient room. She was deemed to have adequate capacity to make this decision. The encounter disposition was recorded as discharged to home against medical advice.

References

1. Blair IV, et al. Implicit (unconscious) bias and health disparities: where do we go from here? Perm J. 2011;15(2):72.
2. Matthew DB. Chapter 5, Implicit bias during the clinical encounter. In: Just medicine. A cure for racial inequality in American health care. New York: New York University Press; 2015. p. 118–22.
3. Tweedy D. Chapter 5, Confronting hate. In: Black man in a white coat. New York: Picador; 2016. p. 105–28.
4. Katie HR. Couric: sexism is more common than racism [Internet]. New York: NYDailyNews. com; 2008 Jul 23 [cited 2017 Dec 19]. Available from: http://www.nydailynews.com/entertainment/tv-movies/katie-couric-sexism-common-racism-article-1.349096.
5. Gender Discrimination in Medicine [Internet]. Chicago (IL): American Medical Association; 2017 [cited 2017 Dec 21]. Available from: https://www.ama-assn.org/delivering-care/gender-discrimination-medicine.
6. Fretté J. Why women are mean to women [Internet]. New York: Huffington Post; 2012 Sept 26 [cited 2017 Dec 19]. Available from: https://www.huffingtonpost.com/juliette-frette/jealousy_b_1914374.html.
7. Nasca TJ. (Chief Executive Officer, Accreditation Council for Graduate Medical Education). Letter to: Members of the graduate medical education community. 2017 Feb 2. 2 p. Available from: https://www.acgme.org/Portals/0/PDFs/Nasca-Community/Nasca-Letter-Immigration-2-2-17.pdf.
8. Farouk A. Taking steps to prevent violence in health care workplace [Internet]. Chicago (IL): American Medical Association; 2016 Jun 14 [cited 2017 Dec 21]. Available from: https://wire.ama-assn.org/ama-news/taking-steps-prevent-violence-health-care-workplace.
9. Heblich S, et al. The effect of perceived regional accents on individual economic behavior: a lab experiment on linguistic performance, cognitive ratings and economic decisions. PLoS One. 2015;10(5):e0124732. https://doi.org/10.1371/journal.pone.0124732.

Chapter 50
Tattooed Doctor

**Marcus L. Martin, DeVanté J. Cunningham, and
Emmanuel Agyemang-Dua**

Case Scenario

Ms. Janice Jones is a 20-year-old African-American female approximately 28 weeks pregnant who presents with mild abdominal pain, possibly in labor. She is gravida 2, para 1, and abortus 0. She has one living child who is 2 years of age. Triage nurse Betty Brown conducts a patient assessment including fetal exam. There is no vaginal bleeding. While waiting for the physician, nurse Brown and Ms. Jones conversed about their shared Christian faith and discussed biblical names to give the unborn child.

Dr. William Merritt, a white male emergency medicine resident (PGY2), working the overnight shift in the emergency department (ED), introduces himself to Ms. Jones and inquires about her chief complaint. He is wearing a scrub top with multiple tattoos visible on both arms. Among the tattoos are images of a mermaid, a heart "mom" tattoo, and a red Hindu swastika with four dots. While he was an undergraduate student, Dr. Merritt converted to Hinduism and got the tattoo as a symbol of well-being. As a medical student, Dr. Merritt contemplated surgical removal of his tattoos. Healthcare providers often face negative perceptions because of exposed skin modifications [1].

Ms. Jones, visibly uneasy, asks Dr. Merritt, "Can I see another doctor, please?" Confused by the sporadic request, Dr. Merritt asks, "Why?" Ms. Jones becomes

M. L. Martin (✉)
University of Virginia, Charlottesville, VA, USA
e-mail: mlm8n@virginia.edu

D. J. Cunningham
Clinical Psychology, Montclair State University, Montclair, NJ, USA
e-mail: cunninghamd3@montclair.edu

E. Agyemang-Dua
University of Virginia, Charlottesville, VA, USA
e-mail: ea9cf@virginia.edu

© Springer International Publishing AG, part of Springer Nature 2019
M. L. Martin et al. (eds.), *Diversity and Inclusion in Quality Patient Care*,
https://doi.org/10.1007/978-3-319-92762-6_50

353

increasingly irritable and uncomfortable and asks for the doctor in charge of the ED. Dr. Merritt complies and calls for his attending, Dr. Amy Austin. Dr. Austin establishes good rapport with Ms. Jones. Ms. Jones shares with Dr. Austin her concerns about Dr. Merritt's tattoos. She wonders if Dr. Merritt is a racist because of the "swastika." The rest of the assessment is conducted without Dr. Merritt present.

Review of Symptoms

Mild abdominal pain; possibly in labor, but no vaginal bleeding – All other systems reviewed and are negative

Past Medical History

G 2, P 1, A 0, past anxiety

Family History

Noncontributory

Social History

Occasional alcohol prior to pregnancy, does not smoke

Physical Exam: Triage Nurse Assessment

Fetal heart tones appear normal

Vital Signs BP 140/90, pulse 70, and respiratory rate 20

HEENT Normal exam

Cardiovascular Heart rate normal

Respiratory Lungs clear

Abdomen Gravid

Extremities Normal, no pedal edema, and reflexes are normal

Skin Normal

Neck Supple

Questions for Discussion

1. What are the attitudes/assumptions?

Attitudes/Assumptions: The Patient

(a) This doctor is a racist because he has a swastika tattooed on his body.
(b) Ms. Jones feels threatened by the symbolism of the tattoos.
(c) This doctor is not professional.
(d) She is concerned about the doctor's ability to attend to her.
(e) She feels that she will not get the best care.

Attitudes/Assumptions: The Physician

(a) Why is this patient refusing my service?
(b) Is she uncomfortable with me as a male doctor?
(c) It may be my attire. Since it is an overnight shift, wearing scrubs is appropriate.
(d) It may be my tattoos. They may be an issue for the patient.
(e) I should not be scrutinized for expressing myself through body art; it does not make me incompetent or unprofessional.

2. What was done?

(a) Dr. Merritt calls for the attending, Dr. Austin, to see the patient instead of him.
(b) Ms. Jones shares her concerns about Dr. Merritt's tattoos with Dr. Austin.

Pearls and Pitfalls

Pearl Dr. Merritt was compliant with the patient's wishes and did not appear to be offended by her request. She received appropriate medical care.

Pitfall Dr. Merritt was perceived by the patient to be a racist because of the visible tattoos. He was unaware of the potential cultural backlash his Hindu swastika could create.

Physicians are often confronted with cultural issues in all aspects of health delivery. A patient's culture will generally prevail when at odds with the medical establishment [1]. This often puts a strain on physician-patient relationships. More so, this dynamic shifts the burden of cultural awareness on the physician and the medical establishment rather than the patient. Cultural awareness or sensitivity is defined as, "The knowledge and interpersonal skills that allow providers to understand, appreciate, and work with individuals from cultures other than their own" [1]. Cultural sensitivity involves an awareness and acceptance of cultural differences, but also knowledge of a patient's age, gender, sexual orientation, education level, socioeconomic status, faith, profession, and disabilities. The burden of cultural awareness and sensitivity can also fall on the patient. Uninformed patients can misunderstand the cultural identity of healthcare providers [2].

The swastika is an ancient Sanskrit symbol that has surged in multiple variations to be used by many civilizations from the Egyptians, to the Vikings, to the Native Americans, and then the Hindus. In Hindu culture, the swastika is a symbol of well-being and peace [3]. In 1920, however, the meaning was perverted by the Nazi regime to be a symbol of Aryan dominance and conquest and as a homage to their Aryan ancestors [3, 4]. Over time, the world has come to contextualize and understand the swastika as a symbol for hate and racism, rather than for peace and well-being. A person with a swastika tattoo may be perceived negatively both for having a tattoo and for it being a swastika [2]. A patient's perception of a physician can influence how they interact or accept care [2]. A patient may refuse care or even report experiencing low quality of care due to their perception of the healthcare provider. People often engage in more avoidance behaviors with tattooed employees rather than non-tattooed ones [5]. Hospitals should review and have policies in place related to employees with visible tattoos [2, 6, 7]. Research based on facial expression ratings concluded that occupations are a factor in how tattoos are perceived; visible tattoos on mechanics compared to physicians are perceived more favorably [5].

In this case, it is apparent that the physician, Dr. Merritt, was not immediately self-aware of the impression his tattoos made on his patient. This lack of awareness contributed to the confusing interaction he had with his patient.

Case Outcome

The attending doctor, Amy Austin, a white female, comes to see Ms. Jones, orders an ultrasound and lab work, and eventually sends Ms. Jones to the labor and delivery unit for monitoring. The ultrasound reveals no complications with the pregnancy.

Later, Dr. Austin and a few other emergency physicians have a conversation with Dr. Merritt about cultural awareness and his swastika tattoo being displayed in the workplace. In this conversation, Dr. Merritt emphasizes that his red Hindu swastika with four dots around the edges symbolizes "universal welfare." "This differs from the 'hooked cross' symbol employed by Nazis for their evils during WWII," he added [8]. Dr. Merritt decides to no longer wear short sleeves and is further contemplating tattoo removal because of misinterpretation of the Hindu swastika.

References

1. American College of Obstetricians and Gynecologists. Cultural sensitivity and awareness in the delivery of health care. Committee opinion no. 493. Obstet Gynecol [Internet]. 2011 May [cited 2017 Nov 8]; 117(5): 1258. Available from: https://www.acog.org/Resources-And-Publications/Committee-Opinions/Committee-on-Health-Care-for-Underserved-Women/Cultural-Sensitivity-and-Awareness-in-the-Delivery-of-Health-Care.
2. Resenhoeft A, Villa J, Wiseman D. Tattoos can harm perceptions: a study and suggestions. J Am Coll Heal. 2008;56(5):593–6.
3. Schmidt N. Reclaiming the symbol. Index Censorsh [Internet]. 2009 Feb 21 [cited 2017 Nov 8]. 34(2):52–53. Available from: http://www.tandfonline.com/doi/full/10.1080/03064220500157798.
4. Cassaro R. The ancient secret of the swastika (pt. 1 of 2) [Internet]. [place unknown]: Richardcassaro.com; 2012 Apr 15 [cited 2017 Nov 8]. Available from: https://www.richardcassaro.com/the-ancient-secret-of-the-swastika-the-hidden-history-of-the-white-race-p-1-of-2.
5. Baumann C, Timming AR, Gollan PJ. Taboo tattoos? A study of the gendered effects of body art on consumers' attitudes toward visibly tattooed front line staff. J Retail Consum Serv. 2016;29:31–9.
6. Linkov N. How tattoos in the workplace affect healthcare jobs [Internet]. Piscataway, NJ: American Institute of Medical Sciences & Education; 2016 May 14 [cited 2017 July 20]. Available from: https://www.aimseducation.edu/blog/tattoos-in-the-workplace-healthcare-jobs-appearance-policies/.
7. Timming AR. Visible tattoos in the service sector: a new challenge to recruitment and selection. Work Employ Soc. 2015;29(1):60–78.
8. Campion MJ. How the world loved the swastika-until Hitler stole it. BBC News Magazine [Internet]. 2014 Oct 22 [cited 2017 Aug 23]. Available from: http://www.bbc.com/news/magazine-29644591.

Part V
Nurses, Staff, and Advanced Practice Provider Cases

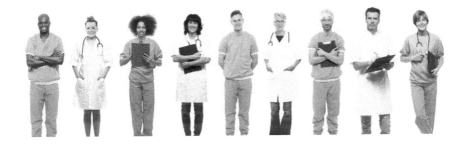

Chapter 51
Ancillary Staff to Nursing Instructor Barriers and Bias

Jamela M. Martin

Case Scenario

Mrs. R, a 63-year-old Caucasian woman with colorectal cancer, is admitted to a post-op recovery and bariatric surgery unit after an ileostomy placement. The patient is known to have mental health issues and has required around-the-clock supervision. A GI surgeon, the staff nurse, and a nursing student are caring for the patient. On post-op day one, the patient complains of shortness of breath to her nurse and the nursing student. The primary nurse tells the nursing student: "Yes, I know. It's been difficult to discern which of her complaints are real versus imagined. She's been a tough patient. Let's watch and wait." When the complaints of difficulty breathing are unaddressed by the primary nurse, the nursing student decides to remain at the patient's bedside to observe and keep Mrs. R company. When the student recognizes worsening circumoral cyanosis and decreased level of consciousness, she immediately calls for help. Mrs. R's respiratory status continues to deteriorate into full respiratory arrest, requiring resuscitation. Post-resuscitation chest x-rays are ordered by the attending physician. The X-ray technician arrives and, recognizing that he will need to reposition the patient, calls for help. The nursing student is still in the room.

Review of Symptoms

Abdominal pain over 14 days, blood in stool, difficulty stooling; post-op ileostomy day one secondary to colorectal cancer; post-op day one difficulty breathing.

J. M. Martin
Old Dominion University, School of Nursing, Norfolk, VA, USA
e-mail: Jm1marti@odu.edu

Past Medical History

Schizophrenia, depression, limited range of motion relative to arthritis, learning disabled, asthma.

Family History

Unable to obtain.

Social History

The patient is learning disabled, unable to care for self, and lives in an assisted living facility. There is no history of alcohol or drug abuse or smoking. No visits from family or friends.

Physical Exam

General The patient is oriented to person only. She is drowsy and responsive to voices, but with limited verbal communication.

HEENT PERRLA, tongue and lips pink but dry, O_2 via facemask.

Cardiovascular RRR

Respiratory Crackles bilaterally in bases.

Abdomen Soft, non-tender.

Extremities Limited range of motion upper and lower extremities, capillary refill brisk.

What Was Said?

After calling for help to reposition the patient for chest X-rays, the X-ray technician looks surprised to see a presumably young African-American woman, dressed in blue scrubs, arrive at the bedside. The African-American woman briefly speaks with the nursing student and then proceeds to help the technician reposition the patient for imaging. As the technician is about to take the first X-ray, the African-American woman comments, "Wait, the patient looks rotated. Let me adjust her shoulders and hips." With a look of surprise on his face, the technician asks, "How did you know that? You're a student."

After speaking with the nursing student and gathering a brief status report on the patient, the African-American woman introduced herself by first name only, assuming the technician was familiar with her role as an instructor.

What Was Done?

The nursing instructor explained to the X-ray technician that despite her age and attire, her background was sufficient to understand X-ray positioning. The X-ray technician, while taken aback, was respectful and apologetic to the nursing instructor once he became aware of her role. The situation was not reported. X-rays were completed and the nursing student and instructor continued to provide care to the patient and document the events surrounding the respiratory arrest.

Question for Discussion

1. What are some attitudes and assumptions?

Attitudes/Assumptions: The Technician

The technician questioned why/how the African-American woman would have knowledge about proper patient positioning for X-rays. The technician erroneously assumed that the young-appearing African-American woman in scrubs was a nursing student.

Attitudes/Assumptions: The Nursing Instructor

The nursing instructor was dressed in blue scrubs and, having just left another patient room, overheard the technician asking for help with the X-ray. She did not put on her white lab coat nor her badge before entering the room to help the technician. She spoke briefly with the nursing student. She introduced herself to the technician by her first name and proceeded to offer her assistance. The nursing student instructor, having worked and taught on that unit for three semesters, was staggered that the technician would presume incompetence. She had previously worked in the ICU setting and was familiar with proper X-ray positioning.

Gaps in Provider Knowledge

(a) Lack of knowledge regarding staff and student roles in the clinical setting. Providers should be aware that students and staff of all levels might be present on a care unit in the hospital learning environment.
(b) Lack of knowledge of disparities/discrimination. African-Americans who serve in leadership roles commonly encounter the assumption from unfamiliar persons that they are employed in lower-tiered positions, based on racial stereotypes.
(c) Lack of knowledge of disparities/discrimination. Preconceived gender and age stereotypes might contribute to personal biases when encountering unfamiliar people in the clinical setting.
(d) Relying on medical attire customs to delineate rank. Beware of relying on old or outdated customs to distinguish a person's role in the clinical setting. This can lead to erroneous assumptions about a person's knowledge and abilities. Interprofessional practice, changing social mores, educational reform, and advances in professional development have led to diluted traditions regarding white coats, scrub color, and other attire.

Cross-Cultural Tools and Skills

(a) When working with providers unknown to you, presume competence.
(b) Do not assume a person's level of education or role based on race.
(c) Do not assume a person's level of education or ability based on age or gender.
(d) Do not assume a person's role based on his/her attire in the hospital setting.

Pearls and Pitfalls

Pearl The nursing student recognized that symptoms were worsening and trusted the patient's complaint of shortness of breath, despite the patient's history of mental health issues.

Pearl The nursing instructor responded to requests for assistance from the nursing student and X-ray technician, providing general support and assistance on the unit during the busy post-resuscitation time frame.

Pearl The nursing student and X-ray technician collaborated to accurately position the patient for X-rays, but, when unable to, called for additional help.

Pearl The nursing instructor addressed the X-ray technician's questions with respect and a calm tone. The technician was apologetic and respectful and the situation did not escalate.

Pitfall The X-ray technician made assumptions about a young African-American woman (nursing instructor) being "just a student" and assumed she had limited knowledge of X-ray positioning and radiology.

Pitfall The nursing instructor did not differentiate herself with clothing or a badge that indicated her level of expertise and/or role on the unit.

Case Outcome

There are several implications in this case. First, from the patient care perspective, it is imperative that complaints of shortness of breath and difficulty breathing be taken seriously with all patients, despite the patient's history of mental health issues or learning disabilities. Had the primary nurse taken the patient's complaints seriously and intervened early, respiratory arrest could have potentially been avoided. Implicit bias toward persons with disabilities might have underscored her lack of response to the patient's complaints [1]. Second, likely based on age, gender, and racial biases, the X-ray technician assumed that the nursing instructor was a student. Implicit bias, while it can be unintentional, has been shown to strongly correlate with lower quality of care [2]. Finally, the nursing instructor's choice to wear scrubs (similar in appearance to her students) could have contributed to the technician's erroneous assumptions. Clothing norms, while subtle, often indicate status, education, authority, and role in hospital settings [3, 4]. Respectful communication surrounding implicit biases can lead to positive outcomes.

References

1. Institute of Medicine (US) Committee on Crossing the Quality Chasm. Adaptation to Mental Health and Addictive Disorders. Chapter 5, Coordinating care for better mental, substance-use, and general health. In: Improving the quality of health care for mental and substance-use conditions: quality chasm series. Washington: National Academies Press; 2006.
2. FitzGerald C, Hurst S. Implicit bias in healthcare professionals: a systematic review. BMC Med Ethics. 2017;18:19. https://doi.org/10.1186/s12910-017-0179-8.
3. Jenkins TM. Clothing norms as markers of status in a hospital setting: a Bourdieusian analysis. Health (London). 2014;18(5):526–41.
4. Thomas CM, Ehret A, Ellis B, Colon-Shoop S, Linton J, Metz S. Perception of nurse caring, skills, and knowledge based on appearance. J Nurs Admin. 2010;40(11):489–97.

Chapter 52
Black Nurse

Edward Strickler and Jamela M. Martin

Case Scenario

This is the case of a 43-year-old woman in-hospital patient following abdominal hysterectomy to remedy endometrial hyperplasia and menorrhagia: currently, post-op day one.

Review of Symptoms

The patient is expected to be discharged in the next 48 h pending clarification of transportation issues. The patient states she feels nauseated and hungry. She is on a clear liquid diet and did not feel like eating breakfast because her throat "felt scratchy," but plans to eat lunch today. She complains of moderate pain at a 4/10 in her lower right and lower left abdominal quadrants near the surgical site. She states she has difficulty shifting and rolling over in the bed due to pain and tenderness at the incision site. She has no complaints of headache, vomiting, diarrhea, swelling in the extremities, back pain, or difficulty urinating. The patient was out of bed with help from the nurse twice in the evening to use the bathroom. No blood in urine was noted throughout the night. Her last bowel movement was the morning of the day of surgery. She has been unable to have a bowel movement today. All other systems are noncontributory at this time.

E. Strickler (✉)
Institute of Law, Psychiatry and Public Policy, University of Virginia,
Charlottesville, VA, USA
e-mail: els2e@virginia.edu

J. M. Martin
Old Dominion University, School of Nursing, Norfolk, VA, USA
e-mail: jm1marti@odu.edu

© Springer International Publishing AG, part of Springer Nature 2019
M. L. Martin et al. (eds.), *Diversity and Inclusion in Quality Patient Care*,
https://doi.org/10.1007/978-3-319-92762-6_52

Past Medical History

The patient has a history of menorrhagia related to menstrual cycles. Onset of menses was at age 13. Menstrual cycles have typically been regular for 5 days until after the birth of her second child. Cycles have become irregularly spaced, occurring anywhere from every 3 weeks to every 5 weeks. Cycles with very heavy bleeding contribute to low hemoglobin and hematocrit. Transvaginal ultrasound revealed endometrial hyperplasia; biopsy is negative for cancerous cells. Progestin-only treatment to reduce endometrial lining has been unsuccessful in controlling excessive bleeding. The patient felt she was out of options but wanted bleeding controlled and opted for hysterectomy. The patient had two spontaneous miscarriages (one at age 22 and one at age 23), followed by two live births.

Family History

The patient lives with her husband, who is self-employed as a truck driver and the sole support for the family. Two daughters, ages 16 and 18, are in high school. Daughters live at home and do not drive.

Social History

The patient has worked occasionally and part time only at the Family Dollar store in the small town where she lives. The patient lives more than an hour away, and staff have not been able to reach her husband or children to ensure transport to home.

Physical Exam

Vital Signs 98.9, BP 136/85, pulse 90.

General Patient is well-appearing, overweight Caucasian female. Awake and interactive during exam, though sleepy.

Head PERRLA

Neck Soft non-tender; lymph nodes non-palpable; trachea and thyroid midline, soft, non-tender.

ENT Nares patent; mucous membranes moist and pink; mild oropharyngeal reddening likely minor post-intubation irritation.

Cardiovascular Regular rate and rhythm; no murmurs, thrills, or rubs.

Respiratory Breath sounds clear to auscultation bilaterally.

Abdomen Soft, mild distention, tender to palpation around incision; low transverse incision with edges well-approximated; no edema, warmth, or reddening; small amount of serosanguinous discharge on wound dressing.

Extremities Warm; non-edematous; brisk capillary refill all four extremities.

Skin Noncontributory.

Neuro Alert and oriented × 4.

What Was Said?

The patient talks on the phone several times each morning and again several times in the afternoon with her daughters or husband (it has not been clear which) and appears during each call to raise her voice to say, "I've told them not to have no lazy dumb black nurses tending to me. They sent some nurse in here to measure something and I said 'No, get another nurse.'"

A nurse of color came in to check the monitors and the patient ordered the nurse to leave stating, "Send a white nurse next time."

What Was Done?

The nurse talked with her supervisor about the incident. After the second time this happened, the nurse came in to ask the patient to "keep your voice down please because others can hear you," implying other patients but also meaning other nurses. After the fourth or fifth time, the nurse came in and said more directly, "Please speak quietly so not to disturb other patients or to disturb nurses."

Questions for Discussion

1. What happened, what is happening?
   The patient has repeatedly, and apparently with purpose, offensively defamed nursing staff with racial stereotyping.
2. What are the impact(s) on providers?
   Nurses have experienced turmoil and disruption in the care of other patients. They have attempted to address the patient's concerns and quiet the patient.

3. What did providers do or try to do?

   First, nurses exercised their authority – specifically referring to the need to care for all patients – by requesting the patient "keep [her] voice down." Later, nurses exercised their authority – specifically referring to the need to avoid disturbances to both other patients and other nurses – by requesting the patient "speak quietly."

4. What impact(s) on providers did this action have? What else might providers do?

   Nurses were able to intervene in a way that showed self-respect and respect for the entire team of nurses. Intervention also protected other patients, and their visitors, from disrespectful language.

Attitudes/Assumptions: The Provider

While the providers did attempt to exercise their authority by quieting the patient's disrespectful behavior, they may have inadvertently ignored the underlying emotional issues that led to the behavior in the first place. Providers may have assumed the patient's attitude was primarily associated with a racist perspective. Because the patient is a relatively young woman experiencing a total hysterectomy, providers should expect there to be some level of accompanying emotional trauma. It is unclear whether the patient was offered counseling in advance of the procedure, whether she has been fully evaluated to determine her level of grief associated with the hysterectomy, and whether the nurses attempted to discuss the underlying issues with her.

Attitudes/Assumptions: The Patient

The patient assumed that since the nurse was African-American, she was lazy, dumb, and unable to provide quality care. The patient also assumed that the hospital would desire to meet her request to replace the current nurse with a Caucasian nurse.

Gaps in Provider Knowledge

Providers must recognize the emotional distress that often occurs for patients who have experienced a hysterectomy. Though there can be relief associated with reduced symptoms, depression can occur after the procedure if the patient feels a loss of self-worth related to womanhood and childbearing and is experiencing stress regarding possible or likely changes in her marriage relationship.

Pearls and Pitfalls

Pearl   The nurse team avoided a pitfall by not stereotyping the patient. This allowed for disclosures by the patient of mental health issues and safety and well-being concerns in her household.

Pearl   The nurse team used a forthright approach to establish and ensure a respectful workplace for the team and a respectful place of care for other patients and their visitors. Involving the disruptively disrespectful patient in their forthright approach provided a channel, defined by respectful relationships, for the patient to disclose important information.

Case Outcome

In the evening, the nurse found the patient crying, and when asked, the patient said that she was "sorry to hurt anyone's feelings" but her husband had told her to "keep away from 'n-word nurses.'" The patient also stated that she had been feeling very sad about having a hysterectomy. Even though she did not have plans to have more children, she felt a sense of loss. She explained that her sadness may have also caused her to lash out. The patient said that she could not say "n-word" but wanted her husband to know that she was obeying him. Later, when hospital social services visited to find out how to get in touch with the patient's husband or other relatives/ caregivers who could ensure she got home safely, the patient said that her oldest daughter had a mixed-race boyfriend early in her high school years. Her daughter had become pregnant (although the patient suggested that the father of the unborn infant was not the mixed-race boyfriend), miscarried, and been sick afterward. She missed a year of high school and cost the family a lot of money, partially because of the patient being unable to keep her part-time job. The patient's husband was continually angry against people of color since then and kept their daughters close to home, and because his work took him away for days at a time, he kept them from driving.

What Happened, What Is Happening?

The patient has revealed information critical for understanding her disrespectful behavior. This information may also be informative when planning for discharge with the patient and her family.

What Are Impact(s) on Providers?

After hearing the patient's story, further questioning by appropriate staff may be necessary. Considerations include how to note the conversation in the records, how to ensure information is known to other staff planning the patient's discharge, and how to conduct or to request screening for possible violence or other hazards to the patient.

In this case, providers encountered racially offensive language by the patient. Providers intervened to reinforce self-respect and respect for the entire team and to protect other patients. Care providers should also consider additional resources that could be used to de-escalate the situation, while keeping the patients and providers safe and comfortable. In this case, the nurse could have consulted with her direct supervisor, unit manager, physician team, or hospital administration to obtain help in resolving the issue. Additional options include obtaining a Spiritual Services consultation to help the patient deal with emotional grief or a social work referral to assess for issues in the home regarding potential emotional abuse.

Intervention not only impacted individual providers and the provider team but also elicited a response from the patient that importantly informs her in-hospital care, discharge planning, and possibly continuing care. The clinical team involved in the patient's hospital care and discharge planning may request a consultation with mental health and social work to discuss appropriate responses to suspected or possible abuse of the patient or others in the patient's household.

In this case, we observe the dynamics of behaviors harmful to the human dignity of providers intersected with behaviors in the patient's family. Intersecting behaviors harmful to human dignity are inherent to many experiences of violence and oppression. Intersecting behaviors may also be iterative: one offense to human dignity generating further, or different, offenses.

One discussion of how providers should incorporate recommendations from the US Preventive Services Task Force describes these intersecting and iterative dynamics and includes attention to the physical, sexual, verbal, psychological, economic, and other aspects of coercive violence, attention to stages and cycles of coercive violence, and attention to evidence for effective prevention and intervention: "Healthcare providers must seek to empower victims to understand the destructive nature of an abusive relationship and its negative effect on their health" [1]. In this case, they must also understand intersecting impacts on providers.

A recent systematic review, including 35 studies, found that while "providers commonly acknowledged the importance of [family] violence screening they yet often used only selective screening," resulting in "a great deal of variability in regard to provider screening practices" [2]. The systematic review found that a majority of studies investigated provider factors – including provider attitude, beliefs, and perceptions of screening – to explain this variability. "Studies elicited several key provider-level factors: provider level of knowledge, comfort, self-efficacy, level of enculturation, and sense of responsibility or role in screening for intimate partner violence. Low levels of these factors were connected with lower rates of screening and limited responses."

References

1. Collett D, Bennett T. Putting intimate partner violence on your radar. JAAPA. 2015;28(10):24–8.
2. Alvarez C, Fedock G, Grace KT, Campbell J. Provider screening and counseling for intimate partner violence a systematic review of practices and influencing factors. Trauma Violence Abuse. 2016. https://doi.org/10.1177/1524838016637080.

Chapter 53
Black Female PA

Jacqueline S. Barnett and Kenyon Railey

Case Scenario

A 52-year-old male patient (Mr. P) presents as a walk-in to the primary care clinic for evaluation of a persistent rash. He was seen in the same clinic 5 days ago, diagnosed with contact dermatitis, and prescribed triamcinolone 0.1% cream. The medical assistant notes on the intake form that "the rash itches less, but is spreading, and now draining pus." The provider, who happens to be an African-American female, enters the exam room and introduces herself as a physician assistant (PA). The patient immediately states, "I don't want to see no black female PA." The PA replies, "I am sorry you feel that way." She politely leaves the room and returns with her supervising physician. The physician explains that he is currently occupied but could see the patient during his first available appointment later in the afternoon. The physician further states, "This clinic values the diversity of our patients and providers, and patients are not assigned to providers based on race. The PA has worked in infectious disease for several years and is considered an expert at this practice diagnosing and managing rashes and infections. She is just as capable to treat your rash as I am." The patient reluctantly agrees to see the PA and the PA resumes the history and exam.

J. S. Barnett (✉)
Department of Community and Family Medicine, Duke University School of Medicine, Durham, NC, USA
e-mail: Jacqueline.barnett@duke.edu

K. Railey
Department of Community and Family Medicine, Office of Diversity and Inclusion, Duke University School of Medicine, Durham, NC, USA
e-mail: Kenyon.railey@duke.edu

© Springer International Publishing AG, part of Springer Nature 2019
M. L. Martin et al. (eds.), *Diversity and Inclusion in Quality Patient Care*,
https://doi.org/10.1007/978-3-319-92762-6_53

Review of Symptoms

The patient complains of itchy rash over torso, groin, and lower extremities. All other review of symptoms is otherwise negative.

Past Medical History

Diabetes for 10 years, controlled with Metformin 500 mg twice daily.

Family History

None relevant to the case.

Social History

Patient is married, with three sons, ages 3 (adopted), 20, and 26. He is a lawyer and is one of the partners at a local law firm. He denies alcohol, drug, or tobacco use.

Physical Exam

Vital Signs Temp, 98.6 F; pulse, 75; BP, 130/80; respirations, 18.

General Awake, alert, no apparent distress.

Cardiovascular Normal S1 and S2, regular rate and rhythm, no murmurs, rubs, or gallops.

Respiratory Clear to auscultation bilaterally.

Skin Excoriated, erythematous papules/pustules over groin, lower extremities, anterior and posterior torso; no other rashes or lesions noted.

What Was Done?

The PA consults with the physician and advises him of the patient's request. The physician supports his colleague, and the patient agrees to see the PA. The PA diagnoses and treats the patient for probable *Pseudomonas folliculitis* with second-ary *Staphylococcus aureus* infection. The PA has a long discussion with Mr. P regarding the probable etiology and risk factors related to his rash. Mr. P regularly used a hot tub over the previous 2–3 months, placing him at risk for folliculitis. The PA explains that his history of diabetes, ongoing hot tub use, scratching, and steroid treatment may have contributed to the exacerbation and secondary infection. The patient thanks the PA and leaves the room.

Question for Discussion

1. What was said by whom, to whom? The patient told the PA, "I don't want to see no black female PA."

Attitudes/Assumptions: The Patient

(a) Advanced practice providers (APP) such as PAs and nurse practitioners (NPs) are inadequately trained.
(b) Seeing an APP leads to substandard care.
(c) He would receive better care from a gender/race-concordant provider.

Attitudes/Assumptions: The Provider

(a) The patient is acting on privilege due to his background and socioeconomic status.
(b) The patient is biased against providers of color or women providers.
(c) The patient is biased against nonphysician providers.
(d) The patient is rude and should not be able to refuse care.

Gaps in Provider Knowledge

Many providers do not realize that informed consent rules and common law battery give patients the right to refuse care from unwanted healthcare providers for almost any reason [1]. When care is refused because of the provider's race/gender, it can be uncomfortable and create many issues in the healthcare setting. Although much has been published (and rightly so) regarding the discriminatory treatment of patients leading to disparities and poor patient outcomes, less has been written about racially intolerant patients and the potential distress they cause to providers, the healthcare team, and the organization [2].

Cross-Cultural Tools and Skills

Having a diverse and supportive healthcare team is vital to improving cross-cultural relationships and team success. The supervising physician showed strong support for the PA by complementing her clinical practice and patient care skills to the patient and advising the patient of the inclusive culture of the practice. The physician's interaction with the patient and strong support of multiculturalism was vital to this case. Institutions must provide the necessary resources and training to help employees address bias, stereotypes, and discrimination in the workplace.

Pearls and Pitfalls

Pearl The PA remained professional and courteous despite the patient's refusal to see her.

Pearl The supervising physician showed strong support for the PA by complementing her clinical practice and patient care skills in front of the patient.

Pitfall It may be difficult for providers to remain professional when a patient insults them. However, becoming defensive or unprofessional when a patient is perceived as rude or unreasonable can damage therapeutic relationships and place organizations at risk.

Pitfall Although the supervising physician was supportive in this incident, what happens when colleagues and supervisors are not supportive? The cumulative effects of patient rejection, along with unsupportive colleagues, can be emotionally damaging and degrading, causing despair and burnout especially for minority healthcare workers/providers [3].

It remains unclear whether the primary reason the patient initially refused care was because the provider is a woman of color or because the provider is a PA. Patients often refuse care from providers for various reasons, and institutions typically honor patient requests for a different provider, even when the preference is due to the provider's race/ethnicity [1]. It is also true that physicians, PAs, nurses, and other employees of healthcare institutions have the right to a workplace free from discrimination as established through Title VII of the 1964 Civil Rights Act [1]. There needs to be a balance between the rights of patients and employees. It seems that accommodating a patient's refusal to see a provider based on race and ethnicity is an absolute antithesis to civil rights law and is the very type of discrimination that civil rights laws were enacted to prevent [1].

It is also possible the patient refused care because he is unfamiliar with the role of PAs and their contributions to increasing access to quality health care. The

Association of American Medical Colleges (AAMC) released a report in 2016 which projected a physician shortage as high as 94,700 physicians by 2025 [4]. The PA profession was created in the mid-1960s during a time of physician shortage to improve and expand access to health care. PAs and other APPs have been shown to provide an equivalent value in caring for common conditions as physicians, thus dispelling perceptions that APPs provide lower-value care than physicians for many common conditions [5]. APPs also manage patients with complicated diseases and have been shown to provide care comparable to physicians to patients with diabetes and cardiovascular disease [6].

As the nation continues to experience an increasingly diverse population, underrepresented minority providers, inclusive of PAs and APPs, can play a vital role in increasing access to quality care.

Case Outcome

Mr. P calls the office several weeks later to see if it is possible to get an urgent appointment for his son with the PA he saw during his visit to the office. His 3-year-old son has been experiencing high fevers while on Tylenol/Motrin, irritability, lethargy, ear pain, and sore throat for about a week. The son was treated recently for otitis media and dehydration but seemed to be getting worse instead of better. The PA evaluates Mr. P's son who exhibited stridor and drooling on physical exam. She orders lateral soft-tissue X-rays of the neck for suspected retropharyngeal abscess. The X-ray supports the diagnosis and she refers the child to the emergency room for emergent care. Establishing good rapport with patients improves continuity and trust. Although Mr. P initially refused to see the PA, it is interesting and very telling that he called back to see if the PA could see his son. This suggests that Mr. P valued the care the PA provided and trusted her to deliver care to his ill son, after he initially refused her care.

References

1. Paul-Emile K. Patients' racial preferences and the medical culture of accommodation [Internet]. [Los Angeles]:UCLA Law Review. 2012 [cited 2017 Jul 5]. Available from http://www.uclalawreview.org/patients%e2%80%99-racial-preferences-and-the-medical-culture-of-accommodation/.
2. Singh K, Sivasubramaniam P, Ghuman S, Mir HR. The dilemma of the racist patient. Am J Orthop Belle Mead NJ. 2015;44(12):E477–9.
3. Paul-Emile K, Smith AK, Lo B, Fernández A. Dealing with racist patients. N Engl J Med. 2016;374(8):708–11.
4. IHS Inc. The complexities of physician supply and demand: projections from 2014 to 2025. Prepared for the Association of American Medical Colleges [Internet]. Washington, DC.: IHS Inc. 2016 [cited 2017 July 30]. Available from https://www.aamc.org/download/458082/data/2016_complexities_of_supply_and_demand_projections.pdf.

5. Mafi JN, Wee CC, Davis RB, Landon BE. Comparing use of low-value health care services among U.S. advanced practice clinicians and physicians. Ann Intern Med. 2016;165(4):237.
6. Virani SS, Akeroyd JM, Ramsey DJ, Chan WJ, Frazier L, Nasir K, et al. Comparative effectiveness of outpatient cardiovascular disease and diabetes care delivery between advanced practice providers and physician providers in primary care: implications for care under the affordable care act. Am Heart J. 2016;181:74–82.

Chapter 54
Provider with Disability "Don't Want That 'Robot' Helping Me!"

Edward Strickler and Marcus L. Martin

Case Scenario

Ray Johnson is a 19-year-old male admitted to a rehabilitation hospital following ankle surgery. The patient's rehabilitation therapist uses an electrolarynx[1] and has made one visit to the patient to introduce the work they would be doing together. This morning when the nurse informed the patient of the schedule for the day, he stated emphatically, "I don't want that robot helping me!" The nurse first asked the patient to repeat himself because she "must have misunderstood what you said." The patient replied: "I can't stand to hear that robot voice. It's creepy. Keep that one out of here."

The nurse advised the patient that she would see if a different therapist was available. The nurse later learned that the therapist could not be changed and informed the patient, "We've checked with the therapy team and they can't change therapists today. It is very important for you to start therapy and that therapist is very good. Won't you be able to get used to the voice? It's an electronic voice because the therapist is a survivor of throat cancer. Does that help you understand the reason for the voice?" The patient shouted back: "My real parents are dead and I have to live with people that I hate. I've busted myself up just when I was about ready to move

---

[1] Electrolarynx: electromechanical device that enables a person after laryngectomy to produce speech. When the device is placed against the region of the laryngectomy, a buzzing sound is made that can be converted into simulated speech by movements of the lips, tongue, and glottis.

E. Strickler (✉)
Institute of Law, Psychiatry and Public Policy, University of Virginia,
Charlottesville, VA, USA
e-mail: els2e@virginia.edu

M. L. Martin
University of Virginia, Charlottesville, VA, USA
e-mail: mlm8n@virginia.edu

out. And you want me to 'understand' someone else's problems?! A robot with cancer: really?! Get somebody else."

Review of Symptoms

The current stay in the rehabilitation hospital is two days post-surgery to repair complex ankle injury (distal talofibular ligament third-degree sprain with widening of the ankle mortise) secondary to kicking a door. Additional days stay may be required for the patient to learn to manage pain and to begin occupational therapy. The post-op course is anticipated to involve up to 6 weeks of movement without bearing weight before a second surgery on his ankle and a second 6 weeks of movement without bearing weight.

Past Medical History

This is the patient's first serious injury and first experience with disability. Other past medical history is insignificant.

Family History

The patient's parents are two men (one is a paternal uncle). The parents were recently married after the US Supreme Court decision striking down states' constitutional prohibition of same-sex marriage. The patient was raised by these parents after an automobile accident killed both birth of his parents when he was 16. His uncle is his legal guardian.

Social History

The patient (Ray Johnson) expresses urgency to get out of the rehabilitation hospital and to establish independence from the household where he has lived since age 16 following the tragic loss of his birth parents. Ray Johnson has had several full-time and part-time jobs in retail services. His last employment was at an athletic/outdoor goods retail store, which recently closed. The ankle injury occurred after the store closing. According to his parents, the patient has a history of angry outbursts including hitting them and breaking objects in the home. This injury occurred when the patient kicked through a patio door. The patient reports he "tried to jump onto the patio by kicking open the patio door."

Physical Exam

No remarkable findings, other than ankle injury.

Questions for Discussion

1. What is happening from the patient's perspective?
   The patient declares that he does not want a rehabilitation therapist who uses an electrolarynx helping him because the therapist sounds like a robot.
2. What are impact(s) on providers?
   The nurse talked with the therapy team to inform them of the patient's attitude. Therapy must get started and they cannot substitute another provider today. Nurses have to balance the resistant patient, burdened schedules, assignments of the therapy team, parents whose insurance covers the patient, and effective care planning for/with the patient. At the center of these conflicts is the patient's inappropriate and offensive conduct.
3. What should providers do when encountering a patient whose offensive conduct also threatens continuity of care?

Attitudes/Assumptions: The Provider

The provider team has experienced the patient's unreasonable bias and explicitly rude behavior regarding a team member who has survived cancer and uses an artificial voice box for verbal communication. The team has also experienced agitation and anger from the patient that may be displacement of anger with his family and health circumstances onto the provider with disability.

Attitudes/Assumptions: The Patient

The patient rudely and angrily dismissed a capable provider on the basis of the provider's disability. The patient resisted intervention by other providers to start therapy.

Gaps in Provider Knowledge

Providers heard the patient exclaim, "My real parents are dead and I have to live with people that I hate." The patient used this exclamation when demanding removal of the provider with a disability. Providers' understanding of the patient's outburst would benefit from knowing more about the patient's family life.

Pearls and Pitfalls

Pearl The clinical team followed respectful protocols of working with all departments and services involved with the patient's care. Team members asked for assistance appropriately; for example, nurse team members spoke collaboratively with the therapy team members. The team members also opened dialogue with the patient and the parents of the patient to learn information that they would not otherwise have known.

Pitfall The clinical team must be prepared for a confrontation between the patient and his parents that may jeopardize the patient's access to stable housing and insurance coverage. Housing and insurance coverage are vital for a successful outcome of this surgery and recovery and for success of the next surgery and recovery.

Strategies and resources for managing discriminatory behavior may include:

1. Open the dialogue (with the patient) with empathy.
2. State the values of mutual respect of the healthcare organization.
3. State the clinical team members' concerns with the patient's behavior.
4. Indicate trustworthiness of the clinical team members' clinical expertise, ethical values, and professional care.
5. Inquire about the patient's point of view.
6. Redirect the conversation to confidence in the professional care provided by all clinical team members.

All these steps were accomplished. Nevertheless, the complex needs of the patient, who depends on family for housing and insurance coverage and has a history of emotional and physical violence within a complex family system, may continue to present challenges for the clinical team. Is the team ready for potential violent outbursts by the patient? Are there resources available to help inform the patient about the electrolarynx and persons who use them? Might patient education be accomplished without stigmatizing either the therapist or the patient by having a member of the team whom the patient responds to best do the patient education? Ethical reflection may be part of the clinical team's response and follow-up in a difficult case involving discriminatory behavior.

In the report of an ethics consultation regarding an offensive request by a patient's family, one commentator relates, "Reasons and motives matter. Some patient preferences are more ethically justifiable than others" [1]. In this case, providers may discuss what arises from their individual and group ethical reflection. For example, is the burden of appearing to endorse the patient's offensive stereotyping by rearranging already difficult therapy schedules a significant ethical burden? Would such ethical burden persist in some damaging way – damaging to provider morale, for example – if schedules are rearranged to accommodate the patient, who will be personally out of sight (if not out of mind) upon discharge? Damaging impacts may be generated, such as anxiety and depression, "when a member of particular group is confronted with the possibility of reinforcing a negative stereotype. The anxiety that is produced subsequently results in lower performance" [2]. Providers may reflect about "stereotype threat": Is the construct of stereotype threat meaningful in this case? Can providers identify when this may have happened within their team, in their service, or in their clinic? Do providers regard the offensive stereotyping related to a disability similarly or differently from that of race or ethnicity?

Another framework for ethical reflection is provided in the report of an ethics consultation with a "difficult patient" [3]. Discussing a case of a patient in serious pain and distress who makes emotional denunciations that providers do not care and demands that provider not touch him, the commentator concludes, "Physicians should view repairing damaged patient-physician relationships as an ethical obligation on par with providing any other medical intervention essential to patient care and should recognize that their greater power relative to patients comes with greater responsibility to repair those relationships." The commentator rests this conclusion on a "duty to treat" that the commentator finds in long-established ethical norms to "do no harm" and "to benefit" the patient that are made real in applying the expertise and skills of the provider. Providers are invited to consider the pain and suffering of the patient and the imbalance of power in the setting of hospital care, in which the patient not only has pain and suffering but also may be experiencing diminished physical ability, mobility, and liberty. This all occurs within a complex system of hospital care, provider routines, and insurance requirements and restrictions. All of these factors may appear to be a sort of captivity or at least a sort of threat. How might this ethical reflection inform the difficult relationship of our patient with the team of nurses and therapists? Is there a duty to repair damaged relationship with the patient? Should providers have additional or special concern for their patient upon recognizing his pain and suffering and the threat(s) he is experiencing? In this case those threats include his injuries, prospective long recovery, need to care at home, and also a possible threat to a safe discharge if his parents will not allow him to return to their home or to continue to cover him on their insurance.

Case Outcome

The parents learn about the missed therapy and the reasons for that. When talking with the nurse in charge during their visit, they:

1. Ask if a different therapist could be assigned.
2. State that they are ashamed of the patient's conduct and will talk with him and ask him to apologize.
3. Confirm that the patient's insurance is through the parent who is his legal guardian and that he has no insurance or other financial resources to pay privately.
4. State that they will remind the patient of what care has cost so far, what it will cost, and that the insurance company may deny coverage for day(s) in hospital in which he does not cooperate with the plan of care.

While waiting for a decision about the therapy schedule, the parents insist that the patient at least apologize for his conduct, saying, "He never apologizes to us, even for hitting us, but by God he'll apologize to you, or he's out of the house and off of our insurance." The clinical team had further discussions with Mr. Johnson, and he apologized and accepted rehabilitation care from the therapist with the electrolarynx.

References

1. Reynolds KL, Cowden JD, Brosco JP, Lantos JD. When a family requests a white doctor. J Am Acad Pediatr. 2015;136(2):381–6.
2. Paul-Emile K. Patients racial preferences and the medical culture of accommodation. UCLA Law Rev. 2012;60:462.
3. Johnson M. Do physicians have an ethical duty to repair relationships with so-called "difficult" patients? AMA J Ethics. 2017;19(4):323.

Part VI
Attending Physician Cases

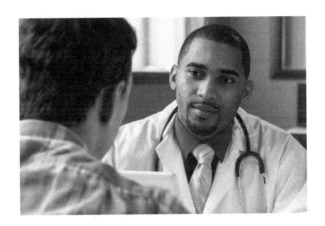

Chapter 55
Black Doctor

Marcus L. Martin, Michelle Strickland, and Stephanie Bossong

Case Scenario

Mrs. April Jameson is an 84-year-old white female who presents to a level 1 trauma center emergency department with the complaint of abdominal pain. The patient has fallen frequently in the past and is currently non-ambulatory. She utilizes a wheelchair. Mrs. Jameson is a widow of 10 years. Her husband, a former truck driver, was killed when his vehicle skidded and overturned, avoiding a head on collision with an African-American male driver of an SUV on a rural roadway during a snowstorm. Mrs. Jameson is accompanied by her only daughter and her daughter's boyfriend. Of note, the daughter's boyfriend is unemployed and has had frequent altercations with African-American males, "colored guys," in their rural community. The attending physician on duty in the emergency department is Dr. William Grady, an African-American male. Mrs. Jameson, her daughter, and her daughter's boyfriend traveled about 1 h from their rural home to this level 1 trauma center. What follows is an interaction between a patient with racist views in the emergency setting where an African-American physician is in charge.

Review of Symptoms

Chief complaint abdominal pain for 5 days.

M. L. Martin (✉) · M. Strickland · S. Bossong
University of Virginia, Charlottesville, VA, USA
e-mail: mlm8n@virginia.edu; ms2yx@virginia.edu

Past Medical History

Cirrhosis of the liver secondary to alcohol abuse, history of schizophrenia, history of bilateral lower extremity fractures secondary to multiple falls, history of bilateral hip dysplasia, and history of wheelchair use for 10 years.

Family History

Noncontributory.

Social History

Drinks alcohol heavily for many years, smokes two packs of cigarettes a day, lives in the rural outskirts of midsize city.

Physical Exam

Vital Signs Temperature normal, blood pressure 140/80, pulse 110.

General Body habitus is generally unkempt.

Neck Supple.

ENT Multiple dental cavities.

Cardiovascular Heart regular rate rhythm.

Respiratory Lungs are clear.

Abdomen Abdomen distended tender right upper quadrant; bowel sounds normal; patient is obese.

Extremities 1+ pitting edema of lower extremities. Clubbing of the fingers.

Neuro Normal.

What Was Said?

Dr. Grady, who happens to be the director of the emergency medicine residency program, introduces himself to the patient who immediately tells him, "I don't want an n-word doctor taking care of me." Dr. Grady states, "I will send in someone else to take care of you and come back later."

What Was Done?

Dr. Grady sends in a resident to complete the examination. The resident is a white female. The resident completes the examination and orders lab work and a CT of the abdomen. Dr. Grady returns later in the assessment after the lab work and the abdominal CT results arrive. Dr. Grady speaks with family members, indicating that he is the person in charge and is supervising the resident's decisions about patient care. Dr. Grady informs the patient and her family that she needs to be admitted because of abnormal lab findings suggesting liver failure. The abdominal CT reveals an abnormal liver but not acute signs of bleeding or masses. The family understands that they have a choice of leaving the emergency department or the patient being admitted to the hospital for further care. Dr. Grady also indicates that an EKG and lab work are concerning for a possible heart attack and that a cardiology consultation will be needed.

Questions for Discussion

1. What are some attitudes/assumptions on the part of the patient and physician?

Attitudes/Assumptions: The Patient

(a) The patient said, "I don't want an n-word doctor taking care of me."
(b) The patient believes she will receive inferior care from a doctor of color.

Attitudes/Assumptions: The Provider

(a) The doctor likely assumes the patient and family are racists, perhaps white supremacists.

(b) The doctor likely assumes there will be a poor outcome for this patient if she refuses admission and treatment.

(c) The doctor likely assumes the patient and family will consider leaving against medical advice.

Gaps in Provider Knowledge

(a) Lack of knowledge about the patient's previous experience with physicians of color or her experiences with cultures different from her own.

(b) Lack of knowledge of the full state of the patient's mental and physical condition, particularly initially, in the absence of laboratory studies.

(c) Lack of knowledge of the patient's family history and beliefs regarding white supremacy.

(d) Lack of knowledge about the full extent of the disability and the patient's activities of daily living.

(e) The provider is not privy to conversations the patient may have had with family members about biases toward people of color.

2. What are some patient issues regarding disability?

Physical disability may be caused by medical illness (infectious diseases or chronic noncommunicable diseases) or trauma. Noncommunicable chronic diseases, including diabetes, cardiovascular disease, and cancer, account for an increasing proportion of disability worldwide. An aging population, dietary issues, alcohol abuse, and lack of physical activity contribute to disability. Those with disabilities face challenges with both their healthcare needs and activities of daily living. Poverty is a risk factor for disability. Healthcare providers may harbor discriminatory and negative attitudes toward the disabled. Physical disabilities bring with them unique medical and psychosocial healthcare challenges for patients. Quality care involves effectiveness, safety, timeliness, and equitable patient-centered care. Patients with disabilities may present to the emergency department for many reasons including lack of a primary care physician providing them regular care. Poorly mobile patients are at increased risk for chronic diseases but also acute pneumonias and thromboembolic disease. Compassion fatigue on the part of the family members who provide care for the disabled can factor in the outcomes. Feelings of depression, hopelessness, and anger can be heightened by stress within families. Once the medical and mental assessment and stabilization have occurred, the patient should be referred to social services to ensure the right support is in place at home and in the community. Developing the best physician-patient relationship possible will increase the overall outcome and future health-seeking behavior for the patient and family [1].

3. What are some patient issues regarding dementia, and mental illness?
   Patients with substance use, dementia, and intellectual and developmental disorders commonly face special challenges because of their mental health conditions. These challenges are further magnified by systematic issues and stigma, resulting in a risk of poor outcomes with elevated morbidity and mortality. Stigma is a pattern of unfair and inaccurate beliefs about a class of persons. Healthcare providers tend to have more negative attitudes and stereotypes than the general populations for patients with schizophrenia and major depression. The attitudes of healthcare providers and staff toward patients with mental illness can affect the ultimate care and outcome. Patients with mental illness also perceive themselves with lower self-esteem, shame, and external fears of social exclusion [1].

Cross-Cultural Tools and Skills

What are some race-concordant considerations?

(a) In a study by Cooper et al., "Race-concordant visits were characterized by higher patient ratings of satisfaction and more positive judgments of physicians' participatory decision-making style" [2].
(b) "Nonwhite [physicians] were more likely to report that discrimination based on race/ethnicity is significant. Nearly 29% of white respondents also believed that such discrimination was very or somewhat significant" [3].

Pearls and Pitfalls

Pearl Mature attending physician decision about having a resident see the patient and then coming back later.

Pearl Healthcare providers must not allow racist comments to detract from providing the best of care, especially in light of a combination of a disability, possible altered mental status, and chronic medical illness.

Case Outcome

Once family members learn of the gravity of the situation, they convince the elderly woman to be admitted to the hospital as per the advice of the African-American attending physician.

References

1. Zun LS, Rozel JS. Chapter 11: Looking past labels: effective care of the psychiatric patients. In: Martin ML, Heron LS, Moreno-Walton L, Jones AW, editors. Diversity and inclusion in quality patient care. Switzerland: Springer International Publishing; 2016.
2. Cooper LA, Roter DL, Johnson RL, Ford DE, Steinwachs DM, Powe NR. Patient-centered communication, ratings of care, and concordance of patient and physician race. Ann Intern Med. 2003;139:907–15. https://doi.org/10.7326/0003-4819-139-11-200312020-00009.
3. Tolbert Coombs AA, King RK. Workplace discrimination: experiences of practicing physicians. J Natl Med Assoc. 2005;97(4):467–77.

Chapter 56
Mexican Doctor

Cynthia Price and Jessica Aviles

Case Scenario

A 56-year-old white male presents to an emergency department with the complaint of chest pain. The resident finishes the exam and sends in the attending, who is a white male, to examine the patient.

Review of Symptoms

Chest pain for 6 h starting at rest, associated with shortness of breath.

Past Medical History

Hypertension, diabetes, hyperlipidemia.

C. Price (✉)
Hartford Hospital, Hartford, CT, USA
e-mail: Cynthia.price@hhchealth.org

J. Aviles
Integrated Residency in Emergency Medicine, University of Connecticut,
Farmington, CT, USA
e-mail: Aviles@uchc.edu

© Springer International Publishing AG, part of Springer Nature 2019
M. L. Martin et al. (eds.), *Diversity and Inclusion in Quality Patient Care*,
https://doi.org/10.1007/978-3-319-92762-6_56

Family History

Myocardial infarction in father at the age of 70.

Social History

Drinks alcohol socially, smokes 1.5 packs of cigarettes a day, lives in the suburbs of a midsize city.

Physical Exam

Vital Signs Temperature normal, blood pressure 160/85, pulse 80.

General Obese middle-aged man in no apparent distress.

HEENT Normocephalic, atraumatic, pupils equal round and reactive to light, normal oropharynx, moist mucous membranes.

Neck No jugular venous distention.

Neuro 5/5 strength in bilateral upper and lower extremities.

Cardiovascular Regular rate rhythm, without murmurs, rubs, or gallops.

Respiratory Lungs are clear to auscultation bilaterally.

Abdomen Obese, soft, non-tender, and non-distended with positive bowel sounds.

Extremities No edema.

Skin No other rashes or wounds.

What Was Said?

The patient states to the Hispanic, female, emergency medicine resident on duty, "I don't want a Mexican doctor." The resident speaks with the patient explaining her level of training and that it is important for her education to see and examine patients. She states that an attending doctor will also be seeing the patient.

What Was Done?

The resident orders labs and an EKG and discusses the case with the attending, who recommends cardiology consult for admission. The attending and the resident return to speak with the patient regarding admission for further workup of chest pain and monitoring in the hospital to arrange a stress test the following day. The attending assures the patient of the resident's ability to provide appropriate care. The patient understands that he has a choice of leaving the emergency department or being admitted to the hospital for further care.

Questions for Discussion

1. What assumptions were made?

Attitudes/Assumptions: The Patient

(a) The patient assumed that because the resident appears Hispanic that her country of origin was Mexico.
(b) The patient may have also thought that the attending was the one ultimately responsible for his care and the resident was no longer involved.
(c) The patient assumed the Hispanic doctor would provide subpar care, demonstrating a potentially unconscious bias.
(d) The patient assumed there was a doctor of a different race/ethnicity available to attend to him. He preferred the white attending doctor.

Attitudes/Assumptions: The Provider

(a) The resident may have felt offended initially but had to overcome personal feelings in order to provide care for the patient.
(b) The provider may have thought the patient was refusing care from a Hispanic person because of racism or as a demonstration of microaggression.

2. The white attending may have felt his presence ultimately satisfied the patient's desire to have a provider of his racial preference as a member of the care team. How far are providers willing to bend to accommodate patient preference and does that affect the trust between patient and provider? Would it be different if it were a Hispanic patient requesting a Hispanic provider?

   Research is often conducted to examine race-discordant relationships with the minority patient experiencing health care provided to them by a nonminority provider. In a study published by Blanchard et al. [1], patients reported perceptions of "unfair treatment because of race and language and believed that he/she would have received better treatment if they belonged to a different race," suggesting the unfair treatment was related to a race-discordant relationship with their provider. The authors tried to ascertain if the patient's negative perceptions could be explained by language barriers, but even when controlled with interpreters, the result was the same. Ultimately, the result was inconclusive as to why patients felt this way – whether it was secondary to culture, time spent with the providers, socioeconomic status, or communication styles.

Unlike the study done by Blanchard, Cooper et al. [2] studied the experience of African-American patients with Caucasian and African-American providers and found that race-concordant visits not only were characterized by higher patient satisfaction but also lasted longer on average. The data also noted that this higher satisfaction was independent of communication style, namely patient-centered communication, thus suggesting that other factors such as patient and physician attitudes or continuity of care were more effective.

Despite the many studies that have found a link between patient-provider race concordance and a more positive patient experience (potentially leading to racial minorities seeking resources related to health care), other studies have demonstrated the opposite. Meta-analyses such as the one performed by Meghani et al. [3] have found that there is inconclusive evidence to support patient-provider race concordance with positive health outcomes. Overall, it seems the literature has not found a particular link to determine if race concordance between patient and provider leads to a positive healthcare experience.

Gaps in Provider Knowledge

The provider did not take the time to inquire why the patient wanted a different doctor or what experiences the patient may have had to lead him to this point.

Cross-Cultural Tools and Skills

Cultural competency training for residents and attendings may have helped the providers in this scenario better explore the patient's rationale for wanting another provider and mitigate the conflict with the patient. Ultimately, directly addressing the patient's concerns may have helped the patient communicate his reservations. This could have led to a better rapport and working relationship, which would help the patient feel more included in his own care.

Pearls and Pitfalls

Pearl The resident explaining to the patient about patient care being a part of her training and not taking the patient's comment personally.

Pearl The attending returning with the resident to discuss the plan with the patient.

Pitfall The resident could have traded the assignment or asked the attending to see the patient independently since the patient was not in an emergent situation.

Case Outcome

The patient ultimately agreed to be admitted for further inpatient workup per the advice of the care team. The resident requested feedback at the end of the shift as to how she could have better handled this particular case. The attending was able to provide feedback. After cultural competency training later that year, the resident learned to explore the patient's concerns and work collaboratively to provide care rather than feeling offended by the remark and avoiding the physician/patient encounter. Ultimately, if a similar situation were to present itself, the resident has learned communication strategies to help optimize patient care and reflect on the subtle impact that microaggression plays in her patient care experiences.

References

1. Blanchard J, Nayar S, Lurie N. Patient–provider and patient–staff racial concordance and perceptions of mistreatment in the health care setting. J Gen Intern Med. 2007;22(8):1184–9.
2. Cooper LA, Roter DL, Johnson RL, Ford DE, Steinwachs DM, Powe NR. Patient-centered communication, ratings of care, and concordance of patient and physician race. Ann Intern Med. 2003;139(11):907–15.
3. Meghani SH, Brooks JM, Gipson-Jones T, Waite R, Whitfield-Harris L, Deatrick JA. Patient–provider race-concordance: does it matter in improving minority patients' health outcomes? Ethn Health. 2009;14(1):107–30.

Chapter 57
Latino Doctor

Steven Nazario and Maria Ramos-Fernandez

Case Scenario

A 52-year-old white male presents to a community hospital emergency department (ED) with a complaint of chest pain. He works as a landscaper.

Review of Symptoms

Chief complaint: Chest pain.

No recent foreign travel, no long car or plane rides, no fever/chills/weight loss, no recent weight loss, and no report of nausea/vomiting/diarrhea.

Past Medical History

None.

S. Nazario (✉)
Emergency Medicine Residency Program, Florida Hospital, Orlando, FL, USA

Emergency Medicine, Florida State University College of Medicine, Tallahassee, FL, USA
e-mail: Nazario@post.harvard.edu

M. Ramos-Fernandez
Emergency Medicine Residency Program, University of Puerto Rico, San Juan, Puerto Rico

Family History

Father died of a heart attack at age 48.

Social History

Drinks alcohol socially and smokes a pack of cigarettes a day. Lives at home with wife and four children.

Physical Exam

Vital Signs Temp 99.6 F, BP 158/100, HR 100, RR 28, Sat 99%.

General Moderately obese male who appears uncomfortable.

HEENT Atraumatic, PERL, IOM, supple neck, no carotid bruits.

Cardiovascular Normal heart tones without murmurs or rubs.

Respiratory Lungs clear.

Abdomen Soft, non-tender.

Extremities 2+ symmetric pulses, no edema, neg Homan's sign.

Skin Warm, dry.

Neuro Awake, alert, oriented with fluent speech, normal gait, moves all four extremities.

What Was Said?

Doctor: "Hi, I am Dr. Martinez and I'm here to take care of you. What brings you
        into the ED today?"
Patient: "Where are you from?"
Doctor, with some restraint: "I'm from New York."
Patient: "No, you're not. Where are you really from?"
Doctor: "I'm from Brooklyn and have lived here my whole life."

Patient, incredulously: "I don't believe you…where are you really from?"
Doctor, derisively: "Do you really wish to play twenty questions about my heritage
or where my 'peoples' are from or do you want me to look into your chest pain?"

What Was Done?

A workup for chest pain reveals a positive troponin and a nonspecific EKG. Dr. Martinez
plans to admit the patient and reviews his concerns with the patient. "I want an American
doctor. I can't trust a foreigner," the patient replies after being advised about his diagnosis of NSTEMI (heart attack) and the need for admission to the hospital. "What difference does it make where I am from? You do understand that you are having a heart
attack." Dr. Martinez tries to control the flutter in his voice as he relays this latest piece
of information. "I want another doctor," replies the now disgruntled patient. Dr.
Martinez states, "Unfortunately, I am the only doctor working the ED tonight. Are you
willing to risk dying from this because of where my family came from?"

Question for Discussion

1. What are the underlying attitudes and assumptions in this case?

Attitudes/Assumptions: The Provider

(a) The patient's prejudice is interfering with his best interests.
(b) The patient is ignorant and needs to realize that Latino healthcare providers
    may have been born and raised in the USA just like him [1]. In addition, provid-
    ers who are trained abroad and working in the USA have the same credential
    requirements as those trained in the USA.
(c) Non-maleficence – in light of the physician feeling slighted, the provider should
    not allow this to affect his treatment of the patient.

Attitudes/Assumptions: The Patient

(a) The doctor (with an ethnic sounding name) is not an American or may not have
    originated from North America.
(b) Since the doctor is perceived to come from another country, he provides less
    than competent care. According to Cajigal et al., ethnicity is the second most
    common reason physicians receive biased comments from patients [2].

Gaps in Provider Knowledge

(a) Lack of knowledge regarding this specific stereotyping
(b) Lack of knowledge of this patient's prior experiences with people of other cultures

Cross-Cultural Tools and Skills [3]

(a) Assume the patient is acting out of ignorance.
(b) Assume the patient is scared that he may die and is in the midst of an emotional crisis.
(c) Assuage the patient's fear or bias by assuring them that they are as qualified as any other healthcare provider.
(d) Assuage the patient's fear through the use of humor.
(e) There are steps on how to deal with discriminatory situations. The first step is to decide if the patient is stable. If so, then assess if the patient has decision-making capacity. If the patient is competent and his request cannot be accommodated, then another member of the staff may wish to engage with the patient and family members. Hopefully the patient and family members will understand and allow treatment, but if not, physicians should state the limits to such unacceptable conduct [3].

Pearls and Pitfalls [1, 3, 4]

Pearl The doctor did not take the comments made by the patient personally, as this patient is in a state of distress. Emergency physicians need to be aware they are particularly susceptible to experience bias, as patients do not get to choose who oversees their care [2].

Pearl The doctor kept the encounter centered on the chief complaint rather than confronting the issue of patient prejudices in the emergency department.

Pearl Offer to transfer the patient's care to another provider. Although 59% of patients who are referred to another physician experience no impact on care, this option may not be available at all times in the emergency room setting if the providers are working a single cover shift [2].

Pitfall The conversation could have degenerated into name-calling or an angry confrontation culminating with the patient leaving the emergency department under less-than-ideal conditions.

Case Outcome

Dr. Martinez has a lengthy discussion with the patient highlighting that the patient always has the option of leaving against medical advice, but in light of his presenting complaint, this would not be the best option. The patient decides to stay in the hospital for further evaluation.

References

1. Whitgob EE, Blackenburg R, Bogetz A. The discriminatory patient and family: strategies to address discrimination towards trainees. Acad Med. 2016;91(11):S64–9.
2. Cajigal S, Schudder L. Patient prejudice: when credentials aren't enough [Internet]. New York: WebMD LLC; 2017 Oct 18 [cited 2017 Nov 20]. Available from: https://www.medscape.com/slideshow/2017-patient-prejudice-report-6009134.
3. Kimari PE, Smith A, Lo B, Fernandez A. Dealing with racist patients. N Engl J Med. 2016;374(8):708–11.
4. Parry NM. How physicians can combat discrimination by patients [Internet]. New York: WebMD LLC; 2016 Oct 26 [cited 2017 Nov 20]. Available from: https://www.medscape.com/viewarticle/871015.

Chapter 58
Jewish Doctor

Taneisha T. Wilson

Case Scenario

A 29-year-old white state correction officer with no significant past medical history presents to the emergency department (ED) complaining of a laceration to the left upper arm. The patient reports receiving the cut from a sharp, crude, metal object. He sustained the injury at work while intervening in a fight among inmates. His injury is located on the left bicep, which is covered by a white bandage. His only other complaint is a pain at his right knuckles. He cannot recall his last tetanus vaccination.

At the end of the interview, the patient politely asks the interviewer (his physician who is a Jewish woman with dark curly hair) that a white male provider, preferably not Jewish, repair his laceration.

Review of Symptoms

Laceration to left upper arm and bruising to the right knuckle; all other systems are negative.

T. T. Wilson, MD, ScM
Brown Emergency Medicine, Injury Prevention Center, Rhode Island Hospital, Providence, RI, USA

Alpert School of Medicine, Brown University, Providence, RI, USA

The Miriam and Rhode Island Hospitals, Providence, RI, USA
e-mail: taneisha_wilson@brown.edu

© Springer International Publishing AG, part of Springer Nature 2019   407
M. L. Martin et al. (eds.), *Diversity and Inclusion in Quality Patient Care*,
https://doi.org/10.1007/978-3-319-92762-6_58

Past Medical History

None.

Surgical History Wisdom tooth extraction.

Family History

Sudden cardiac death of father at 50.

Social History

1/2 pack per day smoker.

Physical Exam

Vital Signs Temp, 98.2 F; pulse, 75; BP, 125/60; respirations, 16; O_2 sat, 99% RA.

General Well appearing; no apparent distress.

Neck Supple; no midline tenderness.

ENT No nasal bone tenderness.

Cardiovascular Normal rate rhythm; no murmurs, gallops, or rubs.

Respiratory Clear breath sounds.

Abdomen Non-distended and non-tender with normal bowel sounds.

Extremities Bruising to right knuckles and scratch to the dorsum of his left hand; laceration as described below; full range of motion in all joints without pain and is neurovascularly intact.

Skin 3 cm superficial laceration to the lateral aspect of the left upper arm; the laceration bisects an iron cross/swastika hybrid tattoo. Unaffected confederate flag tattoo is located on left pectoral muscle. The unaffected tattoo on right pectoral is a "Don't tread on me" flag tattoo with accompanying snake.

Neuro Grossly intact, moves all four extremities, and no visible sign of deficit.

What Was Said?

Patient: "I want a white man as my doctor."
Provider: "Sir, I am your physician today but will not care for you against your will as this laceration is not life-threatening. Let me speak with my supervisor about the options we have for you."
The physician consults the hospital administrator on call. The hospital administrator on call states, "Our hospital policy does not accommodate discrimination from patients or providers. Since this is a non-urgent case, the patient may be provided an option to be treated elsewhere."

What Was Done?

The patient was presented with hospital policies regarding his request.

Questions for Discussion

1. Should the physician comment on the tattoo symbols?

Attitudes/Assumptions: The Physician

(a) The patient is racist and a bigot.
(b) He thinks I am unqualified because I am female and Jewish.
(c) If I care for him, he will find a reason to sue or report me.
(d) These prejudices and discrimination are contributing to my burnout as a female Jewish physician [1, 2].

2. Can the patient request a white male physician for the repair?

Attitudes/Assumptions: The Patient

(a) The provider hates white men.
(b) She doesn't know that my family is German and was ostracized after World War II. My grandfather was a high-ranking Nazi soldier who tried to help, but no one believes that. Because of Jewish people, my family is impoverished.
(c) I have to work in a prison where black men are the majority; they don't respect me, and I don't respect them.
(d) She will not respect my wishes because they are all like that.

(e) Only white men are capable providers.
(f) She only got into medical school because of affirmative action.

3. As she is the only provider available, can the physician refuse to care for the non-life-threatening injury after the patient request?

Gaps in Provider Knowledge

(a) Will refusing or accepting the patient's request violate the EMTALA?
(b) Do I know institutional protocols addressing patient requests based on discrimination?
(c) What are my options?

Cross-Cultural Tools and Skills

Provider Tools

(a) Respecting the patient's autonomy as the patient has decision-making capacity [3].
(b) Must consider the EMTALA (Emergency Medical Treatment and Labor Act) [4].
(c) May offer the patient transfer to another facility if there is no life-threatening injury and the patient's request cannot be accommodated at the institution.
(d) Though it is recommended that institutions do not routinely accommodate requests of bigoted patients, it may benefit physician-patient interaction if these requests are granted.
(e) The patient's beliefs, though unacceptable in our society and dependent on the population served, are not illegal [2, 5]. For example, though it is not socially acceptable that this patient may believe that a male physician is smarter than a female physician, it is not illegal to hold this belief or to request a physician of a different race or gender because of these beliefs.
(f) The patient is not making hateful speech or being disruptive. Deciding to discuss the tattoo with the patient may impact the patient-physician relationship in an already tenuous situation.
(g) The physician has no obligation to discuss this with the patient's employer, and doing so may be a breach of confidentiality.
(h) Discussing the case with colleagues and mentors may mitigate some of the adverse effects. Institutional support is also crucial in providing tools and support when managing these challenging patients [1, 5].

The staff involved in this situation may feel demoralized and stigmatized [5, 6]. Individuals affected may internalize the microaggressions the patient perpetuates. This internalization can contribute to burnout and poor job satisfaction. In these situations, it is imperative that a supervisor exhibits support for the staff member to help mitigate these feelings [6]. Additionally, a supervisor or other supportive personnel should stress to the affected staff that such behavior reflects on the patient and not on them; in other words, they are not at fault. A supportive environment is critical in thwarting the internalization of aggressions such as the ones presented in this case [6].

Some institutions advocate strict interactions with patients who display bigoted or socially unacceptable behavior. In some organizations, this behavior is not tolerated, and individuals' requests are acknowledged but not accommodated. However, some institutions have a policy of acquiescing if possible. Currently, there exists no unified approach to managing this behavior, unless the individual works within a government-run institution such as a Veterans Administration (VA) hospital. A healthcare provider is ensured a safe work environment in the federal health system. The physician would be violating HIPAA with any disclosure to his employer regarding the patient's ED visit. The patient's biases, though socially unacceptable and morally reprehensible, are not illegal.

Pearls and Pitfalls

Pearl Recognize microaggressions, but avoid internalization.

Pitfall Learn institutional policies and procedures for interacting with staff/provider discrimination.

Case Outcome

The patient does not have a life-threatening injury, and the physician has time to consult the administrator on call to discuss her options regarding this patient. She learns from her on-call administrator that their institution has a no-tolerance policy regarding bigotry and that as the patient has no life-threatening injuries, he has the option to seek care elsewhere if he wishes, but the hospital will not offer an alternate provider. The administrator offers to come in to assist the staff in relaying this message. The provider feels comfortable presenting the options to the patient.

Upon learning that the hospital will not entertain his requests and that he has the option of seeking care elsewhere, the patient agrees to stay for care with his current provider. The provider repairs his laceration with her usual expert care. The provider feels empowered during this visit and supported by her institution.

Diagnosis Left upper arm laceration with bruising of the right hand.

Disposition The left forearm laceration was repaired with eight simple interrupted sutures and two deep sutures to aid in the cosmetic outcome. Plain film of the right hand did not reveal a fracture. Tetanus vaccine was updated. The patient was discharged to home after laceration repair with follow-up instruction for wound care and suture removal.

References

1. Corbie-Smith G, Frank E, Nickens HW, Elon L. Prevalences and correlates of ethnic harassment in the U.S. Women Physicians' Health Study. Acad Med. 1999;74(6):695–701.
2. Olayiwola JN. Racism in medicine: shifting the power. Ann Fam Med. 2016;14(3):267–9.
3. Fiester A. What "patient-centered care" requires in serious cultural conflict. Acad Med. 2012;87(1):20–4.
4. Urdang M, Mallek JT, Mallon WK. Tattoos and piercings: a review for the emergency physician. West J Emerg Med. 2011;12(4):393–8.
5. Paul-Emile K, Smith AK, Lo B, Fernandez A. Dealing with racist patients. N Engl J Med. 2016;374(8):708–11.
6. Whitgob EE, Blankenburg RL, Bogetz AL. The discriminatory patient and family: strategies to address discrimination towards trainees. Acad Med. 2016;91(11):S64–9.

Chapter 59
Muslim Doctor

Tareq Al-Salamah and Sarah Sewaralthahab

Case Scenario

A 54-year-old African-American male presents to a community emergency department with the complaint of right ankle pain and deformity after a fall.

Review of Symptoms

The patient complains of pain and deformity to his right ankle. He denies any trauma or pain to any other part of his body and denies hitting his head. The patient also denies numbness or tingling in his extremities. The rest of systems review is unremarkable.

Past Medical History

Hypertension.

T. Al-Salamah (✉)
University of Maryland School of Medicine, Baltimore, MD, USA

Emergency Department, University of Maryland Capital Region Health, Cheverly, MD, USA

Emergency Department, King Saud University, Riyadh, Saudi Arabia

S. Sewaralthahab
Department of Internal Medicine, University of Maryland Medical Center, Baltimore, MD, USA

Internal Medicine Department, King Saud University, Riyadh, Saudi Arabia

© Springer International Publishing AG, part of Springer Nature 2019
M. L. Martin et al. (eds.), *Diversity and Inclusion in Quality Patient Care*,
https://doi.org/10.1007/978-3-319-92762-6_59

Family History

Noncontributory.

Social History

Smokes one pack per day, drinks alcohol occasionally, denies drug use.

Physical Exam

Vital Signs Temperature 37.2, blood pressure 140/80, pulse 95, respiratory rate 18, oxygen saturation 96% on room air.

General Overweight, appears intoxicated.

Head Normocephalic, non-traumatic.

Neck No midline cervical spine tenderness.

ENT Normal.

Cardiovascular Regular rate and rhythm, no added heart sounds.

Respiratory No respiratory distress, lungs are clear.

Abdomen Soft, non-tender to palpation.

Extremities Right ankle deformed, with limited range of motion, no overlying abrasions. Right dorsalis pedis and posterior tibial pulses palpable but slightly weaker than left. Capillary refill in the right foot is <2 seconds. Left lower extremity and bilateral upper extremities are normal. Sensation is intact in both lower extremities.

Skin Warm and dry.

Neuro Normal.

What Was Said?

An American board-certified emergency medicine attending physician, who happens to be a Muslim from the Middle East, performs the physical exam. The patient notices that the attending physician's last name is "Masood" during the secondary survey and states, "Wait! Are you Muslim?! I don't want your kind to take care of me!" The doctor says, "Sir, I don't know what you mean by that, but your ankle appears to be dislocated and possibly broken. I need to finish my exam and ask you more questions to make sure we're not missing anything life or limb threatening, then I'll have an orthopedic specialist come over and speak with you about the next steps." Although appearing very uncomfortable, the patient agrees to continue with the exam but refuses to answer any more questions or engage in any dialogue.

What Was Done?

The physical exam is completed, and the Muslim attending from the Middle East informs the orthopedic physician assistant on duty of the likely fracture/dislocation and the need for completion of the rest of the history. The rest of the history is completed by the Hispanic male orthopedic physician assistant and conveyed to the Muslim attending. No additional interactions occur between the patient and the Muslim attending as the laboratory and imaging tests do not show any abnormalities aside from the ankle fracture/dislocation. The orthopedic physician assistant informs the patient of the plan for admission and operation the next day. The patient agrees with the plan.

Questions for Discussion

1. Why did the patient become uncomfortable when he noticed the physician's name? What were the physician's thoughts about the interaction?

Attitudes/Assumptions: The Patient

(a) I have lost many friends in the military by Muslims, and I do not want a Muslim to take care of me at any time.
(b) There are many non-Muslim physicians out there. Why can't I be treated by a physician I would be comfortable with?
(c) I read an article online about terrorist attacks carried out by Muslim doctors in London and how any Muslim can be a terrorist. I do not know why we still let them in our country.

Attitudes/Assumptions: The Physician

(a) Like my colleagues, I am a medical professional, and my religion does not change how I manage any of my patients.

(b) Trying to find another physician to satisfy this patient's prejudice will just waste more time to definitive care.

(c) I am licensed by a governmental body to practice medicine in the United States. I should not be perceived as a threat to anyone, especially as a physician working in a hospital.

2. How likely is something like this to happen in a hospital setting? What are the patient's rights? What are the physician's rights?

Cross-Cultural Tools and Skills

Encountering a patient with strong negative biased views is more likely nowadays given the increasing diversity of the physician population in the Western world. This is significantly compounded by the upsurge in discrimination against Muslims in general, including healthcare workers, since the events of September 11, 2001 (9/11) [1]. These encounters can be challenging. On one hand, the patient is protected by the Emergency Medical Treatment and Labor Act (EMTALA) [2] and has the right to autonomy. On the other hand, physicians are protected by Title VII of the 1964 Civil Rights Act [3], which guarantees a workplace free from discrimination based on race, color, religion, sex, and national origin.

A number of Muslim physicians face cultural trauma in either overt or covert forms of discrimination. Direct and blatant overt discrimination consists of racial slurs, jokes, or patients requesting a non-Muslim physician, while covert discrimination results in avoidance and exclusion by colleagues and neighbors [4].

3. What impact does the sense of discrimination have on care providers?
   The negative bias often portrayed by the media, general public, and in the workplace has resulted in a heightened sense of anxiety and fear for life and safety among the Muslim population, as well as feelings of insecurity and loss of social stability. Whereas Muslims once found solace in each other and in their community/mosques, the fear of guilt by association with suspected terrorists or mosques under surveillance forced a sense of isolation upon hardworking, law-abiding Muslims [5]. Not only did workplaces and schools become minefields of social and professional acceptance, but so did their very own homes and neighborhoods.

4. How important is it for care providers to understand the role of diversity in patient care?
   Although studies have shown that racial concordance was associated with better patient-physician interaction, these studies also highlight the importance of training physicians and patients to engage in high quality communication with racially discordant patients by focusing on improving patient-centeredness and partnership building [6]. Muslim physicians can rise above issues of race and

religion through the use of patient-centered behavior and communication, which has been shown to be more effective than racial concordance in patient outcomes [7].

5. What can Muslim providers do to overcome such interactions that may negatively impact their work experience and their well-being?

It is difficult for Muslim physicians to augment or change certain negative ideologies of patients in the workplace; hospitals are not a suitable venue to engage in political or societal dialogue, nor do treating physicians have the time or capacity to tackle such complex issues. There are, however, mechanisms and activities that Muslims, physicians, and non-physicians alike can engage in to cope with psychological stress resulting from discrimination. Political engagement and public service involvement have shown to have a positive effect. Opening channels of dialogue with coworkers, family, and friends about personal concerns raises awareness of the issues, their scope, and how detrimental they can be personally, professionally, and communally. Muslim physicians may also choose to join existing groups of individuals with similar background/job/status who struggle with comparable feelings of discrimination and ostracism, such as the Association of Physicians of Pakistani Descent of North America (APPNA), the Islamic Medical Association of North America (IMANA), and the American Muslim Health Professionals (AMHP). These organizations allow physicians with similar backgrounds and beliefs from different parts of the United States to discuss and perhaps resolve common concerns [4].

6. What went well in this case? What should be avoided in similar interactions?

Pearls and Pitfalls

Pearl The attending physician explained his main concerns and limited his interaction to what was medically necessary and asked the orthopedic physician assistant to complete the history.

Pearl The attending physician did not react negatively or inappropriately to a comment by a patient who may have very limited exposure and interaction with Muslims and people from the Middle East.

Pitfall Engaging in political or racial discussions/arguments in the emergency department when the absolute focus should be on patients' well-being.

Pitfall A limited history may be detrimental to patient care, but if the patient refuses to engage and interact, ask your colleagues and other medical staff to help where possible.

Case Outcome

After the attending explained his main objective and concern for the patient's well-being, he limited interaction with the patient to the most important aspects of the evaluation. The attending physician completed what was necessary by asking the orthopedic physician assistant to complete the history. The patient's management proceeded appropriately with an ankle reduction in the emergency room by the orthopedic physician assistant and admission for surgical intervention the next day.

References

1. Rousseau C, Hassn G, Moreau N, Thombs B. Perceived discrimination and its association with psychological distress among newly arrived immigrants before and after September 11, 2001. Am J Public Health. 2011;101(5):909–15.
2. Centers or Medicare & Medicaid Services. Emergency Medical Treatment and Labor Act (EMTALA) [Internet]. Baltimore, MD: Centers or Medicare & Medicaid Services; [updated 2012 Mar 26; cited 2017 Nov 3]. Available from http://www.cms.gov/Regulations-and-Guidance/Legislation/EMTALA/index.html?redirect=/EMTALA.
3. U.S. Equal Employment Opportunity Commission. Title VII of the Civil Rights Act of 1964 [Internet]. [Washington D.C.]: U.S. Equal Employment Opportunity Commission. [Cited 2017 Nov 3]. Available from http://www.eeoc.gov/laws/statutes/titlevii.cfm.
4. Abu-Ras W, Senzai F, Laird L. American Muslim physicians' experiences since 9/11: cultural trauma and the formation of Islamic identity. Traumatology. 2013;19(1):11–9. https://doi.org/10.1177/1534765612441975.
5. Abu-Ras W, Abu-Bader S. The impact of the September 11, 2001, attacks on the well-being of Arab-Americans in New York City. J Muslim Ment Health. 2008;3(2):217–39. https://doi.org/10.1080/15564900802487634.
6. Cooper LA, Roter DL, Johnson RL, Ford DE, Steinwachs DM, Powe NR. Patient-centered communication, ratings of care, and concordance of patient and physician race. Ann Intern Med. 2003;139(11):907–15. https://doi.org/10.7326/0003-4819-139-11-200312020-00009.
7. LaVeist TA, Nuru-Jeter A. Is doctor-patient race concordance associated with greater satisfaction with care? J Health Soc Behav. 2002;43(4):296–306.

Chapter 60
Foreign Doctor

Kumar Alagappan and Jan Hargrave

An emergency physician, raised and trained in the United States, was born in India but has never lived there. His father served with the United Nations, and his family moved to New York City from Bangkok when he was 4 years old. He attended the UN International School in the city and lived in Queens, probably the most diverse of New York's five boroughs. Queens' residents speak more than 160 languages, and half of the US citizens who live there were born in other countries. His parents are of South Indian origin, and, like them, he looks very "Indian," yet his English is impeccable and he speaks without a discernable accent (other than, perhaps, a certain New York inflection). Given his multicultural upbringing, he grew up with little awareness of his racial difference. Only when he headed to a university in the Midwest did it become obvious that his background was quite different from that of most of the students on campus.

As a newly minted doctor, he worked in an emergency department at a teaching hospital in Queens. One evening, he had a heated telephone exchange with a young resident and demanded that he come down to the emergency department to see a patient. The resident came reluctantly and was very vocal with the staff there (including the Indian attending doctor – Dr. JV) about the particulars of the conversation he had just had. He did not know the Indian doctor was the attending he had just spoken with. Once introduced to the attending, the resident became extremely apologetic, saying, "I did not know that I spoke to you." What he really meant was that he did not recognize the Indian attending as the person whom he had spoken

K. Alagappan · J. Hargrave (✉)
The University of Texas MD Anderson Cancer Center, Houston, TX, USA
e-mail: jan@janhargrave.com

© Springer International Publishing AG, part of Springer Nature 2019
M. L. Martin et al. (eds.), *Diversity and Inclusion in Quality Patient Care*,
https://doi.org/10.1007/978-3-319-92762-6_60

with on the phone because, on the basis of Dr. JV's appearance, he expected the attending to have an "Indian" accent.

Case Scenario

In the same emergency department, Dr. JV encountered the patient for this case study, a young white female who was complaining of lower abdominal pain. When the attending first met her, she was sitting upright on the stretcher in the middle of a bustling emergency department, wearing a gown and separated from her neighbor by one thin curtain.

By necessity, the medical history interview included numerous personal questions about her sexual activity and menses, which the attending asked in a matter-of-fact, unemotional manner. Because the attending also had to examine her lower abdomen and perform pelvic and rectal exams, he had a chaperone accompany him. He was careful to ensure that the patient was comfortable during the entire encounter. He was extremely aware of her body language and constantly assured her while he spoke with her, before he touched her or further examined her. He maintained constant eye contact with her and spoke in a soft tone.

Review of Symptoms

Lower abdominal pain

Past Medical History

Unremarkable

Family History

Unremarkable

Social History

Single female; sexually active

Physical Exam

Abdomen Mild tenderness lower abdomen

Pelvic Exam Negative

Rectal Exam Stool heme negative; no tenderness

What Was Said?

The attending advised her to follow up with her regular doctor. She informed him that she did not have one and asked if the attending could recommend someone, but not a foreign doctor with a long and unpronounceable name. She then asked the attending if he had an office practice, and he joked with her that she was in his office now. She suddenly realized that he had a long name unpronounceable to her and that he was not a white doctor. She had forgotten that the attending was of a different background, even though she was looking right at him.

What Was Done?

Dr. JV ignored her faux pas, but the patient nonetheless began to fidget uncomfortably when she realized that she had been impolite. She apologized profusely, and the attending assured her that it was all right and told her not to worry. He arranged for her to follow up with a provider in her neighborhood.

Question for Discussion

1. What are some attitudes and assumptions in this case that affect the provider-patient relationship?

Attitudes/Assumptions: The Provider

The aforementioned incident validates the importance of a physician's experience in monitoring reactions, both his or her own and those of the patient. Effective people skills, reflective listening competencies, nonverbal cue recognition, and empathy mastery during patient encounters can deeply affect patient perceptions and even health outcomes.

Attitudes/Assumptions: The Patient

Patients consistently articulate their desire for a physician whom they trust, one who has their best interests in mind and one who understands and takes into consideration their social context. Emergency room physicians, on the other hand, do not have that option. While attitudes concerning stereotyping of others are difficult to address, patients should increasingly recognize the physician-as-a-person concept. Physicians who elicit psychosocial and biomedical communication during the emergency room visit can influence the patient's satisfaction with his or her medical care. When patients and physicians form a personal bond, patients view their physician as not only clinically competent but also supportive and engaged.

Gaps in Provider Knowledge

Self-awareness and self-management enable physicians to recognize their own and other people's emotions and to manage and adjust the environment to achieve their goals. Skillfully employing these emotional intelligence qualities to guide one's thinking and behavior confers a superb advantage in dealing with clinical encounters and day-to-day circumstances.

Empathy for others is another vital trait of the skillful clinician. In the clinical context, empathy is the physician's ability to identify and understand a patient's situation, feelings, motives, and emotions, so as to facilitate a more accurate diagnosis and more caring treatment. Empathy is simply about connecting with others. In a 2012 study, Hojat et al. [1] analyzed the health outcomes of more than 20,000 patients with diabetes who were assigned to three different groups of physicians (pre-evaluated for their levels of empathy). The physicians who demonstrated the highest degrees of empathy achieved the best results from their patients, who had statistically significantly lower levels of diabetic complications compared with patients whose physicians scored lower in empathy. Physician empathy improved the odds of successful health outcomes.

In medical settings, employing empathetic behaviors can alleviate so-called doorknob moments [2]. Doorknob moments occur when, as the doctor prepares to leave, hand wrapped around the doorknob, the patient asks one more question or mentions one more detail about his illness that changes everything. Clinicians who pace themselves, monitor reactions, supply therapeutic touch, and employ directed gaze techniques may stave off such doorknob moments.

A thorough understanding of nonverbal communication cues and recognition of the value of empathy in the clinical setting is directly related to patient satisfaction. Keep these pointers in mind when attempting to connect with others.

Cross-Cultural Tools and Skills

When entering the room or otherwise approaching the patient:

1. Establish eye contact. When you look directly at another person, you show interest in them and communicate their importance to you. Clinicians who constantly face away from patients while inputting information into a computer decrease the amount of direct eye contact, further adding to the patient's sense of hurried, uncaring, and ineffective communication. Maintaining eye contact 60–70% of the time will indicate interest without seeming aggressive.
2. Adopt a positive facial expression. A genuine smile communicates warmth and confidence and is appropriate in all but life-or-death situations. Patients will be more receptive to you if you enter the room with a positive expression.
3. Offer a sturdy handshake. Shaking hands establishes physical connection and conveys a sense of security and a wealth of psychological information. Extend your hand in a vertical position (neither palm up nor palm down) to create a feeling of equality between parties.

Pay attention to your own body language:

4. Angle your body toward the patient. Facing your patient and leaning toward them will indicate that you are fully present and totally aware of the conversation. To communicate effectively at the same eye level, pull up a chair next to the patient's bed.
5. Position your head intentionally. Keeping your head straight will make you appear self-assured and authoritative. To come across as friendly and open, tilt your head slightly.
6. Keep your hands visible. Your hands need to be seen; that is how others begin to trust you. Arms can be crossed or folded over your chest so long as your hands are visible; this position signals contemplation and evaluation. Tucking your hands behind your crossed arms communicates disinterest or disagreement. Resist the urge to put your hands in your pockets.

Be aware of verbal and nonverbal cues:

7. Listen with your ears, eyes, and heart. Pay attention to body language, tone of voice, and hidden emotions behind what the patient is saying. Calling the patient by name says that you have paid attention from the start of the conversation, and paraphrasing shows understanding. Research indicates that, on average, physicians interrupt patients within 18 seconds of beginning to listen to their medical issues [3]; constantly interrupting a patient or answering abruptly seemingly dismisses his or her concerns.
8. Practice patience. Do you repeatedly glance at your watch or answer your cell phone? Satisfied patients who feel that their physician is committed and fully present during the medical encounter typically perceive their visits to be two minutes longer than they actually are.
9. Notice what the patient *doesn't* say. Ninety-three percent of the message that a person communicates to another person is conveyed by tone of voice and body

language, not by actual words. Does the patient look down as he describes his illness? Does the patient wring her hands or refuse to meet your gaze? What might his facial expression be telling you? Awareness of nonverbal gestures and affect can provide important information about the patient's emotional state.

Patients judge your intelligence, aptitude, genuineness, and even leadership ability by the actions that accompany your medical advice. The easiest way to make a positive first impression is to demonstrate immediately that the patient, not you, is the center of action and conversation. Empathy is essential for establishing trust, the foundation to a good doctor-patient relationship.

Pearls and Pitfalls

Pearl A direct relationship exists between patient satisfaction and provider empathy.

Pearl Unlock the emotional intelligence skills of self-awareness and self-management when dealing with other individuals.

Pitfall Empathy is not sympathy. Putting yourself in another's shoes during a conversation is empathy.

Pitfall A nonverbal gesture does not stand alone; clusters of similar gestures together give true meanings to body language.

Case Outcome

Ultimately, the patient's labs revealed a urinary tract infection that could be treated with oral antibiotics. She was relieved that she was not pregnant, did not require surgery, and did not have any other complicating pelvic infection. The patient was started on antibiotics and referred to a physician near her home. The attending did not hear from her again.

References

1. Hojat M, Louis DZ, Markham FW, Wender R, Rabinowitz C, Gonnella JS. Physicians' empathy and clinical outcomes for diabetic patients. Acad Med. 2011;86(3):359–64.
2. Harpham W. Wendy Harpham on healthy survivorship [blog on the Internet]. [Texas]: Wendy Harpham. [24 Jan 2008]. Doorknob moments. 2011 Sep 20 [cited 24 July 2017]. Available from: http://wendyharpham.typepad.com/healthy_survivorship/2011/09/doorknob-moments.html.
3. Boodman SG. How to teach doctors empathy [Internet]. Washington: The Atlantic Monthly Group; 2015 Mar 15 [cited 24 July 2017]. Available from: https://www.theatlantic.com/health/archive/2015/03/how-to-teach-doctors-empathy/387784/.

Chapter 61
Race/Ethnicity Concordant Provider

Kenyon Railey and Michael Railey

Case Scenario

A 45-year-old African-American male patient presents to the clinic to establish care. He reports he has a history of hypertension and obstructive sleep apnea (OSA). It has been several years since the patient has seen a primary care provider. The patient recalls running out of his blood pressure pills "a few months ago." He recently attended a healthcare screening at his church, and his blood pressure was "160 something." As a result of this and the urging of his significant other, he says he is "ready to get back on track." The patient mentions that he has been resistant to scheduling a visit because "Each time I go to the office, somebody adds more medication. I don't want to be on so many pills." He also comments that it took him longer to find a provider because "I didn't want to see a white provider." He goes on to say that he thinks racism and stress have played a role in why his blood pressure is so elevated. He comments that "a white provider has no idea what it's like to be black in this country. I really want someone I can relate to." The patient also recalls a bad experience with his mother who passed away a few years ago. He felt that the care the family received was suboptimal and possibly contributed to his mother's death: "Although my mom didn't go to college, she raised four children; all with advanced degrees. Everyone in the hospital treated us like we were poor and stupid. I lost a lot of faith in the system as a result of that experience."

K. Railey (✉)
Department of Community and Family Medicine, Office of Diversity and Inclusion,
Duke University School of Medicine, Durham, NC, USA
e-mail: Kenyon.railey@duke.edu

M. Railey
Family and Community Medicine, Student Affairs and Diversity, Saint Louis University
School of Medicine, St. Louis, MO, USA
e-mail: Railey.michael@health.slu.edu

© Springer International Publishing AG, part of Springer Nature 2019
M. L. Martin et al. (eds.), *Diversity and Inclusion in Quality Patient Care*,
https://doi.org/10.1007/978-3-319-92762-6_61

Review of Symptoms

The patient denies any exertional chest pain, shortness of breath, abnormal heart-beats, dyspnea on exertion, paroxysmal nocturnal dyspnea, lower extremity swelling, or loss of consciousness or diaphoresis. In addition, the patient denies any cough, wheezing, hemoptysis, or exercise intolerance.

Past Medical History

Patient was diagnosed with hypertension 8 years ago; the patient cannot recall names of medication he used. He thinks he was on "a water pill." He was diagnosed with OSA 5 years ago and uses CPAP "most of the time."

Family History

The patient's mother died at age 71 from CVA. She had a history of hypertension, CHF, and CKD. Father is healthy with "prostate problems" but no cancer. He has four siblings, two brothers, two sisters; both brothers have HTN, otherwise healthy. His children are healthy.

Social History

The patient is married and has two children, aged 17 and 14. He is a software engineer. He does not smoke, drink alcohol, or use illicit drugs.

Physical Exam

Vital Signs Temp, 98.4 F; pulse, 84; BP, 160/100; respirations, 20; O_2 Sat, 99% on room air; weight, 220 pounds; height, 5'10"; BMI, 31

General No apparent distress

Cardiovascular Regular rate and rhythm, normal S1 and S2, and no murmurs

Respiratory Normal work of breathing and clear in all lung fields

Extremities Warm, well perfused, and no edema is noted

HEENT Normocephalic, atraumatic; pupils equally round and reactive to light and accommodation, extraocular movements intact, anicteric, moist mucosa

Neck No jugular venous distensions and no carotid bruits noted

Neuro Alert and oriented; cranial nerves 2–12 intact; strength and sensation are normal; gait is normal

Questions for Discussion

1. Why would it be difficult for a patient to find a provider of color? What is the evidence regarding race concordance in healthcare settings?

   Although diversity in the United States is increasing, the number of racial and ethnic minority providers has remained relatively stable over time. For one group in particular (African-American males), the number of applicants to medical school has actually decreased in the last three decades [1]. White and Asian providers continue to represent the largest percentage of medical school graduates. Approximately 4% of the faculty at academic institutions are underrepresented minorities [2], and only about 8.9% of all physicians in the United States identify as black or African-American, American Indian, Alaska Native, Hispanic, or Latino [3]. A lack of diversity among medical providers has long been recognized as a major contributor to healthcare disparities in the United States [4].

   It is a reasonable desire for a minority patient to seek a medical provider of the same racial/ethnic background. Creating race concordant patient encounters has been proposed as one of many potential methods to combat health inequities. However, multiple investigations and systematic reviews over the last few decades have not shown consistent evidence that race concordance actually improves outcomes or perceptions of communication [5–7].

2. How could mistrust and perceived discrimination affect patient satisfaction?

   Patient satisfaction and healthcare quality are inexorably linked; higher satisfaction is associated with higher physical and mental function as well as improved health status [8]. Patient satisfaction is influenced by many factors, one of which is trust. For African-American patients, mistrust in the healthcare system is deeply rooted in the historical memory due to slavery, Jim Crow, segregation, ethical violations (e.g., Henrietta Lacks), and experimentation (e.g., Tuskegee Syphilis Study). These historical abuses create environments of care where trust in the medical provider is not guaranteed [9].

   Past personal experiences with discrimination also contribute to poor patient satisfaction and likely to poorer outcomes. Perceived racial discrimination has been shown to negatively impact trust and satisfaction with care [10] as well as lead to worse health for minority and majority populations [11].

Understanding the importance of trust in the healthcare encounter will be a key component of improving patient-provider relationships and outcomes for vulnerable populations.

3. What are some of the potential barriers to a successful visit in this scenario?

Attitudes/Assumptions: The Provider

(a) Only providers of color can relate to patients with concerns regarding racism.
(b) The patient may be playing the "race card" regarding previous encounters, attributing poor outcomes to intentional acts of discrimination rather than individual acts of poor communication or lapses in professionalism.
(c) The patient is a so-called "difficult" patient.

Attitudes/Assumptions: The Patient

(a) Only providers of color can relate to patients with concerns regarding racism.
(b) Having a provider that is the same race/ethnicity improves the quality of care.
(c) Previous bad experiences in care were the direct result of racial biases, not errors in communication or professionalism.
(d) Lifestyle modifications are often not sufficient to prevent further medication use.
(e) The risks of untreated hypertension are not well understood.

Gaps in Provider Knowledge

(a) Lack of understanding of the structural racism and health inequities present in the United States.
(b) Lack of understanding of the health consequences of racism, bias, mistrust, and discrimination.
(c) Lack of understanding of patient-centered care, which is appropriate in all encounters despite racial or ethnic background.
(d) Lack of understanding of an individual patient's health literacy, which is variable.
(e) Lack of understanding that although race concordance does not necessarily improve outcome, it can improve perceived patient satisfaction.

Cross-Cultural Tools and Skills

Difficult patient encounters are common in medical care. Although the presence of mood disorders, anger, fear, high symptom severity, and grief are all likely to increase the possibility of a "difficult" patient encounter, language barriers or cross-cultural issues can also make for challenging interactions [12]. Empathy and compassion are cornerstones to successful clinical encounters, no matter the race/ethnicity of the provider or patient. In addition, good interpersonal communication skills and an awareness of one's own biases are crucial components of culturally appropriate care. The reality is that the healthcare team is often multidimensional. The evidence regarding outcomes in race concordant patient/provider visits is not conclusive. Therefore, as the United States becomes more diverse, all members of the healthcare encounter (including staff) should be open to interactions that are discordant in multiple aspects of identity. At the same time, however, students and providers alike should work to understand the structural causes of health disparities, while institutions simultaneously work to diversify the provider workforce. These and other tools will allow the clinicians of the future to manage diverse patient populations while maximizing patient satisfaction and potentially improving outcomes.

Case Outcome

The patient establishes care with the new medical provider, who empathizes with the patient regarding his difficulties in past encounters. The provider has a long discussion with the patient about lifestyle modifications and the importance of adherence to CPAP for his OSA. The patient is placed on an appropriate antihypertensive medication, and a follow-up visit is scheduled in 1 month. He returns in 1 month and has lost 3 pounds with lifestyle modifications. His blood pressure is now at goal.

References

1. Altering the course: Black Males in Medicine [Internet]. American Association of Medical Colleges; 2015 [cited 1 Aug 2017]. Available from: https://members.aamc.org/eweb/upload/Black_Males_in_Medicine_Report_WEB.pdf.
2. AAMC Facts & Figures 2016: Diversity in Medical Education [Internet]. American Association of Medical Colleges; 2016 [cited 1 Aug 2017]. Available from: http://www.aamcdiversityfactsandfigures2016.org/.
3. AAMC 2014 Diversity in the Physician Workforce [Internet]. American Association of Medical Colleges; 2014 [cited 1 Aug 2017]. Available from: http://aamcdiversityfactsandfigures.org/.
4. Institute of Medicine Committee on U, Eliminating R, Ethnic Disparities in Health C. Smedley BD, Stith AY, Nelson AR, editors. Unequal treatment: confronting racial and ethnic disparities in health care. Washington (DC): National Academies Press (US).
5. Meghani SH, Brooks JM, Gipson-Jones T, Waite R, Whitfield-Harris L, Deatrick JA. Patient-provider race-concordance: does it matter in improving minority patients' health outcomes? Ethn Health. 2009;14(1):107–30.
6. Shen MJ, Peterson EB, Costas-Muniz R, Hernandez MH, Jewell ST, Matsoukas K, et al. The effects of race and racial concordance on patient-physician communication: a systematic review of the literature. J Racial Ethn Health Disparities. 2018;5(1):117–140. doi: 10.1007/s40615-017-0350-4.
7. Sweeney CF, Zinner D, Rust G, Fryer GE. Race/ethnicity and health care communication: does patient-provider concordance matter? Med Care. 2016;54(11):1005–9.

8. Hung M, Zhang W, Chen W, Bounsanga J, Cheng C, Franklin JD, et al. Patient-reported outcomes and total health care expenditure in prediction of patient satisfaction: results from a national study. JMIR Public Health Surveill. 2015;1(2):e13.
9. Murray TM. Trust in African Americans' healthcare experiences. Nurs Forum. 2015;50(4):285–92.
10. Benkert R, Peters RM, Clark R, Keves-Foster K. Effects of perceived racism, cultural mistrust and trust in providers on satisfaction with care. J Natl Med Assoc. 2006;98(9):1532–40.
11. Hausmann LR, Jeong K, Bost JE, Ibrahim SA. Perceived discrimination in health care and health status in a racially diverse sample. Med Care. 2008;46(9):905–14.
12. Hull SK, Broquet K. How to manage difficult patient encounters. Fam Pract Manag. 2007;14(6):30–4.

Chapter 62
Female Doctor

Taryn R. Taylor

Case Scenario

A 6-year-old male is brought by his mother and father into the pediatric emergency department for evaluation. The chief complaint as reported to the triage nurse is "dehydration." Upon entering the exam room, the female attending physician observes that the child is sitting on the exam bed playing games on a tablet. The physician introduces herself and reaches to shake hands with the parents. The father immediately stands up and shakes the physician's hand but then positions himself in front of the mother, such that the physician cannot extend her hand toward the mother. The physician then sits at the foot of the bed, next to the patient. The father remains standing and provides very curt, abrupt answers to the physician's questions about the medical history. He avoids eye contact, appears agitated, and interrupts the mother when she attempts to provide additional details. Eventually, the father explodes, "I am done talking to you. I need a male physician to take care of my son."

Review of Symptoms

The patient had loose, watery, non-bloody stools for the last 2 days. He had a normal appetite until this evening at dinner, when he had onset of nausea and vomiting. He had three episodes of non-bloody, non-bilious emesis. He has been afebrile over

T. R. Taylor, MD, MEd
Emory University School of Medicine,
Atlanta, GA, USA
e-mail: Taryn.Taylor@emory.edu

© Springer International Publishing AG, part of Springer Nature 2019   431
M. L. Martin et al. (eds.), *Diversity and Inclusion in Quality Patient Care*,
https://doi.org/10.1007/978-3-319-92762-6_62

the course of the illness. The remainder of the history is difficult to obtain, as the father refuses to answer additional questions.

Past Medical History

The patient has a history of asthma but has never been hospitalized. He had tympanostomy tubes placed bilaterally at age 2.

Social History

He is in the first grade, where multiple children have had "the stomach flu." The father refuses to provide any additional information pertinent to the social history, demanding, "Why does all this matter?"

Family History

The father refuses to provide additional history.

Physical Exam

Vital Signs Temperature 37.6 °C, Pulse 98, RR 19, BP 98/57, O_2 Sat 98% on room air.

General Healthy-appearing young male child, who is resting comfortably, engaged in a game on his tablet, appears well hydrated.

The remainder of the physical exam cannot be obtained.

What Was Said?

Prior to the physician being able to examine the patient, the father demands that his child be treated by "a male doctor." The female attending physician replies calmly, "It seems as if you are upset, sir. Please tell me your concern about having a female physician." The father angrily replies, "I don't need this!" He grabs his wife and child and attempts to leave the emergency department.

What Was Done?

Before the family exits, the male charge nurse talks with the father and promises to find a male physician to care for his son. The family returns to the examination room and a male attending physician evaluates the patient, diagnoses him with an acute gastroenteritis, and discharges him to home with a prescription for Zofran.

Questions for Discussion

1. Why did the patient's father demand a male physician?

Attitudes/Assumptions: The Father

(a) Male physicians are smarter and more competent healthcare providers.
(b) Males are the authoritarian figures in his family, and his son should see this leadership modeled in his environment.

2. Why did the charge nurse and second physician acquiesce to the father's demands without discussing expectations with him or providing verbal support to the original female physician?

Attitudes/Assumptions: Charge Nurse and Second (Male) Physician

(a) Pleasing the patient/customer is the highest priority.
(b) This experience, although an annoyance, will not have any lasting effect on the female physician.

3. How could the female physician have improved the interaction with the patient's father?

Attitudes/Assumptions: Female Attending Physician

(a) If I am polite enough to the father, he will see that I am trying to help his son, and he will become more reasonable.
(b) If I openly acknowledge his concern about having a female physician, we can then start a dialogue about his concerns; this improved communication will improve the patient encounter.

Cross-Cultural Tools and Skills

(a) Ask questions to elicit patient/parental preferences. From the beginning of this patient encounter, the father displayed nonverbal cues that indicated his disapproval. The female physician used tactics, such as sitting on the patient stretcher, which she assumed would be viewed as conciliatory. Rather than speculate about patient preferences, one should inquire in a respectful and direct manner.

4. Are there additional steps the female physician could have taken to help prevent similar situations in the future?

Attitudes/Assumptions: Female Attending Physician

(a) These patient encounters will "come up from time to time" and "that's just the way it goes."
(b) There are no helpful resources for situations like these, so "I just have to deal with it."

Gaps in Provider Knowledge

(a) Lack of knowledge of specific strategies to address bias in others
(b) Inability to recognize institutional cultural challenges

Pearls and Pitfalls

Pearl The mature physician recognizes the nonverbal cues that indicate a patient or family member may be experiencing displeasure. One should define his or her personal and professional boundaries in order to manage surrounding conflict without being manipulated by it [1].

Pearl During an encounter with a difficult patient or family member, it is important for the physician to remain calm, be empathetic to their needs, and try to engage them in conversation to determine a mutually agreeable solution to the problem [1].

Pitfall One will likely not change the cultural beliefs and practices of a patient/family member in a single encounter. It is important to manage your own expectations as well as the patient's.

Pearl Team dynamics play a critical role in the healthcare setting. Rather than dismissing the opinions or value of a team member, as noted in this case by the nurse manager and male physician, providers should have open communication and define shared goals such that each team member is supported.

Pearl While there are many studies that explore physician gender bias toward their patients, the literature is less robust with respect to the gender bias of patients toward their providers. Some studies suggest that communication between patients and doctors of the same gender is more satisfactory. However, female physicians have been noted to engage in more patient-centered communication, and their decision-making styles have been described as more participatory [2, 3]. These strengths of women providers should be acknowledged and leveraged in the healthcare setting to optimize patient care.

Case Outcome

The patient was discharged to home with the prescription for Zofran. The female attending physician was notified by emergency department leadership that the father filed a complaint about her to the hospital patient representative and submitted a negative patient satisfaction survey. The physician spoke with her direct supervisor, who recommended she seek additional support and resources offered by the Office of Equity and Inclusion.

References

1. Hull S, Broquet K. How to manage difficult patient encounters. Fam Pract Manag. 2007;14(6):30–4.
2. Cooper-Patrick L, Gallo JJ, Gonzales JJ, et al. Race, gender, and partnership in the patient-physician relationship. JAMA. 1999;282(6):583–9. https://doi.org/10.1001/jama.282.6.583.
3. Roter DL, Hall JA. Physician gender and patient-centered communication: a critical review of empirical research. Annu Rev Public Health. 2004;25(1):497–519. https://doi.org/10.1146/annurev.publhealth.25.101802.123134.

Chapter 63
Gay Doctor

Michael K. Brown and Joel Moll

Case Scenario

A 64-year-old male presents to a rural community emergency department with a chief complaint of 1 day of abdominal pain, vomiting, and dyspnea. The patient reports onset of symptoms 1 day prior, which acutely worsened today. He has a history of type II diabetes mellitus (DM) but does not take his insulin as prescribed. Blood sugar at home was 550; blood glucose has been in the 300's the past 2 days. There is no history of diabetic ketoacidosis. He had a recent upper respiratory illness 2 days prior to onset of symptoms.

Review of Symptoms

Epigastric abdominal pain, nausea, non-bilious vomiting, dyspnea, polyuria, and polydipsia. He denies fevers, chest pain, dysuria, and diarrhea. All other systems are reported negative.

Past Medical History

Hypertension, hyperlipidemia, insulin-dependent type II DM, obesity

Past Surgical History Cholecystectomy, appendectomy

M. K. Brown · J. Moll (✉)
Department of Emergency Medicine, Virginia Commonwealth University,
Richmond, VA, USA
e-mail: joel.moll@vcuhealth.org

© Springer International Publishing AG, part of Springer Nature 2019
M. L. Martin et al. (eds.), *Diversity and Inclusion in Quality Patient Care*,
https://doi.org/10.1007/978-3-319-92762-6_63

Medications Amlodipine, HCTZ, simvastatin, insulin lispro with meals, and insulin NPH

Family History

DM, hypertension, coronary artery disease

Social History

Drinks four to five beers daily for the last 20 years, smokes one pack of cigarettes per day, denies illicit drug use

Physical Exam (per Attending Physician)

Vital Signs Temp, 98.2 °F; pulse, 130; BP, 95/60; RR, 35; O_2 sat, 94% on 2 L nasal cannula

General Obese male; moderate distress

Cardiovascular Tachycardia, no murmurs, gallops, or rubs

Respiratory Tachypnea, moderate respiratory distress, clear breath sounds, and no wheezes

Abdomen Moderate epigastric tenderness, no guarding or rebound, and negative Murphy's sign

What Was Said?

During the examination by the resident physician, a PGY3 on his local community emergency medicine rotation, the patient notices that the resident doctor is wearing an iWatch with a rainbow-colored wristband. The patient grimaces and states, "I don't want no faggot touching or treating me." The astute young physician, who also bears a wedding band on his left hand from his newlywed husband, politely replies, "Sir, I do not appreciate the use of such harsh language. I am a proud gay male, and I have just as much experience as any other physician, and you will get the same treatment from me as you would from anyone else. I believe you are in diabetic ketoacidosis (DKA), and you are very sick right now. I would like to help you by examining you, ordering lab work, and giving you insulin and IV fluids. If you aren't treated, you could die from this condition." The patient rips off his nasal cannula and states, "Get out, or I will."

What Was Done?

The resident physician politely acknowledges the patient's request and exits the room. He updates the attending physician outside of the room, and the attending then enters the room to complete the rest of the history and exam. The attending physician exits the room after examining the patient and reports findings as above to the resident physician. The attending then advises the resident, "It probably would have been better to just acknowledge the patient's frustrations, and maybe you should not have told him you are a 'proud gay male.' I will take care of the patient from here to avoid any more disputes." The resident apologizes and continues to see other patients.

Questions for Discussion

1. Why did the patient become so combative?

Attitudes/Assumptions: The Resident Physician

(a) I am a doctor, and I have many years of training and schooling in my past. My sexual orientation should not be relevant to my care of the patient, and I know what is best for the patient.
(b) The patient is from a rural area, and he probably grew up in a town and family who are very conservative.
(c) The patient may not have the appropriate medical literacy to know what is best for his care and health.
(d) I probably should have just lied to the patient and said I was a straight male.

Attitudes/Assumptions: The Patient

(a) I have lived for 64 years, and I know what is best for my health. I can choose who I don't want as my doctor.

(b) This resident doctor is too young to be a doctor. He doesn't know what he's talking about.
(c) I don't want this gay doctor touching me; he may find me attractive or may have AIDS.

Attitudes/Assumptions: The Attending Physician

(a) This whole confrontation could have been avoided if the resident physician didn't wear the rainbow-colored watch.
(b) I've worked 30 years in medicine; the resident should say what the patient wants to hear because it's easier, and he should not have worn the rainbow iWatch band.

2. Was the communication between the attending and resident physician appropriate?

Attitudes/Assumptions: The Resident Physician

(a) I hope this experience won't have an effect on my evaluation by the attending.
(b) The attending must think I am less of a doctor because of this experience and the fact that I am a gay male. Does the attending perhaps share the same feelings as the patient?

Gaps in Provider Knowledge

(a) There is little to no formal education provided in medical schools to medical students about LGBT issues [1], and some heterosexual physicians have negative attitudes about caring for LGBT patients or working with LGBT coworkers [2].
(b) The lack of education in most medical training may lead to many attending physicians feeling uncomfortable working with LGBT patients and providers. In one study from 2011, physicians reported that they received no formal education in medical school on lesbian and gay content (61% for lesbian women, 49% for gay men) [2]. Less is known about graduate medical education. A study of emergency medicine training found that only 33% of programs

provided any LGBT education [3]. The average amount of time provided in programs who did participate was less than an hour [3].

(c) Gaps in provider knowledge have likely resulted in certain negative workplace experiences. In the same study cited above, 65% of responders experienced hearing disparaging remarks about the LGBT population, and 36% have witnessed discriminatory care of an LGBT patient [2].

(d) Medical school is a critical time for shaping future physicians' attitudes and treatment toward sexual minorities. Only 8.3% of medical schools teach comprehensive topics in LGBT health [1]. One study from 2015 found that a significant number of medical students had some type of bias toward gay and lesbian individuals (45.8% exhibited explicit bias, and 81.5% exhibited implicit bias) [4].

(e) Resources to provide education in LGBT patients and providers may be available within the medical school, such as a diversity office or diversity officer. In addition, many specialty organizations have diversity groups at both a local and national level.

Pearls and Pitfalls

Pearl The resident physician remained calm and polite to the patient during the entire encounter.

Pearl The resident physician did not take being called a derogatory term personally. He explained to the patient that his competency was not related to his sexual orientation and continued working and seeing other patients.

Pitfall The conversation between the attending and resident was rushed. The attending should have acknowledged the resident's frustrations and sat him down to listen to him.

Pitfall The resident is worried that his performance evaluation may be negatively impacted by this experience, and in some instances, this could be true.

Case Outcome

The attending physician completes the work-up and management of the patient's DKA. The patient improves after IV fluids and insulin and is admitted to the medicine service.

References

1. Obedin-Maliver J, Goldsmith ES, Stewart L, White W, Tran E, Brenman S, Wells M, Fetterman DM, Garcia G, Lunn MR. Lesbian, gay, bisexual, and transgender related content in under-graduate medical education. JAMA. 2011;306(9):971–7.
2. Eliason MJ, Dibble SL, Robertson PA. Lesbian, gay, bisexual, and transgender (LGBT) physicians' experiences in the workplace. J Homosex. 2011;58:1355–71.
3. Moll J, Krieger P, Moreno-Walton L, Lee B, Slaven E, James T, Hill D, Podolsky S, Corbin TL, Heron SL. The prevalence of lesbian, gay, bisexual, and transgender health education and training in emergency medicine residency programs: what do we know? Acad Emerg Med. 2014;21(5):608–11.
4. Burke SE, Dovidio JF, Przedworski JM, Harderman RR, Perry SP, Phelan SM, Nelson DB, Burgess DJ, Yeazel MW, van Ryn M. Do contact and empathy mitigate bias against gay and lesbian people among heterosexual first-year medical students. Acad Med. 2015;90(5):645–51.

Chapter 64
Interaction with a "Foreign Doctor"

Ugo A. Ezenkwele

Case Scenario

During an evening shift in a level 2 emergency department (ED), the phone rings, and a clerk announces that there is a call for an attending physician from a local nursing home. The nursing home doctor, Dr. Rembi, wants to transfer in a patient. Dr. Smith, an ED attending on duty who is Caucasian, picks up the phone and proceeds to get the details.

Dr. Smith answers: "What, what? Excuse me. What? Speak English. In this country, we speak English." A few seconds later, Dr. Smith looks at Dr. Clark, the other attending on duty, in exasperation, mutters under his breath, and hands him the phone. Standing next to Dr. Smith is a charge nurse, who is looking at both physicians. Dr. Clark answers, "Hello, Emergency Department." Dr. Clark hears a voice with a thick, raspy Southeast Asian accent that is difficult to understand. The conversation that follows is Dr. Clark's interpretation of what was said.

Dr. Rembi: "Allo, I 'ave a 84 year ol' who is beeding and sen' to you."

Dr. Clark: "Excuse me? What?"

Dr. Rembi: "Patient goin' to you."

Dr. Clark: "What happened? Is the patient stable? What are the vitals? How long?"

Dr. Rembi: "Soon."

Dr. Clark: "What happened?"

Dr. Rembi: "Started beeding dis moning...found by noise. Has ucer on bak. Blod pessur lo. We sen to you. Okay."

Dr. Clark: "Excuse me? Did you say blood pressure is low? How low? What did you do?"

U. A. Ezenkwele, MD, MPH
Department of Emergency Medicine, Mount Sinai Queens, Mount Sinai School of Medicine,
New York, NY, USA
e-mail: Ugo.ezenkwele@mountsinai.org

Dr. Rembi: "70 somthin. Flouids givn. Shuld be dere soon..."
Dr. Clark: "What?"

As Dr. Clark tries to understand what was said, he hears sirens getting louder and approaching the ambulance bay. Is this the patient? Dr. Clark tells the charge nurse who is waiting to hear what the notification is about: "I think there might be a GI bleeder coming in. Sounds like he might be unstable..."

Dr. Smith looks at Dr. Clark and states, "Those foreign docs. Don't know what they are doing. Always killing patients..."

The doors to the ED open and in comes a stretcher with a pale elderly man who is unresponsive. EMS is performing cardiac compressions and Dr. Clark rushes over. The medic looks at him and states, "84-year-old man who was found bleeding from a decubitus ulcer. Two large bore IVs were started and fluids given at the nursing home. We can't feel a pulse. Doc, he is lying in a pool of blood. He definitely bled out."

Dr. Clark goes into hyper mode, rushes the patient over to the critical care room, asks a colleague to establish a definitive airway, tells the nurse to place the patient on the monitor, and has a tech take over compressions. Next, Dr. Clark asks the clerk to initiate the massive transfusion protocol and tells them to send the initial two units of unmatched red blood cells to the ED as quickly as possible. Dr. Clark asks the paramedics for any written report from the nursing home, which the paramedic states was given to the triage nurse.

Vital signs are unable to be obtained. The patient is in pulseless electrical activity, and with compressions, a pulse in the 70s is generated. Several rounds of epinephrine are given. The patient is intubated and placement of the tube confirmed. Packed red blood cells are immediately initiated along with ongoing crystalloids. Surgery is notified and on their way. The blood bank notifies the attending that more products, including platelets, have been prepared and are on the way. Eventually, Dr. Clark notices an organized rhythm on the monitor, and the nurse informs him that she feels a pulse. Compressions are stopped and a strong pulse is felt. Dr. Clark's surgical colleagues arrive, the patient is turned, and the source of the bleeding is identified (a vein that is oozing from a sacral decubitus ulcer) and manually controlled with sutures. The patient is stabilized and eventually taken to the operating room for further exploration. From there he is transferred to the intensive care unit.

Dr. Smith states, "Those foreign doctors really don't know what they are doing, especially those from outside the country."

What Was Said?

A local nursing home doctor, Dr. Rembi, calls a level 2 emergency department to inform them that he is transferring a patient. Dr. Smith answers the phone and discovers that Dr. Rembi has a thick accent. Dr. Smith is overheard saying, "What, what? Excuse me. What? Speak English. In this country, we speak English." After becoming frustrated, Dr. Smith hands off the call to his colleague Dr. Clark who proceeds to speak with Dr. Rembi and obtains the history that an 84-year-old patient is being sent to the ED with a gastrointestinal bleed. After Dr. Clark informs the ED staff of the incoming patient, Dr. Smith says, "Those foreign docs. Don't know what they are doing. Always killing patients."

What Was Done?

The best history obtainable is procured from the nursing home doctor. Although fragmented and difficult to understand, Dr. Clark makes an effort to obtain the history instead of giving up in exasperation. Upon presentation, the patient was stabilized and admitted to the intensive care unit.

Questions for Discussion

1. What attitudes or gaps in knowledge interfered with the patient's care?

Attitudes/Assumptions: Dr. Smith

(a) Doctors who don't speak English well are foreign.
(b) Doctors who are foreign kill patients.
(c) Foreign doctors are improperly trained.

Attitudes/Assumptions: Dr. Rembi

(a) I have a sick patient who needs emergency care. I will have to speak with the ED staff and give a history even though they may have a hard time understanding what I am saying.

Gaps in Provider Knowledge

(a) Lack of knowledge regarding communication and how it impacts patient care: Poor communication does not obviate the need to obtain necessary information and prepare for patient care. Learn to recognize critical signs and address as necessary.

(b) Lack of knowledge regarding proper handoff of clinically unstable patient: Management and stabilization of patient supersede communication barriers.
(c) Lack of knowledge regarding foreign-trained doctors: Beware of generalizations. Learn about the process for foreign medical graduates to work in the USA [1].
(d) Lack of knowledge regarding the training of doctors outside the USA: Avoid stereotypes. Difficulty understanding language does not imply improper training [2].

2. What could the providers have done differently in this scenario?

Cross-Cultural Tools and Skills

(a) Assume that foreign sounding doctors are competent and know what they are doing.
(b) Assume that foreign sounding does not mean foreign trained.
(c) Obtain the best history using multiple modes of communication if verbal is difficult to understand.
(d) Understand that foreign-trained doctors are as competent as US medical graduates [3].
(e) Diversity education/sensitivity training may be helpful to Dr. Smith.

Pearls and Pitfalls

Pearl Obtain the best history that you can. Seek a written report if verbal communication presents a barrier.

Pearl Treat the patient as you would in any critical case.

Pitfall Communication barrier from thick accent and improper transfer of critical information.

Understand that in an emergency situation, depending on time of day, perhaps another attending physician would not be available to assist and the initial physician would have had to take the details of the pre-notification.

Case Outcome

Dr. Clark discusses the case with his colleague, Dr. Smith, and informs him that the best path would have been to get as many details of the case as possible, ask the notifying physician to prepare a written report to be sent as soon as possible electronically, and then prepare to receive the patient. Furthermore, Dr. Clark informs Dr. Smith that although a communication barrier exists, it does not indicate that the notifying provider is foreign trained or incompetent.

References

1. Chen PG, Nunez-Smith M, Bernheim SM, et al. Professional experiences of international medical graduates practicing primary care in the United States. J Gen Intern Med. 2010;25(9):947–53.
2. Coombs AA, King RK. Workplace discrimination: experiences of practicing physicians. J Natl Med Assoc. 2005;97(4):467–77.
3. Tsugawa Y, Jena AB, Orav JE, et al. Quality of care delivered by general internists in US hospitals who graduated from foreign versus US medical schools: observational study. BMJ. 2017;356:j273.

Chapter 65
Implicit Bias Illustrated by Attending-to-Attending Bias and Attending-to-Patient Bias

P. Preston Reynolds and Robert E. O'Connor

Case Scenario

GTA serves as the medical director of a local jail and also has an appointment as a full-time professor of medicine at the nearby medical school. She has been the medical director of the local jail for 2 years. The clinical staff of the jail includes a full-time nurse practitioner (NP), one registered nurse, and a dozen licensed practical nurses. In addition, there is a full-time Ph.D. nurse with specialty training in mental health, a part-time forensic psychiatrist, and a part-time dental team. Since GTA assumed this leadership role, the jail has implemented an electronic medical record (EMR); the clinical staff has revised all of the disease management protocols and has been trained in these updated protocols. In addition to GTA's oversight of the medical needs of the inmates, she oversees the dental program and works collaboratively with the psychiatrist and Ph.D. nurse specialist in the delivery of comprehensive mental health services. The jail recently received full accreditation by the Department of Corrections with a score of 100% for its medical, dental, and mental health care. Previously, the medical director was a male who had a joint appointment in the Department of Emergency Medicine at the nearby medical school.

GTA is called by the jail's NP to evaluate an inmate who is complaining of abdominal pain. GTA learns that AP, a 37-year-old woman who was arrested 2 months ago, started developing abdominal pain yesterday afternoon. Since the pain persisted, AP asked to be seen by one of the nurses, who after evaluating her, moved AP to the medical area of the jail just before GTA was called. GTA is on the way to the jail for weekly rounds and asks the nurse practitioner to get AP ready so she can be evaluated as soon as GTA arrives. The NP has seen her and shares that

P. Preston Reynolds (✉) · R. E. O'Connor
University of Virginia, Charlottesville, VA, USA
e-mail: pprestonreynolds@virginia.edu; reo4x@virginia.edu

© Springer International Publishing AG, part of Springer Nature 2019
M. L. Martin et al. (eds.), *Diversity and Inclusion in Quality Patient Care*,
https://doi.org/10.1007/978-3-319-92762-6_65

AP's pregnancy test is negative, she is febrile, and her abdominal examination is notable for rebound tenderness in the right lower quadrant.

AP tells GTA that her abdominal pain is getting worse, so much so that she now needs to curl up and remain very still to get any relief. AP describes the pain as 10 out of 10, the worst pain she has ever experienced. On examination, GTA notes that the inmate is febrile, tachycardiac, and has severe right lower quadrant pain with guarding and rebound. GTA is concerned the inmate has appendicitis and arranges for AP to be transferred to the emergency department at the nearby medical school. GTA calls the emergency physician on duty and speaks with a physician because she wants to be sure that the treating physician has background information in case this individual needs to be taken urgently to the operating room.

On the phone, GTA is greeted by a faculty colleague, who is well respected by other physicians, residents, and students. She communicates to the ED physician her physical examination findings of AP, the inmate, and her concern that AP may need surgery. Out of courtesy, GTA offers to send paperwork documenting her physical examination findings.

GTA is surprised when the ED physician shares he is not accustomed to thinking of a woman serving as the medical director of a jail. He questions her examination findings and need for urgent evaluation. He then says, "I wonder if the inmate is faking pain in an attempt to get out of the jail and into the hospital where she can get pain medications. It is very suspicious that this patient who has been arrested is now complaining of abdominal pain."

GTA realizes quickly that the ED physician's comments reflect his feelings about people who have been arrested and his concerns about her ability to serve in her role, but she knows she must ensure the safety of her patients who are incarcerated. GTA decides to page the chair of the Department of Emergency Medicine because the clinical situation demands the attention of a physician who will treat her patient, an inmate, with a commitment to excellence and professionalism.

Review of Symptoms

General AP last saw a primary care physician 2 years ago for a urinary tract infection. She believes she is up to date with her vaccinations. She complains of feeling febrile and noted last night that she had chills and sweats.

HEENT No visual changes, hearing loss or tinnitus, or seasonal allergies. She has had several months of dental pain. She has never seen a dentist and has not allowed the dentist in the jail to examine her teeth.

Cardiovascular No chest pain, palpitations, or lower extremity edema.

Respiratory No asthma, wheezing, shortness of breath, hemoptysis, cough, or pneumonia.

Abdomen No constipation, diarrhea, or bloody stool. The abdominal pain started yesterday afternoon and is getting worse. She is beginning to feel nauseous. She has not taken anything by mouth in 24 h.

Extremities No history of fractures, no loss of strength, no joint swelling, and no neck pain. She has low back discomfort that has been present since she was in a motor vehicle accident 3 years ago.

Neurological No history of seizures or headaches. She has had symptoms of previous drug withdrawal, usually from cocaine, but no hospitalizations for drug overdose.

GU No history of sexually transmitted diseases and no knowledge of HIV or Hep C status. She has never had a PAP smear. She denies performing sex acts in exchange for drugs. She denies any sexual activity in the past 2 months while incarcerated.

Skin History of acne during adolescence; no history of skin abscesses.

Past Medical History

She has a history of hypertension that required medication to control. With a 25-pound weight loss several years ago, her blood pressure returned to normal.

Past Surgical History None.

Family History

No history of inflammatory bowel disease, cancer, diabetes, hypertension, or coronary artery disease; there is a positive family history of mental illness, mostly bipolar disease complicated by alcohol and drug addiction.

Social History

She was living with her boyfriend when arrested. She uses cocaine regularly, and sometimes smokes marijuana to help her sleep. She denies the use of opiates or benzodiazepines. She has had a problem with alcohol in the past, but has been abstinent for the past year.

Tobacco One pack per day, before being incarcerated, and 15 pack-year history. She thinks smoking calms her nerves.

Children Two children, ages 10 years and 14 years, both of whom live with their father.

Education Graduated from high school.

Employment She has not been able to keep a regular full-time job, but when she is doing well, she works as a waitress at a nearby diner.

Physical Exam

Vital Signs BP = 158/96, T = 103.3, P = 112, R – 20, O_2 sat = 98%

General She appears very uncomfortable and in pain as she lays curled up trying not to move.

HEENT PERRL, EOMI, no cervical or supraclavicular lymphadenopathy, and neck supple. Mucous membranes are somewhat dry.

Cardiovascular Tachycardiac, S1, S2, no murmurs, rubs, or gallops.

Respiratory No wheezes, rhonchi, or rales; no pain on deep inspiration.

Abdomen Guarding with rebound on palpation of the right lower quadrant, diminished bowel sounds throughout, and increased pain with extension of right leg when lying on the left side.

Extremities 5/5 strength in upper and lower extremities; full range of motion.

Skin Hot, flushed, intact without signs of IV drug use, and no track marks or abscesses.

Neuro Cranial Nerves II–XII intact; normal reflexes throughout.

What Was Said?

GTA informs the ED physician that she needs to ensure the safety and care of her patients in the local jail and is concerned enough with his comments that she believes she needs to ask for additional help. GTA calls the chair of Emergency Medicine, BE, whom she knows well. She and BE worked together to improve emergency care of people injured and brought to the jail who needed to be transferred to the hospital first. Safe transfer and quality care have been their priority as they have worked on several community-health system initiatives.

GTA speaks with BE, who agrees that the statements made by the ED physician were not appropriate and offers to stop over in the ED. He is in a meeting and asks GTA to page him when the inmate leaves the jail so that he can meet the patient when she arrives.

What Was Done?

BE calls the ED physician, who agrees to evaluate the patient in the ED, and reaffirms the need for urgent surgical consultation because of the possibility of an impending rupture of her appendix. A CT confirms the presence of an inflamed appendix with fluid. The surgical team sees the patient and agrees to take AP to the operating room. During surgery, the surgeons find an inflamed, non-ruptured, appendix that is then removed. AP is sent to the floor for post-op care and pain medications. Her post-op course is uneventful, and after 48 h, she is returned to the jail where she is housed in the medical area since she is still requiring narcotic pain medications.

GTA decides to talk with BE about the comments of the ED physician. They discuss the unprofessional behavior, both the comments about GTA's appointment as medical director of the local jail and derogatory reflections about the patient. GTA has recently recertified in internal medicine and serves as a tenured, full-professor in the medical school where she is active as a clinician and teacher of medical students, residents, and faculty. BE and GTA brainstorm on how the unprofessional lapses can be addressed in a way that may help the ED faculty and staff.

GTA is a member of the medical school's diversity consortium and also serves in a leadership role in her department on issues of diversity and professionalism. She is aware of implicit bias training offered through the medical school's Office of Diversity and Inclusion, which faculty members in her own department are required to take. She suggests the ED faculty could be invited to participate in this training. GTA also knows the authors of the Implicit Association Test, an online test that assesses individual biases, and offers to ask if they are interested in creating a test that examines attitudes toward incarcerated persons.

BE thinks basic training on implicit bias would be a good start since he has heard that the workshop offered through the Office of Diversity and Inclusion has been appreciated by faculty in other departments in the medical school. He thinks, however, that everyone in the ED, including the staff and residents, should be encouraged to do the training.

For almost a decade, GTA has been conducting a longitudinal series of workshops on professionalism with the residents in her department and recently integrated implicit bias training into her introductory seminar on professionalism, which also addresses the topic of professional lapses. She asks BE if his faculty might be interested in a session on race conscious professionalism. She shares that she has found the residents' self-awareness of their own biases and a deeper understanding of professionalism in clinical medicine has improved the overall learning climate in internal medicine and the residents' ability to be effective role models, especially with students and other residents.

BE thinks GTA's ideas are a good beginning and decides to bring up the topic of implicit bias training and professional lapses at the next departmental meeting. He also offers to talk directly to the ED physician because he knows that his comments about the jail inmate and GTA's new role as medical director of the jail are inappropriate.

Questions for Discussion

1. Is implicit bias relevant in academic medicine? In higher education [1, 2]?

   (a) Does implicit bias serve as a barrier to hiring, recruitment, or academic advancement of women? At what levels: students, residents, fellows, faculty, and/or administrative leaders such as deans, provosts, and chief operating officers?
   (b) Does implicit bias serve as a barrier to hiring, recruitment, or academic advancement of minority persons in the health professions? At what levels: students, residents, fellows, faculty, and/or administrative leaders such as deans, provosts, and chief operating officers?

2. Does implicit bias impact clinical care provided to patients [1, 3–6]?

   (a) Does this impact occur in acute care settings, in ambulatory settings?
   (b) Is there evidence that implicit bias impacts the care of patients seen in an emergency room?
   (c) Are there certain types of patients that are impacted more by implicit bias, such as minorities, elderly persons, disabled persons, or incarcerated persons? What populations of patients experience worse clinical outcomes because of implicit bias?
   (d) Are younger generations of physicians protected against implicit bias and its impact on clinical decision-making [4, 7]?

3. What training is necessary for the medical director and the clinic staff of a jail?

   (a) Does GTA need to obtain additional training since all of the patients in the local jail are adults and she is board certified in internal medicine?
   (b) What other healthcare professionals should be part of the team of providers who care for inmates?
   (c) What training should this group of health professionals have to ensure quality care is provided to inmates of a jail?

(d) What type of relationships should the medical staff of the jail establish with local providers?

(e) Should local physicians be expected to provide care to inmates if inmates need expertise beyond the training of the jail medical, mental, or dental health staff?

Attitudes/Assumptions: The Patient

(a) Inmates of local jails have the right to health care.

(b) Incarcerated persons should be treated the same as all other persons seeking medical, mental health, or dental care.

(c) Inmates of local jails should be able to receive pain medications post-op, such as opiates, when they are returned to the jail from a hospital.

(d) Persons who are incarcerated should be able to see specialists in the community if they are diagnosed with a disease requiring specialized care?

Attitudes/Assumptions: The Physician

(a) The ED physician demonstrated bias toward the female medical director of the local jail.

(b) The ED physician demonstrated bias toward the inmate patient.

(c) The ED physician responded appropriately to coaching related to an unprofessional lapse in conduct.

(d) The ED physician addressed his internist colleague with appropriate communication and insight related to unprofessional lapse in conduct and communication

Gaps in Provider Knowledge

GTA, a board-certified internist, is qualified to care for inmates in the jail, with the exclusion of persons who are pregnant. The jail policy is to refer all inmates for specialty care when their conditions warrant specialized services. This also includes advanced dental procedures. The jail psychiatrists are trained in the care of the mentally ill and in forensic psychiatry. The nursing staff, beyond skills in nursing, are trained in the use of protocols. The NP and the medical director are available 24/7 to assist the nursing staff if any questions arise.

Pearls and Pitfalls

Pearl Professional lapses are common and most often result from stresses in the clinical environment along with unawareness of inherent biases and skills in managing challenging situations. They are best addressed immediately and professionally with a focus on behaviors the individual would like to demonstrate, along with expectations for professional conduct, skills in helping an individual become more aware of their biases, and ways to reduce the impact of biases in clinical decision-making. [8].

Pitfall Professional lapses are breaches of professional conduct that do not reflect a health professional's character, but instead reflect the culture of an institution, inherent biases, and a lack of skills training in self-awareness and self-correction [8].

Case Outcome

AP returned to the medical area of the jail where she was housed for 3 days. She received narcotic pain medication for another 48 h and then transitioned to ibuprofen. She remained afebrile, tolerated all foods and fluids, and maintained a normal bowel regimen. She returned to the women's area of the jail once signs of illness were gone. She was released shortly thereafter.

BE spoke with the ED physician about his lapse in professional conduct. The ED physician admitted that he knew what he said was wrong as soon as he had spoken. It had been a particularly stressful day, and while he had been unusually busy in the ED that evening with a trauma involving several people, he knew his comments about GTA's role as a woman physician serving as medical director of the jail and the medical needs of her inmate were not what he really meant to say [1, 2, 8, 9]. He offered to call GTA, which he did. GTA thanked her colleague for his call and for his encouragement of her in her new role. She was able to express her appreciation for the care he provided her patient once she was transferred to the ED since the jail is limited in what the clinicians are able to do, especially in any acute situation. They shared the challenges of maintaining ideal professional behaviors in stressful situations, and both hoped there were not any medical students or residents around who might have overheard his comments [7].

BE also decided to move forward with implicit bias and professionalism training and reached out to GTA and the Associate Dean for Diversity and Inclusion for guidance. BE and GTA's collaboration continued in an effort to improve the safety and quality of care in their own institution.

References

1. Project Implicit; c2011 [cited 2017 Dec 7]. Available from: https://implicit.harvard.edu/implicit/takeatest.html.
2. Lewis D, Paulsen E, editors. Proceedings of the diversity and inclusion innovation forum: unconscious bias in academic medicine. 2014 Diversity and Inclusion Forum, 2014 June. Washington: AAMC; 2017. 105 p. Jointly published by The Kirwan Institute for the Study of Race and Ethnicity.
3. Dividio JF, Penner LA, Albrecht TL, Norton WE, Gaetner SL, Shelton JN. Disparities and distrust: the implications of psychological processes for understanding racial disparities in health and health care. Soc Sci Med. 2008;67:478–86.
4. Green AR, Carney DR, Pallin DJ, Ngo LH, Raymond KL, Iezzoni LI, Banaji MR. Implicit bias among physicians and its prediction of thrombolysis decisions for black and white patients. J Gen Intern Med. 2007;22:1231–8.
5. Smedley BD, Stith AY, Nelson AR, editors. Unequal treatment: confronting racial and ethnic disparities in healthcare. Washington: National Academies Press; 2003. 780 p.
6. Schulman KA, Berlin JA, Harless W, Kerner JF, Sistrunk S, Gersh BJ, et al. The effect of race and sex on physicians recommendations for cardiac catheterization. N Engl J Med. 1999;340:618–26.
7. White-Means S, Dong Z, Hufstader M, Brown LT. Cultural competency, race and skin tone bias among pharmacy, nursing and medical students: implications for addressing health disparities. Med Care Res Rev. 2009;66:436–55.
8. Levinson W, Ginsberg S, Hafferty FW, Lucey CR. Chapter 11 When things go wrong: the challenge of self-regulation. In: Understanding medical professionalism. New York: McGraw-Hill Education; 2014. p. 243–75.
9. Risberg G, Johansson EE, Hamberg K. A theoretical model for analyzing gender bias in medicine. Int J Equity Health. 2009;8(28). https://doi.org/10.1186/1475-9276-8-28.

Chapter 66
Faculty Toward Faculty Barriers and Bias

Amy Cohee and Michael D. Williams

Case Scenario

An associate professor of endocrinology, Dr. Bayley, is scheduled to a see a new patient in the clinic for establishing diabetic care. As the patient is being placed in a room, Dr. Bayley receives a call that his 10-year-old son needs to be picked up from school due to vomiting. Dr. Bayley's wife frequently travels for business and is not often available for urgent childcare issues. Dr. Bayley turns to one of his partners, Dr. Winstead, and says, "I apologize for the inconvenience, but my son's school just called and said that he needs to be picked up immediately because he is vomiting. Do you have time to see a new patient that is on my schedule?"

Dr. Winstead declines and says, "Why can't your wife pick him up? You shouldn't have to deal with things like that."

Dr. Bayley speaks to his scheduler and cancels the rest of his appointments for the afternoon. Dr. Bayley speaks with the patient in the clinic and lets her know that their visit will be shortened today due to a personal emergency. He offers to see her when he returns to the office in half an hour. She agrees and waits. Dr. Bayley picks up his son, brings him to his office, sees the patient, and then takes his son home for the rest of the day.

A. Cohee (✉)
University of Virginia, Charlottesville, VA, USA
e-mail: asc3zj@hscmail.mcc.virginia.edu

M. D. Williams
UVA Center for Health Policy, The Frank Batten School of Leadership and Public Policy and School of Medicine, University of Virginia, Charlottesville, VA, USA

University of Virginia Health System, Charlottesville, VA, USA
e-mail: mdw9g@hscmail.mcc.virginia.edu

© Springer International Publishing AG, part of Springer Nature 2019
M. L. Martin et al. (eds.), *Diversity and Inclusion in Quality Patient Care*,
https://doi.org/10.1007/978-3-319-92762-6_66

Dr. Bayley receives his quarterly review and is dismayed to find a comment about allowing childcare pickup to interfere with his professional commitments, given that the incident was a one-time occurrence. He worries about his tenure review and whether he is viewed as unreliable or not dedicated to his work.

What Was Said?

Dr. Bayley: "I apologize for the inconvenience, but my son's school just called and said that he needs to be picked up immediately because he is vomiting. Do you have time to see a new patient that is on my schedule?"
Dr. Winstead: "Why can't your wife pick him up? You shouldn't have to deal with things like that."

What Was Done?

Dr. Winstead declined to cover the patient encounter. Dr. Bayley informed the patient of the reason for the delay, canceled the rest of his patient appointments for the afternoon, picked up his son, returned to finish the patient encounter, and then took his son home.

Question for Discussion

1. What attitudes and assumptions are apparent in this interaction?

Attitudes/Assumptions: Dr. Winstead

Dr. Winstead expressed bias in favor of a "traditional" family structure in which the male partner works outside the home and the female partner works inside the home and cares for children. In many modern families, this structure no longer applies. Bias may be applied to a male colleague, as in this case, when Dr. Winstead assumed Dr. Bayley's wife should/could pick up their sick son. In addition, bias may affect a female colleague if someone assumes she will have children and will have personal conflicts due to being the primary caregiver. A further assumption is that Dr. Bayley is married and that the spouse is female.

Attitudes/Assumptions: Dr. Bayley

Dr. Bayley assumes that demands of child-rearing, including the unforeseeable, are valued in his department/practice. As a result of a family-related issue, Dr. Bayley investigates the possibility that his coworker may be willing to help with coverage.

Gaps in Provider Knowledge

Both providers may lack insight into the other provider's perspective, both of which may have value. Healthcare providers must juggle personal and professional commitments, which are both important and legitimate. It is likely that these commitments will come into conflict in the context of one individual's responsibilities or within one's practice, division, or department. Additionally, both parties may be ignorant of the social circumstances of the other, as well as potentially being unaware of the compensation model for each individual in the group that may either encourage or discourage collaboration.

Men and women can experience bias within the workplace based on sex, gender, and/or sexual orientation. Women may experience bias regarding perceived familial responsibilities, as societal "norms" often cast them as the child-rearing parent. Conversely, men may also experience gender bias if they are engaged in household or child-rearing activities. It is increasingly common for men and women to individualize the division of professional and personal labor (i.e., more women work outside of the home in professional, paraprofessional, and labor roles, while more men work inside the home and provide childcare) [1–5]. Same-sex/same-gender couples and single individuals can also experience workplace bias, as "traditional" patriarchal roles do not apply. Long-standing discrimination against those who are perceived as different creates additional layers of bias [3].

Cross-Cultural Tools and Skills

Practicing respectful and clear communication when conflict arises is key to the success of individuals and teams. Every healthcare provider will have conflicts of some kind outside of work during his or her career. Communicating about these conflicts respectfully with colleagues, without making assumptions about family structure or professional availability, is crucial to good patient care and healthcare professional wellness. Achieving professional equity and transparency is also foundational to the short- and long-term success of any professional organization.

Pearls and Pitfalls

Pearl Have workplace policies in place that define contingencies for all employees. Allow for emergency situations, specifically those that do not directly involve the professional employee.

Pearl Build a team-based model into the work environment, such that no single team member's sudden absence cannot readily be overcome.

Pearl Recognize that career advancement, including promotion and tenure, may be influenced by family status. Women and men may both be penalized for events that impair their productivity at work. Examples include foreseeable parenting responsibilities like parent-teacher conferences, school field trips, or performances and the unforeseeable like family emergencies that do not directly involve the parent. This is a difficult balance to achieve, as a medical practice relies on its providers and employees to be predictably and reliably available to deliver professional services in a patient-centric manner. Concomitantly, a practice must offer a professionally nurturing environment to physicians, nurses, and other staff that promotes retention, professional achievement, and well-being all while meeting "bottom-line" targets in order to be sustainable.

Pitfall Do not make assumptions regarding the relationship or parenthood status of fellow team members.

Case Outcome

Dr. Bayley successfully rescheduled his patients. His son missed 2 days of school, and his absence prompted the Bayleys to identify several emergency childcare providers. In addition, they advocated for a system-wide hospital program to help employees cover emergency-dependent care.

Dr. Bayley continued to work diligently in his practice, and despite the critical remark on his quarterly review, he continued to successfully meet targets for tenure consideration.

References

1. Juhn C, Potter S. Changes in labor force participation in the United States. J Econ Perspect. 2006;20(3):27–46.
2. Livingston G. Growing number of dads home with the kids: biggest increase among those caring for family [Internet]. Washington: Pew Research Center; 2014 Jun 4

[cited 2017 Nov 16]. Available from: http://www.pewsocialtrends.org/2014/06/05/growing-number-of-dads-home-with-the-kids/.

3. Vespa J, Lewis JM, Kreider RM. America's families and living arrangements: 2012. Washington: United States Census Bureau; 2013. 34 p. Report No.: P20–570.

4. Laughlin L. Who's minding the kids? Child care arrangements: spring 2011. Washington: United States Census Bureau; 2013. 23 p. Report No.: P70–135.

5. Yu PT, Parsa PV, Hassanein O, Rogers SO, Chang DC. Minorities struggle to advance in academic medicine: a 12-y review of diversity at the highest levels of America's teaching institutions. J Surg Res. 2013;182(2):212–8.

Chapter 67
Pharmacist to Physician: "Are You Really a Doctor?"

Marcus L. Martin, DeVanté J. Cunningham, and Emmanuel Agyemang-Dua

Case Scenario

On New Year's Day, Dr. Michael Wilson, an African-American physician, and his wife, Mrs. Sandra Wilson, traveled to their vacation home in a remote coastal community. Dr. Wilson had grown a heavy beard, as he often plays Santa Claus for his grandchildren. The previous week, the Wilsons were visiting their children and young grandchildren for the holidays. All of the grandchildren had respiratory infections. During that time, Mrs. Wilson began experiencing increased symptoms related to sinusitis and bronchitis. As the Wilsons traveled, Mrs. Wilson's symptoms began to worsen. Based on the symptoms and Mrs. Wilson's respiratory medical history, Dr. Wilson decided to prescribe Mrs. Wilson an antibiotic.

On the evening of New Year's Day, Dr. Wilson stopped at a small pharmacy approximately 20 miles from the vacation home to write a prescription for the antibiotic for his wife. Due to the remote nature of their vacation home, the time of day, and the holiday season, Mrs. Wilson's primary care physician and healthcare facilities were not readily available. Dr. Wilson is a credentialed healthcare provider with current DEA and state medical licensure. He has prescribed medication for his wife on rare occasions in the past and felt that she absolutely needed medication for this illness. Dr. Wilson observed that the pharmacy did not appear busy on this occasion.

M. L. Martin (✉) · E. Agyemang-Dua
University of Virginia, Charlottesville, VA, USA
e-mail: mlm8n@virginia.edu; ea9cf@virginia.edu

D. J. Cunningham
Clinical Psychology, Montclair State University, Montclair, NJ, USA
e-mail: cunninghamd3@montclair.edu

After entering the pharmacy, Dr. Wilson approached the counter and asked to speak with the pharmacist. Dr. Wilson properly identified himself to the white male pharmacist on duty and stated that he would like to write a prescription for his wife for an antibiotic. The pharmacist replied, "You can write the prescription on your pad." Dr. Wilson stated that he did not have his pad and would like to use the pharmacy prescription pad. After a brief conversation, the pharmacist agreed to allow Dr. Wilson to write the prescription on the pharmacy prescription pad.

The pharmacist then began to ask questions to verify the identity of Dr. Wilson. Dr. Wilson provided his business card, DEA card, medical license, and driver's license, as well as his medical insurance card. The pharmacist appropriately looked in his physician database for information about Dr. Wilson and asked him for work phone numbers. Dr. Wilson complied but felt that the pharmacist was inordinately interrogating him about his credentials.

The pharmacist expressed his opinion that it is inappropriate for doctors to write prescriptions for family members. Dr. Wilson indicated that in this situation he felt it was appropriate to write a prescription for an antibiotic and that he would document the treatment in a medical record, as is standard procedure [1, 2].

The encounter with the pharmacist took a long time, so Dr. Wilson indicated that he would be willing to come back the next day, which would require driving 20 miles in both direction, at which point the pharmacist finally filled the prescription. The prescription, Augmentin 500 mg TID disp no. 30, was filled by the pharmacist.

As Dr. Wilson was paying for the antibiotic, he asked the pharmacy technician the name of the pharmacist. The technician replied that the pharmacist's name was Mr. Boxley.

Review of Symptoms (Mrs. Wilson)

Chief complaint: Cough, productive thick yellow spectrum; nasal drainage yellow mucous; symptoms worsened over the past 2 days.
Present illness: Flu-like symptoms for 1 week since visiting with grandchildren; no fever, mild wheezing.

Past Medical History

Sinusitis, bronchitis, pneumonia, pulmonary embolus, breast cancer, hypertension, type II diabetes mellitus, multinodular thyroid goiter.

Medications HCTZ 25 mg qd, Tylenol cold/sinus prn, Albuterol 2 puffs PRN q 4 h, ASA 81 mg qd, KCL 10 meq qd, Calcium +D 600–200 mg 2 tabs daily, Advair Diskus 250–50 mcg/dose 1 puff q 12 h, Prednisone tapered dose (periodically).

Allergy Latex, seasonal allergies.

Family History

Mrs. Wilson is a breast cancer survivor and has been married to Mr. Wilson for over 40 years.

Social History

Noncontributory.

Physical Exam

Head PERRLA

ENT Neck supple, mild sinus pressure to touch, nasal mucous drainage, throat mild erythema, TMs (did not examine), no exudate.

Cardiovascular RRR

Respiratory Mild wheezing diffusely.

Abdomen Non-tender

Extremities Normal, no edema.

Skin Warm/dry

Neuro Alert and oriented.

Diagnosis Sinusitis, bronchitis.

Questions for Discussion

1. What were the attitudes and assumptions during this encounter?

Attitudes/Assumptions: The Physician

(a) I am the husband of the patient. I am not her primary care physician but am knowledgeable about her medical history, and after doing a thorough exam and taking factors into consideration, I believe she has sinusitis and bronchitis.
(b) It is a common practice to treat relatives and family members in case of emergency or in scenarios of isolation where the family member's primary care physician is indisposed.
(c) I am a physician, and I have gone through this process before; I believe it shouldn't be this complicated.
(d) Asking for a prescription pad is an appropriate request.
(e) The pharmacist is being rude. I am taken aback by the extensive request for credentials.

Attitudes/Assumptions: The Pharmacist

(a) This bearded, black man presents as a physician and is arrogant.
(b) I need to assert my clout and vet this man to show him this is my pharmacy and not his to make requests (asking for a prescription pad). It is my obligation as the pharmacist to request several documents of identification to validate this black man's claim that he is a doctor.
(c) This doctor has no choice but to cooperate with my requests if he wants to get this antibiotic prescription for his wife.
(d) I feel threatened by Dr. Wilson asking my pharmacy technician for my name.

2. What was done?

Gaps in Provider Knowledge: The Pharmacist

(a) Lack of understanding of health professions regulations regarding prescriptions for family members
(b) Lack of cultural sensitivity

Case Outcome

Mr. Boxley overheard the request for his name, and on the following day, January 2, he sent a formal complaint to the state Department of Health Professions (DHP), likely retaliatory in an attempt to mitigate in case the physician filed a complaint about his lack of professionalism.

In the pharmacist's formal complaint, he stated, "I guess the best an Afro-American can be in this country is President of the USA [Barack Obama] and that is not good enough? So angry African-American medical license holders are allowed to harass and pull the race card on Caucasian pharmacists." He further stated, "What a total disgrace this man is to his profession."

At no time did Dr. Wilson raise his voice at the pharmacist, "banter" him, or "become arrogant throwing all sorts of cards on the pharmacy counter" as was reported to the DHP by Mr. Boxley. The physician did not pull the "race card" but provided his bona fide driver's license, professional business card, medical license, and DEA number. An investigation was opened on the case by the DHP, and it was deemed that the physician, Dr. Wilson, had done nothing wrong. Dr. Wilson did not file a counter complaint against the pharmacist.

Physicians should not be a regular prescriber of medication for family members. However, in accordance with health professions regulations, medications prescribed to cover a single episode of treatment while in a remote setting with documented records is an ethical practice [1, 2]. Importantly, Mrs. Wilson recovered from severe sinusitis and bronchitis, and she subsequently followed up with her primary care physician.

References

1. Rakatansky H. AMA code of medical ethics available online. Virtual Mentor. 2001;3(4)
2. American Medical Association. AMA code of medical ethics [Internet]. Chicago: American Medical Association; 2017 [cited 2017 Nov 14]. Available from: https://www.ama-assn.org/delivering-care/ama-code-medical-ethics.

Chapter 68
"Send the White Doctor in Charge"

Brenda Oiyemhonlan and Teresa Y. Smith

Case Scenario

A 36-year-old right-handed male presents to the emergency department in police custody for evaluation of right shoulder pain for one day. Per the patient, prior to being apprehended, he was riding his bike when he experienced a mechanical fall. He states that he struck his shoulder on the concrete. He endorses pain at the anterior aspect of the shoulder; however, he denies weakness, numbness, or tingling. The provider is a physician born outside of the United States.

Review of Symptoms

Constitutional: No weight loss, fever, chills, weakness, or fatigue
Positive for anterior shoulder pain. No forearm, elbow, or wrist pain, no back pain or stiffness; all other review of symptoms negative

Past Medical History

Right rotator cuff injury

B. Oiyemhonlan (✉)
University of California, San Francisco, Department of Emergency Medicine,
Zuckerberg San Francisco General Hospital, San Francisco, CA, USA
e-mail: brenda.oiyemhonlan@ucsf.edu

T. Y. Smith
SUNY Downstate/Kings County Hospital, Department of Emergency Medicine,
Brooklyn, NY, USA
e-mail: Teresa.Smith@downstate.edu

© Springer International Publishing AG, part of Springer Nature 2019   471
M. L. Martin et al. (eds.), *Diversity and Inclusion in Quality Patient Care*,
https://doi.org/10.1007/978-3-319-92762-6_68

Family History

No relevant family history

Social History

Patient is unemployed, resides in San Francisco, California, and has an unstable living environment. He endorses tobacco, marijuana, and alcohol use. He denies health insurance and has no primary care provider. Currently, the patient is in police custody.

Physical Exam

Vital Signs Temp, 98.9 C; blood pressure, 120/80; respiratory rate, 20; heart rate, 62; O_2, 98%; glucose, not recorded.

General Alert, sitting up in bed, well appearing and in hospital gown; airway patent; the patient is speaking in full sentences.

Respiratory Breath sounds bilateral; no respiratory distress; no cyanosis.

Cardiovascular Circulation reveals warm dry skin. Normal capillary refill; pulses equal and present throughout.

Extremities No obvious signs of shoulder dislocation; full range of motion at the shoulder, elbow, and wrist joint; able to externally and internally rotate with no discomfort; negative empty can test; 5/5 strength, normal range of motion, and no swollen or erythematous joints.

Skin No bruises, abrasions, or rashes; the skin otherwise warm and dry and no erythematous areas.

The rest of the exam is unremarkable.

Dr. Abadi knocks at the examination room door. "Good Afternoon. My name is Dr. Abadi. I apologize for your long wait, Mr. Brown and officers. How can I help you today?" (Provider washes her hands prior to walking over to the patient and sits on a stool beside the patient.)

Patient: "My shoulder hurts."
Dr. Abadi: "Can you tell me what happened today? When did your shoulder begin to hurt you?"
Patient: "I was riding my bike and I fell on the concrete. I had a previous injury to my shoulder and I wanted to be sure that my shoulder wasn't broken."

Dr. Abadi: "Okay. Are you experiencing any discomfort at this time? Any weakness, numbness, or tingling in your arm?"

Patient: "No."

Dr. Abadi: "May I ask you another series of questions?"

Patient: "Do whatever you need to do."

Dr. Abadi commences and completes the review of symptoms: only significant for shoulder pain.

Dr. Abadi: "May I evaluate your shoulder?"

Patient: "It's here."

Dr. Abadi commences and completes the physical exam.

Dr. Abadi: "Okay, sir. Based on your exam, I believe that you likely have a muscle contusion or bruise. I do not believe that you will require any additional treatment at this time. For your pain and discomfort..." The patient cuts Dr. Abadi off, stating, "I think I need a MRI."

Dr. Abadi: "Is there a reason why you believe that you need a MRI, Mr. Brown?"

Patient: "I think that my shoulder is broken."

Dr. Abadi: "Based on my clinical evaluation, I do not believe that any imaging (i.e., X-ray) is required at this time. Typically, a MRI is ordered if there is a concern for a ligamentous injury or if you continue to have the shoulder pain despite negative plain films and adequate treatment. However, based on the history you shared with me today regarding your shoulder pain and my examination of your shoulder, I do not believe that you have a fracture, dislocation, or ligamentous injury."

Patient: "I want to see a white American doctor. I want to see your boss."

Dr. Abadi: "Is there a reason why you no longer feel comfortable with our current interaction?"

Patient: "I think I need a CT scan or MRI. I just want to see a white doctor."

Dr. Abadi: "I am the attending physician, and the only doctor available to care for you this evening."

Patient: "Whatever."

What Was Said?

The patient requested to be cared for by a white American doctor after possibly not believing that the foreign-born physician was competent or that his medical care might have resulted in a another outcome in some way if the provider was different.

What Was Done?

The provider informs the patient that there is no other physician to care for him and does attempt to understand why the patient no longer has faith in her clinical decision making.

The provider is protected by Title VII of the 1964 Civil Rights Act to work in an environment that is free of discrimination based on sex, race, and religious background [1].

No report was filed about the interaction. The provider did review the diversity and inclusion policy at the institution to determine if there was any guidance on handling these types of scenarios. She also discussed the case with the chief of service of the emergency department to determine if there were any previous clinical encounters similar to this and what resources were available to employees to manage these types of scenarios. She was informed that an Office of Diversity does exist at the health system, and there are support groups available for women and under-represented staff members.

Question for Discussion

1. What might have prompted the patient's request for a different provider?

Attitudes/Assumptions: The Patient

(a) The foreign-born doctor is not competent.
(b) My medical care might be better with another doctor.

The patient is initially cooperative with the examination and allows the provider to evaluate him. When the provider decides not to order the imaging requested by the patient, the patient dissatisfied with his medical care. The patient then requests to be cared for by someone of a different ethnic background. A patient who has the capacity to make decisions has the right to refuse medical care. Under EMTALA, the hospital must provide emergency screening and stabilization for all patients [1].

Gaps in Provider Knowledge

The provider's response is to state that she is the only attending to care for the patient at this time. This may be true due to limited staffing. The gap in provider knowledge in addressing the situation is based on the lack of communication and further discussion with the patient. The provider could further inquire as to why the patient is dissatisfied with his care. This further questioning may allow the provider to discover that it is not the racial or gender difference that makes that patient uncomfortable but the fact that there was no imaging in the assessment of his shoulder pain. In addition, further investigation as to why the patient does not want to be cared for by a foreign-born provider could have been explored.

Patient-physician ethnic concordance may be warranted for religious and/or cultural purposes (e.g., a Muslim female patient who requests to be cared for by a female physician).

Cross-Cultural Tools and Skills

Paul-Emile et al. discuss a strategic algorithm of how to address situations where patients request a change in physicians based on sex, race, or religious background [1]. The authors encourage providers to determine if the request is reasonable first, based on the medical condition of the patient. All patients deemed unstable should be immediately treated by the assigned physician. Those patients who are stable should then be assessed for their decision-making capacity, with those lacking capacity to have treatment by the physician as the situation deems reasonable. But for those patients who are discriminating based on bigotry with no justifiable cause (e.g., the request of concordant language or religious practices), the decision to comply with the request to change assigned physicians should be made based on the impact the reassignment will have on the treating physician. Despite the decision, the hospital should make it clear to the patient that discriminatory practices are not accepted nor tolerated in their facility. Passive compliance with a patient's request for physician transfer based on racial or ethnic background can be viewed as a tepid agreement with discrimination, and thus, in a professional manner, a statement of anti-discrimination should be made [2]. Through this algorithm, discussion, negotiation, and persuasion are used to improve the patient-physician relationship and create an environment that is a compromise for all parties while doing what is best for the medical condition of the patient.

Pearls and Pitfalls

Pearl Healthcare organizations can become more proactive about marketing their diversity and inclusion values. To date, it is unclear how many organizations actively promote and disseminate their institutional diversity and inclusion guidelines. By educating the public on acceptable behavior and attitudes that can be exhibited while accessing care from institutions, we may be able to preempt scenarios discussed above. Perhaps there should be signage in the facility entrance and exit locations and acute care areas that display the hospital's diversity and inclusion principles. They could also be made publicly available on consent to treatment forms. In addition to general information on the facility's diversity and inclusion policies, perhaps there can also be instructions and guidance on acceptable patient interaction and engagement with clinical staff.

Pitfall According to the US Census Bureau, "foreign-born" refers to anyone who is not a US citizen at birth. This includes naturalized US citizens, legal permanent residents, temporary immigrants, humanitarian migrants, and unauthorized migrants. There are over 40 million foreign-born immigrants in the US, and approximately 10 million of those immigrants reside in the state of California. This accounts for approximately 28% of the state population. The other large concentrations of foreign-born immigrants reside in the states of Nevada, Texas, Florida, and New York. Prior to this current time, there have been underpinnings of negative immigrant sentiment in the United States. However, these ideas have recently been given a platform by the executive branch of the federal government, and thus government and non-governmental organizations have needed to double down on their diversity and inclusion policies in order to promote and preserve the previous administration's interest in increasing globalization and US engagement in and leveraging of cultural exchange. Most academic medical centers have developed several institutional diversity platforms and organizational frameworks such as the idea of cultural humility, which is a construct that is defined as having an interpersonal stance that is other-oriented rather than self-focused, characterized by respect and lack of superiority toward an individual's cultural background and experience [3]. This framework is an alternative paradigm to the pervasive cultural competency construct, which relies on privileged groups becoming experts in the plight of underserved or under-recognized communities. In contrast, the aspects of cultural humility include a lifelong commitment to self-evaluation and self-critique, a desire to fix power imbalances, and an aspiration to develop partnerships with people and groups who advocate for others.

The decision to reassign a patient based on their preferences, which may be based on sex, race, and religious discrimination, is a very difficult situation for providers to be placed in. One should examine the circumstances based on the patient's medical condition first and then consider what is reasonable and comfortable for the treating provider. Using the tools suggested above, a provider can further explore, investigate, and examine the reasons behind a patient's request to reassign a provider, which may be helpful toward arriving at a solution that makes all parties comfortable. Ultimately, the hospital must provide emergency screening and stabilization for the patient, while also preventing the provider from being discriminated against. Institutions should consider providing policies that are well displayed that express the wish of the institution to provide medical care to all in an environment that is free of discrimination.

Case Outcome

After the provider responded to the patient's concerns and offered him pain medications, the patient was discharged to police custody.

References

1. Paul-Emile K, Smith AK, Lo B, Fernandez A. Dealing with racist patients. N Engl J Med. 2016;374(8):708–11.
2. Selby M. Dealing with racist patients: doctors are people too. BMJ. 1999;318:1129–31.
3. Hook JN, Davis DE, Owen J, Worthington EL, Utsey SO. Cultural humility: measuring openness to cultural diverse clients. J Couns Psychol. 2013;60(3):353–66. https://doi.org/10.1037/a0032595.

Chapter 69
Female Doctor Referred to as a Nurse

Simiao Li and Michael Gisondi

Case Scenario

A 74-year-old male nursing home resident presents via emergency medical services to a local community hospital with complaint of a fall. The patient is accompanied by his middle-aged son. The female attending physician introduces herself to the patient and proceeds to take a history and perform a physical examination.

The patient endorses feeling lightheaded upon standing for the past week, which is accompanied by transient blurred vision. When he has these symptoms, he usually sits back down and feels better within a minute. He does not have chest pain, palpitations, nausea, or diaphoresis during these episodes. He does not feel lightheaded when walking. On the day of presentation, the patient was observed by a nursing home caretaker standing from his bed quickly and lowering himself to the ground, sustaining an arm injury. He did not have loss of consciousness or sustain a head injury.

Review of Symptoms

Neuro: Lightheadedness.
  GI: Generally low appetite, does not drink a lot of fluids.

S. Li (✉)
Department of Emergency Medicine, The Ohio State University Wexner Medical Center,
Columbus, OH, USA

M. Gisondi
Department of Emergency Medicine, Stanford University School of Medicine,
Stanford, CA, USA
e-mail: mgisondi@stanford.edu

© Springer International Publishing AG, part of Springer Nature 2019
M. L. Martin et al. (eds.), *Diversity and Inclusion in Quality Patient Care*,
https://doi.org/10.1007/978-3-319-92762-6_69

479

Integumentary: Skin tear to right forearm.
Review of systems otherwise negative.

Past Medical History

Hypertension, hyperlipidemia, atrial fibrillation.

Family History

Noncontributory.

Social History

Resides at a nursing home, drinks alcohol occasionally, remote history of tobacco use.

Physical Exam

Vital Signs Temp, 98.4; pulse, 130; BP, 140/92; respirations, 18; O_2 sat, 97% on room air.

General Cachectic pale patient appearing stated age reclining on stretcher.

Cardiovascular Irregularly irregular rhythm, orthostatic vital signs abnormal.

Respiratory Clear breath sounds bilaterally.

ENT Dry mucous membranes.

Abdomen Non-distended, non-tender with normal bowel sounds.

Extremities No pitting edema to bilateral lower extremities.

Skin 7 cm skin tear to right forearm.

Neuro Grossly intact, moves all four extremities, and no obvious sign of deficit.

Neck Supple, non-tender in posterior midline, and no pain on range of motion.

What Was Said?

At the end of the physician's interview, the patient states, "Thank you, nurse. Now when is the doctor going to see me?" The attending responds, "I am the doctor." The patient's son asks whether the physician can help his father use the bedside commode. The attending states she will ask the nurse to assist the patient to use the bedside commode.

What Was Done?

The provider patiently reiterates that she is the attending physician, meaning that she is the senior doctor taking care of the patient. The son is apologetic, but the patient continues to refer to the physician as a nurse on subsequent encounters as she updates him on his test results. The patient's EKG shows atrial fibrillation with a rate of 133, which slows to 110 after a small fluid bolus.

Questions for Discussion

1. What assumptions do the patient and his son make?

Attitudes/Assumptions: The Patient

(a) This woman introduced herself as a physician, but she must have meant nurse.
(b) The typical ER doctor is a man, and I've always preferred a male doctor [1, 2].

2. What actions can be taken by the doctor to provide the optimal outcome?

Cross-Cultural Tools and Skills

The physician politely but firmly reiterates that she is the physician who is taking care of him. Because the patient continues to refer to her as a nurse, she makes sure to also speak with the patient's son to reiterate her concerns with respect to the patient's care plan.

Pearls and Pitfalls

Pearl The attending physician is calm and does not express frustration when the patient repeatedly refers to her as a nurse but rather patiently corrects him.

Pitfall The physician must verify that the patient and son understand that they have been seen by an attending physician.

Case Outcome

The patient's skin tear is repaired. He had symptomatic orthostasis on gait testing which resolved after administration of parenteral fluids. After discussion with the physician and an opportunity to ask questions and review visit findings, the patient and son agree to follow up with an appointment at his primary care physician's office the next day.

References

1. Martin ML. Applicant pool for emergency medicine residency programs: information on minority and female applicants. Ann Emerg Med. 1996;27:331–8.
2. Engleman EG. Attitudes toward women physicians: a study of 500 clinic patients. West J Med. 1974;120(2):95–100.

Epilogue

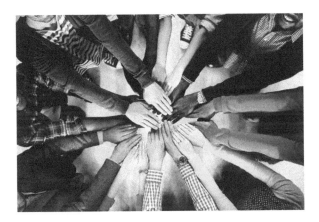

We started the journey of *Diversity and Inclusion in Quality Patient Care: Your Story/Our Story – A Case-Based Compendium* researching and compiling cases related to unconscious bias in health care as a follow-up to our first textbook *Diversity and Inclusion in Quality Patient Care*. The realities of unconscious bias and microaggressions transcend health care and impact sports, justice, law, arts, and many other areas of life. Regardless of culture or community, we are all affected in some way by healthcare biases.

This book is based on real stories with powerful narratives: qualitative data derived from the voices that you have read. This approach perhaps raises more questions than answers. However, we challenge you to consider how *Your Story/Our Story* ties into your own personal experience. We hope the conversation on unconscious biases and microaggressions evolves into a more robust dialogue with solutions that decrease the negative experiences that bias has had and continues to have on society. These conversations could perhaps move patients, providers, and our community to not just consider these biases but act to address them.

© Springer International Publishing AG, part of Springer Nature 2019 483
M. L. Martin et al. (eds.), *Diversity and Inclusion in Quality Patient Care*,
https://doi.org/10.1007/978-3-319-92762-6

Index

CPSIA information can be obtained
at www.ICGtesting.com
Printed in the USA
BVHW01s0746021018
529034BV00021B/97/P